The International Library of Psychology

CONSCIOUS ORIENTATION

Founded by C. K. Ogden

The International Library of Psychology

ANALYTICAL PSYCHOLOGY
In 12 Volumes

I	Studies in Analytical Psychology	*Adler*
II	Complex/Archetype/Symbol in the Psychology of C G Jung	*Jacobi*
III	Psychology of C G Jung	*Jacobi*
IV	Experiment in Depth	*Martin*
V	Amor and Psyche	*Neumann*
VI	Art and the Creative Unconscious	*Neumann*
VII	The Origins and History of Consciousness	*Neumann*
VIII	Jung's Psychology and its Social Meaning	*Progoff*
IX	Religion and the Cure of Souls in Jung's Psychology	*Schaer*
X	Conscious Orientation	*van der Hoop*
XI	Lucifer and Prometheus	*Werblowsky*
XII	The Secret of the Golden Flower	*Wilhelm*

CONSCIOUS ORIENTATION

A Study of Personality Types in Relation to Neurosis and Psychosis

J H VAN DER HOOP

Routledge
Taylor & Francis Group
LONDON AND NEW YORK

First published in 1937 by
Routledge

Reprinted in 1999 , 2001 by
Routledge
2 Park Square, Milton Park, Abingdon, Oxon, OX14 4RN

711 Third Avenue, New York, NY 10017

Transferred to Digital Printing 2007

Routledge is an imprint of the Taylor & Francis Group, an informa business

First issued in paperback 2016

Translated by Laura Hutton

British Library Cataloguing in Publication Data
A CIP catalogue record for this book
is available from the British Library

ISBN: 9780415209472 (hbk)
ISBN: 9781138874930 (pbk)

CONTENTS

PART III

A PHILOSOPHICAL COMMENTARY

PREFACE

THIS book is the product of many years in the practice of psychotherapy. This work constantly reveals to us people in all their complexity. In doing it, one becomes very conscious of the inadequacy of psychological differentiations, to give one a true understanding of this complexity. Psychology has doubtless made enormous advances during recent years, since, primarily under the leadership of Freud, it has forsaken the classroom and the laboratory and has applied itself to the problems of daily life. But medical and pedagogical influences have also led to some confusion, through the propagation from different directions of different principles and schemata on which to base a psychology. This book is partly the product of this conflict, since my personal destiny has brought me successively into close contact with various schools of thought. My attempt to combine in a unified conception certain points of view, as developed by Jung, with the views of Freud and the requirements of phenomenological clarity, finds its origin in my own personal experiences.

In the autumn of 1913 I went to Dr C. G. Jung in Zürich, in order to learn about psycho-analysis, and was analysed by him during a period of six months. I was at that time not aware that a decisive split between Jung's psychological conceptions and those of Freud had recently developed. After my return to Holland I made contact with a group of Freud's followers there, and entered into increasingly lively discussions with them. For a considerable time I remained in touch with Dr Jung; the conflicts between him and Freud were a matter of lively interest to me and formed the main theme of my first book, which appeared in 1921 and was later translated into English.[1] From the outset, the problem of Jung's types appeared to me to be an important amplification

[1] Van der Hoop, *Nieuwe Richtingen in de Zielkunde*, 1921; 2. Ausgabe, 1927; *Character and the Unconscious*, 1923. The concrete descriptions of types in this book are taken from the second Dutch edition.

of Freud's too exclusively dynamic conceptions. The basis of these psychological differentiations was, however, somewhat indefinitely formulated by Jung, and his book, *Psychological Types*, dealt primarily with the opposition between the introverted and the extraverted type. This latter differentiation was also the one chiefly adopted by others, while the classification of the functions of conscious orientation found little acceptance.

The conflict between the ideas of Freud and those of Jung has little to do with these differentiations in the conscious personality. Freud began only later to study the structure of the ego, and his investigations here run in an entirely different direction and have no bearing on the problems of conscious orientation. Psycho-analysis investigates primarily the *contents* of consciousness, and finds behind them influences from the past, which have hitherto received little recognition. In his representation of the origins of the contents of consciousness, Jung has, since the publication of his *Wandlungen und Symbole der Libido*, gone further and further away from Freud. With the latter, the emphasis in the explanation of mental forms rests on childhood experiences, while Jung has displaced it more and more on to the early history of mankind. Jung makes chief use of archaic forms and "collective" psychology to explain the individual and the patient. Although I admit the value of this mode of explanation (as Freud also does), it seems to me that Jung over-estimates their significance, and that he has not fully understood the value of infantile forms. For the observation of the individual, and for the treatment of mental disorders, Freud's standpoint seems to me to be more cautious and more thorough. Although I regret that Freud, by his use of an exaggeratedly sexual terminology, has made it difficult for us to understand the infantile forms, I nevertheless accept "infantile sexuality" as the most important foundation for the psychology of the emotional life. In the treatment of the neuroses I employ mainly the Freudian method, of which I made some years ago a thorough study in Vienna by means of an analysis. I must also confess that the later developments of the Jungian mode of treatment are little known to me, and that the little which has been published concerning it has not enlightened me to any great extent. The method of orientating the individual by collective symbols colours the picture to an ever-increasing degree in the work of Jung and his followers. It is, for example, significant that in the publication issued in honour of Jung's sixtieth birthday there is no mention of typology.

The neglect of typology in the later development of Jungian psychology may have some connection with the fact that his concepts have not been very clearly worked out. My need for precision soon drove me to seek for more definite formulations, and my encounter with phenomenology through Husserl and Heidegger has been of very great assistance to me. Through it I have become aware that my attempt to get a more exact understanding must be regarded as a phenomenological investigation.

During the course of the years that I worked at these problems, it became more and more clear to me how very closely they are bound up with every kind of problem in psychology, psychiatry and philosophy. I am well aware that a real study of these problems would require much greater knowledge than I possess, and much more time than I, as a practising physician, have at my disposal. My contribution cannot be more than an outline of ideas, requiring examination and closer precision in very many directions. I feel, however, that I am justified in publishing my thoughts in this form, because these fundamental questions are important, even when they are for the first time clearly set, and it is not yet possible to answer them fully.

The psychological part of this book was first prepared in the form of six lectures which I gave in November 1929, at the Psychopathic Hospital in Boston. Later it seemed desirable to work out the clinical and philosophical aspects of the subject. The question of the relationship between typological explanation and psycho-analytical explanation has been dealt with in outline in the psychiatric section of this book. In this field also I had to give up the idea of any completeness in my representation, and it was my business first of all to demonstrate the possibilities of the typological point of view.

In this book I have worked out my thoughts in the order in which they have come to me in relation to my practical experience during the course of the years. I think it worth while to emphasize that there is no question here of a system elaborated round the committee table. For readers with a more philosophical outlook, it will, however, certainly prove useful to read the philosophical section first, or immediately after the first part. I fear also that the psychiatric section will offer considerable difficulty to the reader lacking in technical equipment, but I felt it important to demonstrate the possibilities in the way of a practical application of these new differentiations.

In conclusion, I should like to express my warm thanks to all those who have through their interest and their observations encouraged me in the work. This applies first of all to my friends in Boston, Mr and Mrs Tracy Putnam and Dr William Herman, whose premature death is to be so greatly regretted. It was they who by arranging the course of lectures were responsible for the origin of the book: and to Professor C. McFie Campbell who gave me the opportunity to give these lectures in his clinic. Among those who have specially encouraged me I should like to make grateful mention of Professor H. Jordan, Dr Alphonse Maeder, Professor Martin Heidegger, Dr Robert Wälder, Dr Heinz Hartmann and Professor H. C. Rümke. That my grateful recognition includes most of all my two great teachers, Freud and Jung, will surprise many people who know these two scholars only from their more recent conflicting opinions. As regards the danger that I may be attacked by the followers of both schools, I can only say that I hope I have shown in this book that the teachings of both scholars contain complementary elements, capable of reconciliation in a synthesis.

CONSCIOUS ORIENTATION

PART I

PSYCHOLOGY AND THE TYPES OF CONSCIOUS ORIENTATION

CHAPTER I

JUNG'S PSYCHOLOGICAL TYPES

In recent years numerous attempts have been made, especially in Germany, to make the manifold variety in human personalities more comprehensible by means of a description of types. The points from which one may start are so different, that in most cases the results do not coincide with one another, although agreement may be found on some points. The general result is rather confusing, so that it does not seem to me to be a good plan to deal with these various systems side by side.[1] It is, however, of great importance to compare the bases of these various typologies, with a view to recognizing the most vital divergences. As a basis for a theory of types, one must choose characteristics suggesting the main tendencies of the mental structure. For myself, I have, in describing psychological types, taken the classification employed by Dr Jung[2] of Zürich as a starting-point. In the first place, I should indicate why, in my opinion, this classification is preferable, although I can recognize the value of others. At the same time it will become apparent that I have various objections to Dr Jung's conceptions, and that these have led me to formulate rather differently some essential points.

Dr Jung's classification of types has found only slight acceptance. I believe this is partly to be ascribed to its vague and insufficiently systematic description. Another difficulty, however, lies in his peculiar manner of approaching psychological material. The simple observation of mental phenomena, from which most psychologists and psychiatrists set forth, is complicated with him by the conception of the unconscious as the source of some of these phenomena. His standpoint is, in this respect, in accordance with that of psychoanalytical psychology. Here I must explain the significance of this difference in standpoint for our conception of psychological types.

All psychological distinctions are based on peculiarities in the conduct of our fellow-men. We describe and explain that conduct in psychological terms. As this description and explanation become

[1] A clear survey is given by Dr Hermann Hoffmann, *Das Problem des Charakteraufbaus*, 1926.

[2] C. G. Jung, *The Psychology of the Unconscious*, London, 1933; and *Psychological Types*, 1921.

clearer, our terminology becomes more exact, and we become better able to lay down general characteristics, enabling us, under certain circumstances, to predict behaviour. In addition to the external features, by means of which we primarily differentiate our fellow-men, we have learned to recognize certain mental characteristics, giving rise to the concept of temperaments, a term used to designate certain general psychogenic tendencies. Since Galen, in the second century after Christ, differentiated the sanguine, phlegmatic, choleric and melancholic temperaments, these terms have been part of the current speech of many nations. At this stage psychological description remained stationary for a long period. Exact description and classification of phenomena by the natural sciences has in recent times had reference primarily to changes in the constitution of matter. All manner of philosophical speculations, relating to subjective introspective experience, had removed psychology ever farther from exact observation. In the past century the success of the natural sciences induced several psychologists to seek once more a firmer basis for their science in exact observation and description. While experimental psychology sought to find a basis for mental processes in measurable bodily manifestations, men like Kraepelin succeeded in bringing some order into the bewildering field of psychiatry, by means of accurate descriptions. Observation of every kind of phenomenon in mental life, in society and in the individual, in normal and pathological states, in modern as well as in primitive people, has considerably deepened our insight into the life of the mind. The main principles of psychology not only became more comprehensive, but also much more exact. In the field of the differentiation of character-types, Heymans and Wiersma in Holland have sought to deepen current distinctions by means of detailed enquiries of, and communications from, a great number of people. In this work they adopted the differentiations established by Galen, but added further characteristics. The starting-point here, too, was the observation of manifestations as revealed in people's behaviour.

The search for distinguishing characteristics in this field, and their classification into definite systems, has recently been pursued with great zeal, especially in Germany. I need only mention names such as Kretschmer, Klages, Stern, Ewald, Hoffmann, Kronfeld, Spranger, to indicate how scientists are searching from all points of view for useful data for a clearer psychological differentiation of our fellow-men. Klages and Kretschmer, in particular, have contributed a great deal towards stimulating widespread interest in the problem of character-types, the former by careful psychological differentiations, the latter by combining mental and physical types in biological entities. In spite of differences of opinion, all these investigators agree in aiming at exact observation of the forms of expression of an individual, and at an objective comparison of these with those of others. In this, their attitude corresponds directly with that of psychiatrists in their observation and study of their patients. There, too, manifestations, as noted by the observer, form the foundation for scientific description and classification of psychogenic phenomena.[1] From a scientific point of view, this standpoint is unassailable, but it is not always broad enough, because it overlooks a complication which may lead to difficulties in practice, and which seems to demand a more complicated explanation.

To make this clear, let us imagine that a person has been examined and described in accordance with one of these exact methods of classification, and that the result is shown to him. Possibly he will admit that the description, according to the assembled data, is correct, and yet he cannot recognize himself in the character described. The cause of this might be that the observer, in spite of his accurate observation of the details, has nevertheless failed to get a true picture of the total personality, and that the subject himself would prefer to place the accents differently. When it is a question of testing suitability for a certain occupation, or of the diagnosis of a person mentally ill, the subjective standpoint of the individual concerned will not carry much weight. But in the relationship between a teacher and his pupil, or between a psycho-therapist and his patient, it is all-important that the person under examination should be able to share the opinion of the examiner. On this will depend whether an altered point of view will be able to effect a change of attitude, both towards the self and towards the world, and, in consequence, a change in behaviour. Both teacher and psycho-therapist will now discover that the individual in

[1] Here my point of view is no longer a phenomenological one, since I am attempting to describe the various modes of inner orientation as far as possible immediately, without going thoroughly into the views of other investigators. The problem of the mental functions as a whole has not received much attention from other investigators, and it is not possible for me to go into all the details. I will, however, mention a book here, which to some extent deals with the same problem, but in a different way—*Instinct and Intuition, a Study in Mental Duality*, by George Binney Dibblee, which, I regret to say, only came into my hands after I had finished this book. Dibblee quotes the opinions of many philosophers, psychologists and biologists, and he tries to find in the anatomy of the brain a reason for the opposition between instinct and intuition. In that respect his work differs from my psychological investigations, but it may offer important amplifications.

question will readily accept certain views concerning himself, but will repudiate others. This experience will not tempt us, without further evidence, to regard the behaviour and utterances of an individual as consisting of more than one totality. We shall have to differentiate between those manifestations representing his own intentions and opinions and his own conscious personality, and those which he feels to be more or less accidental. Great credit is due to Freud for his increasingly clear emphasis on this distinction, as a result of his own psycho-therapeutic experience. The conscious personality (to which the "pre-conscious" also belongs) provides the origin of some of the mental phenomena, while others must be traced back to unconscious mental processes. A closer study of these unconscious processes revealed that their influence was of much greater importance than had at first been thought. It is well known today that Freud concentrated his researches especially on those manifestations which the patient is not able to recognize as part of his personality. By means of the psycho-analytical method, he sought to make these unconscious sources of psychogenic manifestations conscious, and thereby to bring them under conscious self-control. Through him and his followers this sphere of unconscious mental life has become increasingly better known. In psycho-analytical treatment the patient is confronted with those expressions of his personality which do not correspond with the judgments, opinions and feelings by which he consciously supposes himself to be directed. It is not the doctor who says that certain things are wrong, but contradictions in the patient himself compel him to realize that something is wrong somewhere.

Thus Freud and his followers by no means study the manifestations offered by their patients less exactly than do other scientific psychiatrists, but they offer a more complicated explanation of these manifestations. The difference in this explanation is still further emphasized by the fact that the unconscious, as the source of behaviour, has taken an ever larger place in psycho-analytical conceptions. Originally Freud, like Janet, assumed unconscious mental processes only as the source of certain abnormal phenomena. Very soon, however, he came to the conclusion that in normal people, also, all manner of insignificant disturbances, and other manifestations too, must be explained in the same way. Gradually he came more and more to see in unconscious emotional drives the influence which, in the main, determines human behaviour. As a result, conscious personality with its motives was forced into a subsidiary position in both sick and healthy people. The self believes that it controls, but actually it is controlled. Feelings and aims are usually given a fixed direction in early youth, and they continue to dominate life in the form in which they originally arose.

Anyone who has become to any extent familiar with the practice of psycho-analysis will have to admit that these conceptions are not just taken out of the blue. It may be an amazing and alarming experience to discover to what extent conduct, both in ourselves and in others, is determined by fixated feelings and tendencies. At the same time, one may ask whether the unconscious, as the source of conduct, has not gradually come to occupy too large a place in psycho-analytical conceptions, and does not dominate them too much. As a matter of fact, there has been for some time a reaction, even with Freud and his followers, as a result of which the ego and the personality have come more into the foreground of interest. This reaction had already, at an earlier date, induced two former followers of Freud, the late Alfred Adler and Jung, to separate from him, and their criticism has, without a doubt, had some influence on the changes in psycho-analytical theory. Adler's reaction went farthest. He gave up any explanation of conduct by reference to the unconscious, and made the conscious personality entirely responsible for behaviour. *Individual Psychology* consequently deals exclusively with conscious motives and aims, and has certainly drawn attention to important data in this respect. Where Freud went too far in the assumption of unconscious sources, Adler's work forms a decidedly useful counter-poise. It would, however, be a retrogressive move to abandon the distinction between conscious motivation and unconscious drive.

Jung's criticism of the Freudian conceptions has not gone so far. It is true that Jung, too, as well as Adler, has defended the value of conscious motivation against a too one-sided explanation from unconscious impulses. He has not repudiated the unconscious, however, but has aimed at finding the right relationship between the influence of the conscious personality and that of the unconscious. For that purpose, it was necessary to indicate much more clearly the characteristics which distinguish unconscious adaptation. We had already learned to define the effects of the unconscious more exactly by means of the hypothesis of unconscious complexes.[1] For the conscious guidance of conduct Jung found another standard, namely the motives which a person offers, when accounting to himself for his behaviour. In treating patients, and in ordinary

[1] Some psycho-analysts, e.g. Abraham and Jones, are inclined to consider the conscious personality as determined through fixed complexes. This does not seem correct to me. I shall refer to this point later.

conversation, he observed that there are conspicuous differences in the form of these motives. At first one important distinction in this respect entirely dominated Jung's investigations, namely, the difference between extraversion and introversion.

We will first consider more closely this differentiation of motives. It was observed that some people, in the way in which they consciously seek direction and adjustment in their lives, are almost exclusively guided by objects of the external world. Facts and circumstances, the opinions and feelings of other people, and ideas in current use, determine the adaptations which these people make to life. When in difficulty, they seek support first of all from the external world. Jung calls these people outwardly directed, or extraverted types. Another group of people are guided, in so far as conscious motives are concerned, by entirely different factors; they are primarily conscious of their own subjective reactions to events. They are peculiarly sensitive to these—to what they feel, how they think, about any situation. Where these reactions conflict, they seek to weld them into some sort of harmony of attitude and opinion. In their adjustment to life they thus take as starting-point their own needs and the demands of their own being. They also consult these when in difficulty, and for this purpose they withdraw into themselves. For this reason Jung called them inwardly directed, or introverted types.

A closer investigation shows us that we are here dealing, not with different character-structures, but with typical habits of emphasis, for in everyone we find both forms of adjustment, and it is impossible to say that the one form remains entirely unconscious while the other prevails in consciousness. Under certain conditions, everyone will consciously direct himself towards the external world, while under other conditions he will turn to himself for counsel. Introverted and extraverted states occur in everyone. The only difference is the fact that one person will feel more at home in the one state, while another will find the other more familiar. The extraverted individual will feel much more secure when in contact with other people than when alone. If he reflects too long by himself, everything becomes more confused than if he can guide himself by the opinions of others. The extravert will therefore prefer to maintain contact with others for as long as possible, and if he should find himself in an introverted state, he will soon escape from it. The reactions of others assume more precise and more differentiated forms in his consciousness than do his own.

With introverts, it is exactly the opposite. For them the introverted state is the safest and most agreeable. Alone with himself, the introvert knows exactly what he wants. In contact with others, he loses his sense of security. He finds it an overwhelmingly difficult task to assert himself and to express himself properly. When alone, he feels himself at ease; and when forced into contact with the external world, he has no regrets when the contact is broken and he may withdraw into himself once more. Since an individual of this type is more intensively in touch with himself than with others, he will know his own intentions relatively better than those of other people, and the activities of his own ego will be more differentiated in his mind than those of the external world.

In saying this, it is obvious that contact with both the external world and the self are necessary factors in all living creatures. Even with animals this is evident. If they were to react to external stimuli only, they would become completely exhausted under certain conditions; while under other circumstances they would show no activity at all. If, on the other hand, they were to respond to inner needs without any regard to circumstances, they would probably soon perish. In man both influences are to be found in the conscious personality, but the distinctness with which their effects are seen varies considerably, according to whether the individual is predominantly introverted or extraverted.

Once this difference is recognized, there is usually little difficulty in finding extreme cases of the two types. There are outstandingly extraverted persons, who are almost exclusively led by impressions and impulses aroused in them from the outside. They are, as a result, lively and changeable, and they really do not know themselves at all.[1] On the other hand, extremely introverted people entrench themselves against the external world, and after the slightest contact with it quickly withdraw into themselves again. They impress one as withdrawn and shy.

Even where the general attitude is less marked, it is usually possible, when things are difficult, to note which form of adaptation is the predominating one. The extravert, when uncertain, conforms to the opinion of other people, and immediately becomes more lively and freer in his activity. Under similar circumstances, the introvert is more inclined to withdraw into himself, seeking a solution there. The way in which they take life may also occasion-

[1] A good illustration may be found in *Babbitt*, by the American author, Sinclair Lewis. In his dependence on his environment, he has come to be regarded as a typical product of certain social conditions in the United States. In another book by the same author, *Martin Arrowsmith*, there is a picture of an introvert. Owing to his greater independence of his surroundings, his fate is less typically American than is that of Babbitt.

ally lead us to a correct diagnosis as to type. The extravert seeks, above all things, to remain in harmony with his environment; the introvert seeks harmony in himself.

I think that what I have said will have shown how important is this differentiation as expounded by Jung. Various investigators have pointed out that his introverts and extraverts correspond with contrasts already described by others. If, for instance, we compare Kretschmer's description of the schizoid type with that of Jung's introverted type, many similarities will be recognized. The same holds true of the cycloid (Kretschmer) or syntonic (Bleuler) types and the extravert. There is also an apparent resemblance between the predominance of the primary function (Gross, Heymans, Wiersma) and extraversion, while the secondary function seems to correspond with introversion. This resemblance could be carried still farther. If, however, an attempt is made to equate Jung's differentiation with these other pairs of opposites, the danger arises that its most essential points will be overlooked. It is, accordingly, extremely important that we should proceed to examine rather more closely the special quality of Jung's conceptions.

We saw that Jung took as his starting-point Freud's discovery that only a part of man's behaviour can be deduced from conscious motives, a discovery which has led to the hypothesis of the unconscious. This means the recognition of other important mental factors in addition to the conscious personality.[1] In comparison with other classifications of types, this one is distinctive in regarding the type as an extract from the totality of human capabilities. Moreover, that part of ordinary human experience, which is but little represented in consciousness, is not without effect, although

[1] This conception of the psyche has so influenced Jung that he considers that in their adaptation to the external world extraverts are unaware of the activity of their inner being, while he sees introverts as unconscious of any kind of influence from the external world. We have already noted that this unawareness is only relative, since in certain circumstances all sorts of influences from the other less differentiated aspect may penetrate into consciousness. Here Jung's conception was in contradiction to Freud's earlier idea, that the unconscious contains only repressed material, and that it was impossible, or at least very difficult, to bring this repressed material even partly back to consciousness. Now that Freud has arrived at the view that part of the ego may also remain unconscious, the conflict between his and Jung's views has been considerably reduced. At the same time, it is important to recognize that this reduced awareness of influences from the less differentiated side of the psyche is not to be equated with the Freudian unconscious. Therefore Jung's statement that in the extravert the activities of his inner life are *repressed* appears to me to be inaccurate. It would be truer to say that, as a result of the greater experience and practice gained through a natural inclination in a certain direction, the other side attains only a slight degree of development.

it is expressed more indirectly. Freud gives one the impression that repression of what does not accord with social standards is the only factor accounting for the separation from a general disposition of a kind of conscious extract. Conscious personality, however, is not formed exclusively by repression of what is unserviceable, but also by such development and better adjustment of mental forms as will give more unity and stability to life. I cannot help thinking, therefore, that we should look upon the conscious psyche as primarily an organ for more flexible and more differentiated adaptation. We may most usefully adopt Plato's analogy of a representative government. This image is particularly valuable, in that it also reveals the weak point in such a government. A government which reflects everything pertaining to the life of its people will best be able to provide the advantage of unity in leadership, and to promote quiet and harmony among the people. If, however, a considerable body of the wishes of the people are not understood by the government, an opposition may grow up, giving rise to internal difficulties. A rigid and one-sided attitude on the part of the government may cause the relationship between government and people to be dominated by conflict rather than by cooperation. In the same way, in mental life, harmony or disturbance may exist, according to whether the conscious personality gives scope to the various aspects of the disposition, or represents only a one-sided standpoint.

Now we may take it for granted that it is extremely difficult to find a form of government which is capable of representing all the varied tendencies and interests of the inhabitants of a country. One system of representation will have certain advantages and still be one-sided, while another has advantages and disadvantages of a different kind. So it is with the type of conscious personality, which, as the organ of representation, regulates an individual's adjustments. According to the Jungian classification of types, great differences in personality depend on differences in the mode of adaptation which is adopted.

Where the control exercised by the conscious personality is what it should be, and allows full scope to the subject's whole nature, a state may arise in which his conduct can, in the main, be explained as the product of conscious motives. It will frequently happen, however, that we shall find all manner of manifestations occurring independently of conscious motivation, or even in conflict with it. Here the explanation of conduct from unconscious factors seems justified. If, in such a case, we judge an individual only according to his behaviour, without knowing his motives, we shall interpret all kinds of things in his personality quite differently from what he intends by them.

In order to make this conflict with the more unconscious reactions clearer, I will for the present confine myself to the different emphases provided by introversion and extraversion. Let us take as an example a strongly extraverted person, so much taken up by all manner of claims and demands from his environment, that his personal life is pushed almost entirely into the background and he neglects his own essential needs. Under such circumstances, it may appear to those in his environment that he is very selfish in all kinds of little things, or that he is continually demanding recognition of special merits. Even his readiness to sacrifice himself and to help may to some extent miss the mark, owing to a certain irritability or arrogance becoming evident. While he himself is serenely convinced that he is living entirely for others, they, on the other hand, may feel that this adjustment to external demands is not the only principle governing his behaviour.

As a second example, we may take an introverted person who directs himself entirely according to his own views and principles.[1] In anyone who believes himself to be guided exclusively by an inner aim, it will also be possible to observe in his behaviour manifestations which do not accord with it. It may be evident, for instance, that he is very sensitive to public opinion, and to the impression he makes on the outside world. For the sake of an insignificant success in some direction, he will sometimes unexpectedly overlook matters of principle or his own personal interests. To the outside observer his conduct will then appear to be much more determined by simple forms of adjustment to the external world than would be consistent with his conscious attitude.

In somewhat complicated cases of this kind, neither a description of conduct, nor the subject's own view of the situation, is sufficient for a true understanding, but both behaviour and conscious motives must be compared; when it will become evident that some of the manifestations arise from unconscious factors.

These views of Jung concerning those mental manifestations which are capable of explanation from conscious motives are further complicated by the fact that conscious motivation is determined not only by extraversion and introversion, but also by the mental functions. He considers four functions to be of fundamental importance here: sensation, intuition, thinking, and feeling. Jung

[1] With this form of adaptation, just as with extraversion, highly developed and simple forms may both be found. The introvert's "own intentions" may be selfish, but they may also mean that he is aiming at a high ideal.

has deduced the significance of these functions empirically. At first he differentiated, in addition to introversion and extraversion, only thinking and feeling; later he added intuition, and finally, sensation. Experience with patients and with people in his environment led him to take up this view of the functions. He sees them as products of differentiation from a more primitive and indefinite form of adaptation, which contains, as it were, the germ of all four functions. The functions might almost be regarded as organs of the psyche. Just as in the lower animals certain functions, such as digestion, or perception, are not yet entrusted to specialized organs, so in the primitive psyche there is as yet no differentiation of function. With increasing differentiation in conduct, the functions, as activities directed towards certain modes of adaptation, become more defined. Just as a normal person possesses all the bodily functions, so also everyone has all these mental functions developed to a greater or less degree. Moreover, for a full adaptation to all the requirements of life, none of the functions can be entirely dispensed with: they are complementary to one another.

Sensation includes all the perceptions received through the sense-organs and those relating to the bodily state. It enables us to come into contact with concrete reality. Thinking, as the ordering of objective experience, enables us to recognize things and to form judgments independently of a personal standpoint. Feeling renders the subjective attitude plastic and concrete, and thus develops values and knowledge, referring particularly to personal relationships. Intuition gives rise to spontaneous knowledge and opinions, in the absence of any preceding conscious motivation, and gives a capacity for guessing at the connections and hidden possibilities in any situation.

Any one of these mental functions may be of paramount significance under certain circumstances, but no one is equally at home in all situations. In practice we find that, as a rule, one particular function exercises most influence in conscious mental life. This leads to forms of one-sidedness which may be held largely responsible for the lack of mutual understanding between people. Everyone looks at the world from his own point of view. Persons of the sensation- (or instinctive) type apply themselves simply to the matter-of-fact aspect of things without much reflection; they attach little value to feeling, and possibilities have no allurement for them. They simply stick to concrete facts. Thinking-types, on the contrary, have a particularly ready eye for facts and their associations, provided the data fit into their thought-systems. Anything falling outside the bounds of these leaves them unmoved.

They try to ignore the subjective aspect of the life of feeling. Feeling-types, on the other hand, do not like the impersonal objectivity at which thinking aims, and which seems to them cold and unreal. The individual of feeling-type elaborates facts and possibilities according to his own subjective attitude, and anything outside that sphere has little value for him. Intuitive people are particularly sensitive to possibilities and are guided by inspiration. They are the farthest removed from a materialistic conception of things, since this pre-supposes an attitude of simple receptivity to impressions, which is incompatible with the spontaneous activity upon which intuitive people rely. They have no need for arguments, based on reason or feeling, to discover their motives, for with them conviction comes spontaneously into consciousness, and carries its own certainty with it. We shall later have to study all these characteristics of the functions in greater detail.

The predominance of one of these functions, combined with the impress produced by adjustment to inner needs or to the environment, gives rise to eight different types of conscious orientation. We saw that the conscious personality may be regarded as the organ of representation for the total psyche. It follows that each of these forms of one-sided representation stands in a special relationship to the residual part of the psyche, which remains unaware. This residual part can only express itself inadequately, if it is expressed at all, while the conscious function is in action. This unaware part is thus more or less complementary to the one-sidedness of the conscious personality. The conscious part of the psyche, however, has differentiated and adapted forms at its disposal, so that compensation from the undeveloped and less aware part of the psyche, with its ill-defined and primitive forms, is often very deficient. Its activities may indeed frequently appear more in the form of a disturbance than of compensation, making themselves felt in a tiresome way, and not understood or accepted by the conscious organization, with which they do not harmonize.

In addition to conscious motivation, two unconscious sources of behaviour may thus be postulated: first, manifestations of the less differentiated functions (which in addition often include either internal or external adaptation, according to which form is neglected in the conscious attitude); and second, manifestations of the more involved and more differentiated complexes, which, as a result of repression, have acquired a certain independence.

Taking this view of mental life, we may distinguish two phases in the development of the conscious personality, each involving special difficulties. In the first phase, the personality finds its mode of orientation, i.e. by the differentiated adjustment of its most developed function. From the early, simpler forms of this function, which may give rise to difficulties owing to their violence and extreme one-sidedness, there develop gradually more flexible and more subtle forms, bringing with them increase in versatility and assurance. Anything that is of little use for the prevailing function is gradually discarded, and the conscious personality derives its self-confidence principally from this controlled one-sidedness. In the second phase, the disadvantages of this one-sidedness become apparent. In opposition to a certain rigidity of the personality, influences from the unconscious make themselves increasingly evident, rendering the value of the acquired unity problematical. Insight into the compensating value of activities in the conscious and the unconscious psyche may lead to the search for a broader basis for conscious equilibrium, whereby, if it is found, the one-sidedness of the personality is more or less resolved in a fuller and more mature expression of human nature.

We will now attempt a more detailed survey of the advantages and disadvantages of Jung's classification of types, which has so far been given only in its main outlines. If we compare this mode of approach to the study of mental structure with other classifications, its greater complexity cannot fail to strike us. A similar complexity occurs occasionally in other systems. For instance, Kretschmer's description of certain complicated cases is pretty involved. In Germany this is spoken of as "multi-dimensional diagnosis". Explanation of the totality of the manifestations is sought in a summation of the various data, and the description of these gives rise to great complexity, which is, nevertheless, somewhat accidental. With Jung, however, the complexity is given from the start. It is inseparable from his mode of regarding mental structure, and must be taken into account in every case. This has a great advantage in the more complicated cases, because "multi-dimensional diagnosis" does not give nearly such a clear picture of structure. Moreover, Jung developed his views through the study of complex individuals, whom he treated over a considerable period of time, so that he had every opportunity for studying both their motives and their conduct, as determined by their unconscious. In such cases, as in biographies, and wherever there is complicated material relating to conduct, this method of approach has great advantages.

Against this, it calls for an ability to understand people's conscious motivation; and such an understanding is in many cases not at all easy; not only because many people are not capable of communicating their motives easily, but also because relatively few of them can formulate them clearly, in spite of the fact that they are guided by them from day to day. We are, of course, accustomed to some extent to draw conclusions as to the motives of other people, from their behaviour, and often with success. But in more involved cases we should have to examine such conclusions more closely if we wished to apply them in psychology. For this purpose it may be very important that those whom we are studying should be able to give us an account of how their behaviour appears to them, and what it is that guides them. Adler has clearly shown that fictitious goals may act as a great hindrance to the recognition of our true motives, and Freud has pointed out how we tend to rationalize motives which we are not willing to admit. There are, however, many cases in which it is not difficult to discover the conscious motives by which an individual is being led, and from the study of these in cases in which we are in a position to control our own conceptions by conversations with the individual concerned, we learn to draw more accurate conclusions in those cases where we have only behaviour to go upon. For instance, we may deduce from certain typical motivations, communicated to us as introspective experiences, the activity in the behaviour of other people of certain mental structures which act as a whole. Here the Jungian differentiations and those of the other typologies must needs be combined in due course, when it will be possible to evolve an improved type-diagnosis even on the basis of external characteristics. Understanding of motives will then doubtless add depth to psychological description. This is true not only for teaching and for psycho-therapy, but also for every kind of trend in metaphysics and philosophy, and for scientific, political and religious movements, in all of which both one-sided adaptations and peculiar compensatory influences may be discovered. If Jung's theory of types is to bring about an improvement in mutual understanding, it is to my mind important that his differentiations should be more exactly formulated, and that they should be tested on masses of material, both pathological and healthy. I am, accordingly, well aware that for the moment it is not possible to give more than a rough outline.

In this outline I differ from Jung on some essential points, especially in my account of the functions and in my view of their connection with one another. I will briefly state at this point what these main differences are, and how I have arrived at them. The reader who is not familiar with Jung's conceptions may omit the rest of this chapter, since it will contain only the criticism of those of Jung's views which I reject. My own formulations, to a large extent agreeing with those of Jung, will be dealt with in the succeeding chapters.

Feeling is the function which I formulated differently from Jung some years ago.[1] Jung writes:[2] "Feeling is primarily a process that takes place between the ego and a given content, a process, moreover, that imparts to the content a definite value in the sense of acceptance or rejection ('like' or 'dislike'). But it can also appear, as it were, isolated in the form of 'mood,' quite apart from the momentary contents of consciousness or momentary sensations . . . for a mood, too, signifies a valuation; not, however, a valuation of one definite, individual, conscious content, but of the conscious situation at the moment." In my opinion, this formulation does not give the essential quality of feeling. The attaching of value does not occur exclusively in feeling. Reason also accepts and rejects, distinguishes between valuable and useless mental contents. Intuition attaches great value to every possibility and relationship which it perceives, and rejects everything else. But my chief objection is that the complicated activities which are produced by feeling cannot possibly be explained by like and dislike. This would simply equate emotion and feeling, whereas in my opinion feeling means something much more complicated. I have, indeed, already indicated as the characteristic quality of feeling a certain attitude of mind in which a variety of emotional reactions are combined. I then discovered with pleasure that this conception of mine had already been formulated in similar terms by McDougall and Shand.[3] They also distinguish "sentiments" as a combination of emotions attached to a definite object. Simple emotions they class with instinct. This latter conception has also enforced itself on me, before I came across their opinion. Because I had begun to regard emotion as an expression of instinct, I was no longer able to accept Jung's formulation of the function of perception. Other considerations, too, added to my criticism of this function.

If we try to take mental experience as our starting-point, free from all pre-conceptions, it becomes obvious that emotional reactions are immediately bound up with our sensations. Intellectual considerations, with their retrospective differentiations, have blurred these inwardly perceptible (phenomenological) facts. So-called feeling-tone, together with reactions of liking and disliking, thus

[1] J. H. van der Hoop, *Character and the Unconscious*, 1923.
[2] C. G. Jung, *Psychological Types*, pp. 543-4.
[3] W. McDougall, *Social Psychology*; A. F. Shand, *The Foundation of Character*, 1926.

form, with sensation, a psychological entity. Another fact, which inner perception may reveal, is the association of all kinds of sensations in a single coherent field of experience. Philosophers, in their ideas about sensation, are too apt to start from the point of view of perception, which is quite a different process. Perception is a circumscribed cognitive process, and this limited conception has been transferred to sensation. Jung goes so far as to regard sensation and perception as identical. But perception, in my opinion, is more related to thought, since by it truth [1] is tested. Sensation is a much simpler and more passive mental process, in which it is much more difficult to define the units of the experience. Receptivity and reaction are here still closely related. If, however, sensation and reaction are regarded as a whole, there is an exact correspondence with those manifestations which many biologists describe as instinctive, and which even psychologists like McDougall regard as manifestations of instinct. This instinctive sphere of experience is regarded by the behaviourists as the only real basis for psychology. Although their views relating to conditioned reflexes partly coincide with my ideas about instinct, and although I esteem this field as of great significance in mental life, I hope to make it clear that there are other spheres of mental experience, in which other modes of reaction are current. If, like the behaviourists, we believe we can explain everything as "conditioned reflexes", then there is, in fact, no point in retaining the expression "instinct". But in contrast to mental experiences having a different structure, it is useful to be able to designate this whole field as the instinctive sphere of mental life.

Besides these theoretical considerations, I have been led also on practical grounds to regard the instinctual mode of reaction as characteristic of those people whom Jung calls sensation-types. In studying their mode of adaptation, I saw, in fact, more and more clearly that they were not guided exclusively by their sensations, but by their sensations coupled with their emotional reactions thereto, and, further, by their instinctual needs as well. It seemed, therefore, incorrect to me to regard sensation as the only characteristic factor in this function. The psychological peculiarities characteristic of experience in the instinctive sphere will be expounded in greater detail later. At this stage I should merely like to point out that adaptation is here governed by emphases in regard to emotion and attention in the field of sensations, and that action is also directed by details of a concrete kind.

After these characteristics of the instinctive sphere in the

[1] As expressed in the German word *Wahrnehmung*.

psyche had become more distinct, it also became possible to get a clearer definition of intuition; here it is not details of emphasis, but an attitude to the whole, which from the outset determines the forms taken by adaptation. In this respect I can support Jung's observation, that in intuition "any one content is presented as a complete whole, without our being able to explain or discover in what way this content has been arrived at".[1] Jung's definition, according to which intuition is the mental function "which transmits perceptions *in an unconscious way*",[2] I do not, however, regard as very useful. In the first place, intuition is not felt as perception, nor as a group of perceptions, but as an insight into the significance of the whole of an experience. In the second place, it cannot claim as a characteristic, that it arises in an unconscious way. The expression "in an unconscious way" is extraordinarily vague, and likely to give rise to endless misunderstandings. It is true that intuition does not appeal to arguments, as thought and feeling often (but not always) do. But the certainty of sensation depends just as little on arguments. Moreover, feelings and thoughts may also arise in an unconscious way, without thereby becoming intuitions. This definition, therefore, needs to be amplified by means of clearer mental data, as I shall show in greater detail in the chapter on intuition.

It is not only in my conceptions of the functions that I differ from Jung, but also in my views respecting their mutual interrelationship. According to Jung, the functions stand unrelated, as organs developed for certain forms of adaptation. It is true that he states that sensation and intuition were present at earlier stages in human development than were thought and feeling; but he does not proceed to give any idea why this should be so. This conception of the functions as entirely unrelated suggests that the various types have little in common, and that a basis for their understanding will be extraordinarily difficult to find. The common element would then appear to lie in the unconscious, while it would appear to be the fate of conscious personalities to grow ever farther apart. In this respect I have gradually come to a different point of view, according to which the functions are much more related, and are manifestations of a certain mental structure, developed in the human race during the course of the ages. In its essence this structure is the same in all men, with the reservation that the general stage of development attained may vary. In consciousness, however, one definite field will be more clearly lit up than others, and as a result, the forms which it contains will be more differentiated.

[1] C. G. Jung, *Psychological Types*, p. 568. [2] *Op. cit.*, p. 568.

Later I will treat of my views of this structure of the psyche in greater detail, but since these conceptions have developed out of my professional practice, it seems to me desirable first to define them in rather more concrete form before I discuss the view of mental structure which has resulted. At this stage I do not wish to do more than indicate, after describing my own point of departure, where I feel I must suggest alterations in Jung's typology. These are concerned more with the explanation of the various types than with their description, although I have also striven here to make the latter more plastic and more defined. At the same time, my explanations of the functions and my conception of the nature of the psyche are so different from Jung's views that I can no longer identify my conceptions with his. It will, however, be obvious that, with all my objections, I retain a warm appreciation of Jung's conception of mental life, and of the theory of types which he has developed.

CHAPTER II

INSTINCT AND THE INSTINCTIVE TYPES

(A) *Instinct in Psychology*

To psychologists who seek to derive their science exclusively from observation of behaviour, the concept of instinct does not present any very important problem. For them instinct may be taken in two ways; first, as inborn reactions, not yet influenced by knowledge gained from experience, and second, as fundamental impulses, forming the basis for all human behaviour. In the first case, instinctual reactions can be studied only in the very young child, since at a later age the influence of experience can never be entirely excluded. In the second case, instinct is the stimulus to every human action, and the use of this concept becomes superfluous, since it tells us nothing definite.

I have taken as my point of departure a more complicated basis for psychology, which includes introspection as a special form of experience; and if instinct has any significance in this kind of experience, it must be possible to differentiate it, by means of certain properties, from other forms of conscious experience. It is certainly possible, in any description of our own inner life, or in similar descriptions presented to us by others, to distinguish all kinds of peculiarities. Are there now certain forms of conscious experience which would deserve the designation of instinctual more than others?

There are, to be sure, various ways in which even a simple object, such as a chair, may be experienced in consciousness, and it may be of use to discuss some of these by means of an example, before entering on more elaborate descriptions. We may see a chair without thinking much about it, but with the practical knowledge in our minds of how we use it, how we must walk round it, or how we want to see it used. Also, in observing the chair, we may suddenly get a picture before our minds of how this chair would look in another room. Or a dealer in antiques may suddenly recognize that it is this kind of chair which a certain customer would particularly value. This form of experience we shall later learn to distinguish as intuitive. Yet another way of seeing the chair would be to study its workmanship, or its style, or to consider it from a general philosophical point of view, as an object. In this way it takes its place in some thought-system. On other occasions the sphere of feeling may surround the chair, and may be the most essential factor in our minds. We feel, for example, the friendship of the person who gave it to us, or it gives us a feeling of the atmosphere which pervades our home.

Not long ago, psychologists would have been inclined to explain these differences by means of various associations bound up in our minds with the image of this chair. This has, however, proved to be an inadequate description of what in reality takes place in our consciousness. It has become necessary to describe such mental contents as entities, having their own special structure. For the moment we will direct our attention primarily towards the simplest form of conscious experience. This will nevertheless prove to be pretty complicated, certainly more complicated than it appears at first sight. We are dealing here with a practical form relating to the recognition and use of things, in which sensations play a large part. I propose to call this field the instinctive sphere of conscious experience, pending a more exact justification of the phrase, and I will now proceed to describe its characteristics.

(*a*) In my view, the whole field of simple sensory experience belongs to this instinctive sphere of the mind. There are good reasons why we should here differentiate between sensation and perception. The latter indicates a mental content of greater definition, directed towards a definite object, while sensations are all linked up in one single field of sensory experience. Intellectualistic psychology is inclined to lose sight of this distinction, by regarding the separate sensations as the units from which the totality of our sensory experience is constructed. Closer observation reveals, however, that this totality is felt by us as a coherent unity, in which certain emphases attract our attention, and that it has its own peculiar structure. The fact that our sensory experience has structure is borne out by the *Gestalt* (Configuration) theory. Phenomenologists (Husserl) have already stated this in a different way, by pointing out, for instance, that it is a peculiarity of sensation that objects appear against a background which shifts when we move. In simple sensation, objects stand in close relationship to their environment and have their place in the structure of the field of experience. Many important details in this form of experience still await closer investigation.

(*b*) A second characteristic of instinctive experience may be found in the circumstance that it is impossible to make a clear separation between our own reaction and awareness of the sensation. Association psychology has more or less recognized this fact in stating that a "feeling-tone" is associated with our "perceptions". Perceptions are, however, mental contents of far greater differentiation than the field of sensation which we have in mind, and there is also no reason to include emotional reactions here, since these are from the outset part of the totality of the experience. This emotional reaction may show various degrees, fluctuating indeed between indifference (which is itself a reaction) and a feeling of worthwhileness (Drever), or such special emotions as fear, disgust, wonder, anger, tender feeling, all of which are regarded by McDougall as instinctive. It is a peculiarity of such instinctive emotional reactions that they may be experienced again and again in association with the same objects, and that certain parts or qualities of the object may have great influence as a stimulus to instinct. Desire and emotion may be constantly evoked by the same exciting factors. This is true, not only for instinctual satisfactions in the realms of food and sex, but also for such pleasant reactions as those to a day in spring, with its warm sunshine and the reappearance of flowers and young leaves, or for the satisfaction afforded by physical exercise.

(*c*) Emotional reactions to sensation are frequently accompanied by an impulse to act. In our conscious mind this may assume various forms, e.g. that of a vague inclination to do something, or of a strong, impulsive drive towards certain acts; or there may arise a certain mode of behaviour, determined more or less by habit. All these cases have in common the fact that sensation, emotion and action form a unity, and that action and reaction are directed by emphases in the field of sensation, determining attention and emotion. The forms assumed by action of this kind are remarkably constant—it is as if an unconscious pattern of activity was activated—but the emphases which determine the course of action may, under the influence of experience, gradually shift. In this way, sexual inclinations, for example, may be controlled by different emphases in emotional sensation in different people. It is well known, too, that habits may change with changing circumstances. The existence of a special instinctive mode of learning by means of a gradual displacement of reactions and of emphases in sensation can be well seen in the process of learning a game.

(*d*) In the field of "knowing", too, a definite form may be distinguished which belongs to the sphere of instinct. Although we may know our way about in a forest or a town, we may nevertheless feel at a loss if asked to communicate this knowledge. We possess a practical knowledge, but no articulate expression for it. One often comes across this phenomenon among sporting folk. But we cannot say that this kind of knowing is unconscious. When listening to sportsmen carrying on endless conversations concerning the details of their hobby, one gets the impression that they are speaking in terms of some common experience. Although they would find it difficult to convey this experience to an outsider, they are conscious enough of it themselves. It is impossible to say that this form of knowing is chaotic. It is controlled by fixed associations of sensation and action. The original instinctual interest, lending to things their "primary meaning" (Drever),[1] has led to further experiences, as a result of which fresh emphases in the field of sensation have provided a "secondary meaning", and these points, attracting special attention, are linked up by being associated together in practice.

We now see the sphere of conscious instinctual experience as a mode of conscious orientation, covering various items which nevertheless appear to us, coupled with our emotional and behaviour reactions thereto, as parts of a single experience, bringing with it a practical form of knowledge, inseparable from the sensations involved. It may be useful to realize that experience of this kind is by many people only distinguished with great difficulty, although it is shared by everyone. This is because other functions employ this experience as material for other purposes—as I hope later to demonstrate—and the moment we try to examine the instinctive sphere, these other processes (which do not belong to it) are activated, and the original experience becomes blurred. Hence we must develop in ourselves an, as it were, innocent state of mind, in order to be able to become more aware of this kind of experience, and in this we may be helped by situations which specially involve this mode of orientation. At the time when I was investigating the instinctive sphere, I took up riding again, after a long interval, and it taught me a lot about a state of mind in which more complicated mental activity must be cut out. If I had begun to think too much about it, I should certainly have been in danger of being thrown. If I had given way to feeling, I should have perhaps become anxious or too self-confident, which would have been no more helpful, nor would intuition have got me very far. Yet I was conscious of being intensively active, my attention being riveted on the totality of my sense-experience and my reactions to it. This mental activity, bound up, as it unquestionably is, with emotion, is very difficult to describe. Most certainly I was not

[1] Drever, *Instinct in Man*, 1917.

unaware, although this sphere is not the one in which one is, as a rule, most conscious of experiencing mental activity. Once we have become aware, however, of this mode of orientation, we can experience it often enough. For example, when going about a familiar city, coping with its traffic, and in so doing constantly making use of our practical knowledge, our state of mind is certainly conscious, although it would be difficult to describe it or to fix it in memory.

In this discussion I have so far only sought to establish certain differentiations in our conscious experience which are capable of confirmation by means of introspection, our own and that of others. If others tell me that they in their conscious experience perceive the same form, having the same properties, I tend to assume that this differentiation may be regarded as holding good for human psychology in general. I accordingly objectify my own experience, assuming that it occurs in others in the same form. We are all of us accustomed to look upon such a projection of our own mental experience as commonplace and natural. The psychologist is, however, well aware that in doing so he must guard against various possibilities of error. One guarantee is to verify our conclusions by discussing them with the person under observation. Another is to correct and verify introspection, both in ourselves and in the person under observation. Since this is in many cases impossible, we may employ a rougher, more or less collective form of control, by noting the regular association of certain modes of behaviour and expression with certain mental contents. Thus we regularly associate with certain modes of behaviour the mental states of being cross, or in love. When we fail to be able to attach a particular psychological label in this way to a particular mode of behaviour, we are very ready to call the person concerned abnormal or crazy, and are content to do so, so long as most people are of the same opinion as ourselves. Official psychology takes the same course in many cases, the result being merely that it tries to describe behaviour in a more objective and more subtle way. Occasionally it appears to be quite forgotten that there are other forms of control through introspection, as seems to be the case with the behaviourists.

Among the psychological differentiations, based on visible behaviour, there are also to be found forms of behaviour which, in ordinary speech and by a few psychologists (McDougall, Drever), are described as instinctive.[1] Such forms are characterized by an impulse to action, in an emotional situation which is the product

[1] In this case no rigid distinction is made between experience of behaviour and introspective experience, a characteristic of those who believe it to be possible to found a psychology exclusively on the former.

of some sensory experience, and in which motivation and insight seem to play no part. I believe that the state of mind which is presupposed as the source of such behaviour corresponds pretty closely with the state of mind which I have described as the instinctive sphere of conscious orientation. I venture to affirm that the characteristics of this state of mind, viewed introspectively, would on closer examination prove to be determined in the manner which I have described. The visible form of behaviour corresponding with this conscious experience appears to me to be characterized by the following peculiarities:

(1) There is here a closer connection between certain emphases in sensation and the mode of reaction.

(2) The reaction appears to be according to a more or less fixed pattern.

(3) To the observer behaviour seems to be motivated by instinctual wishes, by blind impulse, or by habit; reason or conscious motivation appearing to have little influence.

(4) A change in the pattern of behaviour, or an adaptation to circumstances, takes place gradually and empirically, by means of a shifting of the emphases (trial and error).

Thus we have now before us a certain sphere of conscious experience, and beside it certain modes of expression of a kind to suggest that they are the forms of conscious experience giving rise to this sphere. The advantages of this psychological differentiation will become more evident as we study the other modes of conscious orientation. But even now our insight into the structure of this mode of conscious orientation will be able to render good service in the differentiation of certain character-types.

These instinctive influences are active in everyone. They form the foundation of mental life. But it makes a great difference whether the superstructure erected upon this foundation conceals it entirely and dominates the mental structure, or whether the foundation itself remains the most important element in the psyche. This latter event does not necessarily indicate a primitive nature—as one might perhaps expect—but it does probably imply a closer contact with the primitive side of the psyche. It may bring about a considerable degree of development in the instinctive function, so that, in spite of the altered conditions in modern life, it is still able to direct life. Inter-action between sensation and impulse is maintained, although the original instinctual reactions would be scarcely suitable in the modern world to which the individual belongs. But the instinctive person is able to make good use of these very changes to attain gratification of his needs. He has all the advantages of a technique in this sphere, and he will make use of them to extract the last ounce from his capacity for enjoyment and to get what he wants. His technique is for him, as it were, an organ, given to him for the purpose of fulfilling his instinctual needs.

What are the outward and visible signs of this predominance of instinct in the psyche? Instinct is pre-occupied with the concrete, and is usually controlled by details, without any clear awareness of connections with the whole, or of purpose. Where instinct is in control, there is, therefore, great capacity for perception of details and for practical evaluations based on them; further, there is the power to make sound estimations in regard to usefulness, serviceability, health, and even in regard to the value of simple forms of beauty. But instinct has no use for great complexity; it likes to see all round a thing. Where there is complexity, it quickly becomes confused. On the other hand, it is able to absorb an immense number of simple facts, and to have a relationship with every one of them. Further, for instinctive evaluation, impressions must be neither too new nor too strange; for instinct works in a familiar environment, and is hence conservative in nature, better able to deal with variations in the known and with fixed habits, than with what is entirely new. There is an exception with things with which instinct is by nature associated, such as varieties of landscape, or food, or even sexual gratification. Here what is new seems less alien to instinct than would be, for instance, an entirely fresh social environment.

Where instinct predominates, judgment by reason is closely bound up with the perception of facts, and deals with concrete and practical problems, without worrying much about theories. Feeling is also just as little able to develop to any great independence, and is chiefly expressed as emotion coinciding with certain sensations. Action is in the main reactive and related to instinctual impulses; so that it may be intensive in one domain and feeble in another. If instinct is aroused, a tremendous energy, of a driving kind, may be developed.

In describing instinctive people, it will be found useful to differentiate the extraverted and introverted types.

(B) *The Extraverted Instinctive Type*

The life of the instinctive extravert is determined by impressions received from without, to which he reacts with his instinctual impulses. In children of this type it is possible to observe at a very early age that sensations are for them of particular significance, and that they very quickly become at home in the world of facts and things. At the same time, they are strongly reactive. If an object catches their attention, they at once seize hold of it, or they go after it, and study it from all sides. They will, moreover, repeat this reaction again and again over a long period of time. Such a child needs to have a world of forms, colours and tones. He wants to sniff at every flower, and can with difficulty restrain his impulse to gobble up the things that tempt him. At a later age, also, facts perceived through the senses remain for people of this type the only reality. They never linger over reflections and principles; they are, to an extreme degree, realists. Nor do they feel any need to evaluate their experiences in any systematic way, but their reactions drive them from one sensation to the next. They are thus strongly influenced by their environment, but are nevertheless not entirely passive within it; for both in the manner in which they are affected, and in their reaction, there is some personal activity of their own. The purposes of this activity are usually only known to them in so far as it is a question of intentions which can be fulfilled in practice. It would also not be true to say that instinct leads exclusively to personal satisfaction of sensuous desires. For an individual is also bound by his instinctual life to the group to which he belongs, and under certain conditions it will drive him to dedicate his powers to its service, or even to sacrifice himself for it. In the case of a woman, one thinks of the instinctual aspect of her love for her children; in the case of a man, of his urge to fight on behalf of his family. This instinctive aspect in adaptation to the community is also expressed in the faithful maintenance of custom and tradition, for here lies, as in instinct, a wealth of ancestral experience. For an instinctive person it is particularly dangerous to break loose entirely from them, for they provide him with a special kind of support in the ordering of his life, owing to the fact that he understands the meaning of these traditional forms better than do individuals of other types, and indeed he can only with difficulty develop other modes.

A great many so-called "ordinary" people belong to this type. If they do create any impression, it is more owing to their success in making an art out of life than to any special qualities. They feel at home in the world, accept things as they are, and know how to adjust themselves to circumstances. Since their acceptance of things as they are extends to themselves, they are occasionally a little too easy-going towards their own faults; but, on the other hand, they do not readily overvalue themselves. They have, in fact, a tendency to expect too little of themselves, since they are very little aware of their aims and possibilities. They are most impressed by facts, and their originality finds expression in a truer and less prejudiced view of these than others take, with the result that they may also discover fresh facts. The phrase "matter-of-fact" describes this attitude very clearly. They fight somewhat shy of ideals. They stick to experience, are empiricists *par excellence*, and are in general conservative in their practical life, if they see no prospect of advantage in change. They are pleasant people, good comrades, and jolly boon-companions. They often make good observers, and they make good practical use of their observations. They are frequently good story-tellers. They are most suited to practical callings, such as those of doctor or engineer. Their fondness for knowing a multitude of facts is related to a preference which they occasionally show for collecting objects of scientific or aesthetic interest. One may also include in this type many people of good taste, who have developed appreciation of the subtler pleasures of life into a fine art. Such people are often well able to discuss problems and theories of life, but in this case it is more for the pleasure of the discussion than out of interest in the actual problems. For the sake of some special sensation, they will take up all kinds of things which otherwise would not interest them. For people of this type are not satisfied with a simple pursuit of instinctual gratification. They seek intense and unusual sensations, and by no means only those which are pleasant and easily attained.

Here, as with the other types, there may exist great variety within the bounds of the type. But the ideals of such people are directed almost exclusively towards the external side of life. They are well dressed, live in comfortably appointed houses, eat and drink well, have pleasant manners, and a reasonable variety in their conversation and mode of life. They take pleasure in the possession of a house and garden, and in looking after them; their usual preference is for natural pleasures such as physical exercise and sport. In uncomplicated people of this type, the inner life plays practically no part. Anything emanating from this side of life, which might disturb the happiness of their life, is rejected as morbid. Feelings and thoughts are identified with emotions and perceptions. Their activity is primarily reactive. They will do no more than is necessary to procure those sensations which offer them pleasure, and this will mean much or little, according to circumstances.

More complicated forms of this type occur where a second function is developed up to a certain point. Where reason is developed, it will, in these people, be affected by the predominating function, i.e. in this case by outwardly directed instinct. The result is that reason is directed chiefly to facts, and limited to the empirical. It accepts, for its classification of facts, the thought-systems in current use. Thought is thus unoriginal and avoids any complexity, but is solid and practical. In simple, practical matters, judgment is accurate and very reliable.

Feeling may also exert some influence within the limits set by the type. In this case the sensual aspect of feeling is reinforced by instinctual activity, while the result of extraversion is a dependence on sensation. As a result, feeling is to a high degree controlled by the external appearance of the object, and demands expression in tangible form. Concrete facts, such as the presence and possession of the object, play a large part here. Anyone who is absent for a long time will, for example, find it difficult to arouse strong feelings in a representative of this type. Their feelings embrace the sphere of their lives as a whole. An instinctive person will love his wife, for example, not because of his personal contact with her, but primarily because she is his wife, and the mother of his children. Similar feelings are also aroused in him by the house which he has known from childhood, and by the objects which it contains, by the people of his home town and by his native soil. In their love-relationships sex plays a large part with these people; in fact, any feeling can with them attain satisfactory development, only if it can be expressed in the ordinary affairs of daily life.

Intuition is the least effective function in the instinctive individual, for, with its spontaneous, unfounded convictions, it is far removed from the instinctual mode of orientation, proceeding, as this does, empirically and step by step. These people find it impossible to understand how anyone could attach value to inspiration, but they can appreciate intuitions in the form of wit or jokes, both in themselves and in others. The things that can only be grasped intuitively, however, such as the vast order of the universe, and a realization of their own potentialities and of the meaning of their lives, may easily pass them by. They are not only suspicious of any complexity, but find it difficult to perceive possibilities in the way of action and development, unless chance circumstances lead them right into them.

(C) *The Introverted Instinctive Type*

The instinctive introvert is ruled by his emotions and impulses. These form the subjective side of instinctual life, just as sensation represents its objective side. The attention of the introvert is not directed primarily to the source of sensation (as communicated to him through his sense-organs), but to its so-called "feeling-tone", and to his own impulses. It depends upon the extent to which he is stirred, whether a given experience will make a big impression on him, not upon the intensity of the sensation itself. This aspect of susceptibility to emotion may occasionally, under certain conditions, prevail in anyone, but here it dominates all the other functions. Inherited disposition and early experience have produced a certain susceptibility to impressions and a certain need for emotional experience, and in these cases the whole mental life is directed by these two factors. Adjustment along these lines may, under favourable circumstances, provide for such people a satisfying existence, so long as these needs are met. Since in most cases there is little external evidence of this inner satisfaction, the lives of these people may sometimes appear to others as anything but happy, arousing compassion, for which there is no real reason.

Children of this type are frequently noted for a certain gentleness and receptiveness, but also for periods of timidity and monosyllabic reserve. There is something a little vague and passive about them. They are attached to people in their environment who are kind to them. They love nature, animals, beautiful things, and an environment with which they have become familiar. Anything strange or new has at first no attraction for them; but they offer little active resistance to it and soon learn to accept the good in it. They are often friendly and easy to get on with, but a little lazy and impersonal. When older, too, these people usually give an outward impression of being reserved, quiet, and somewhat passive. Only in rare cases, for example, in artists, does the distinctive and personal quality of their inner emotion come to expression. In other cases, however, their whole behaviour reveals their peculiar characteristics, although it is not easy to define these.

People of this type have well-developed sense-organs, but they are particularly receptive to anything having lasting value for human instinctual needs. This lends to their lives a certain solid comfort, although it may lead to somewhat ponderous caution, if instinct becomes too deeply attached to all kinds of minor details. The advantages and disadvantages of this type are well brought out in the reserved and conservative farmer, with his care for his land and his beasts, and his tendency to carry on everything, down to the smallest detail, in the same old way. The same is true of the sailor. He also shows a passive resistance to anything new, which can only be overcome by absolutely convincing experience. Other examples of this type are the naturalist, devotedly observing in minutest detail the lives of plants and animals, the lonely collector of beautiful or interesting things, the worker in applied art, and the painter, who manage to express a deep experience in the presentation of ordinary things.[1] In their own field these people are usually very much at home, having a good mastery of the technical side of their calling, but without regarding this as any special merit. They accept both what they can, and what they cannot, do, as simple facts, but they tend on the whole to under-estimate rather than to over-estimate themselves. Pretence and bluff in others may irritate them to the point of protest, which is probably connected with their own difficulty in understanding their own potentialities and worth. These people usually strike one as very quiet and somewhat passive. Except in relation to persons and things in their own immediate sphere, to which they are bound by their instinctual reactions, they show little inclination to activity; they never readily depart from their routine. If anything gets in their way, they put up a peculiarly passive resistance, although under exceptional circumstances there may be an outbreak of wrath. If their environment is not favourable, they will nevertheless try to adapt themselves to it; in such circumstances, they are inclined to regard their emotions, in so far as they differ from other people's ideas, as morbid. At the same time, they feel extraordinarily helpless and inferior. Or they may turn away from the world and give themselves up entirely to their own emotions. Where this is the case, they see any adaptation to other people as a mere pretence, and may develop remarkable skill in belittling the motives and ideals of others.

The development of reason also follows the same lines here as the general attitude to life. Facts are its point of departure, and particularly certain fundamental facts, which are subjected to exact and thorough investigation. Observations and ideas are matter-of-fact and clear. There is nothing contemplative about people of this type. Moreover, they prefer to stick to the familiar, and find it difficult to adopt anything new. This is connected with their need to see things in a clear setting. If they can bring themselves to accept anything new, they tend to occupy themselves with it until it has become absolutely clear to them. Here is revealed the obstinacy of instinct, with its ever-renewed attack until it has learned to control its object. Circumstances, however, have to be favourable. In more abstract matters, they find it difficult to form an opinion of their own, and follow those authorities

[1] I regard the Dutch painter Vermeer as an introverted instinctive, while that master in the expression of every human emotion, Jan Steen, seems to me to be an extravert of this type.

which, by a knowledge of facts, give them the impression of being thorough. Even so, they do not feel any confidence, and are easily upset if drawn into discussion in this field, or if the value of their authorities is questioned. On the other hand, they have few prejudices, and their view of things is calm and temperate.

Feeling may also make itself felt here, in which case it is, by the influence of instinct, attached to concrete objects. But the emphasis does not rest on the object, as with the extravert of this type, but on its feeling-tone, on the reactions of the subjective personality. Here there is something compulsive in the reaction. It appears as something unalterable, and the feelings which arise therefrom are also experienced as something unavoidable, and are accepted with a certain fatalism. The attitude is, "I was born that way, and I cannot change my nature". As a result, those people and circumstances are sought out which are congenial to them, and no attempt at adaptation is made if this search is not immediately successful. Feelings are therefore specially developed within a personal sphere to which the individual is attached and which reminds him of home. Within such a sphere, these people may occasionally be able to emanate a certain warmth and cosiness around themselves, and their love is frequently concentrated on beautiful things and on animals within this sphere. If they do not succeed in creating such a personal sphere for themselves, they may become very depressed and unhappy. In the realm of sex their feelings are strongly coloured by sensual manifestations, with the result that they may become deeply attached to the object of their attraction. This predominance of the sexual instinct causes sexual attraction to play a larger part in their sentimental relationships with the opposite sex than is the case with people of other types. Masculinity and femininity are accordingly strongly emphasized in the emotional life of such people.

As regards intuition, it is a concept which this type of instinctive individual also finds very difficult to grasp, and he regards its activity in others with misgiving. He cannot take it seriously. At the same time, the intuitive views of leading spirits on matters, for example, of religion and politics are accepted by him, provided they appear in traditional form. The somewhat passive attitude towards life of these people then exerts an influence, in that factors of predestination and fate are likely to play a large part in their philosophy. This latter is not much affected by their personal life, since abstract vision and practical adaptation are for them two entirely different things. This lack of a comprehensive vision, and their introversion, stand in the way of a satisfactory external adaptation. They are less able than the extraverts of this type to make use of helpful circumstances, and in this respect they have, as a rule, to get help from others, who, recognizing their good qualities, manage to find an environment for them where these can come to expression.

CHAPTER III

INTUITION AND THE INTUITIVE TYPES

(A) *Intuition in Psychology*

MOST psychologists have some objection to intuition as a scientific concept, although they frequently enough make use of the word in practice. The reason for this is partly the very vague and mystical significance attached to the term in philosophy, the consequence being, that psychologists overlook important manifestations, well worth their consideration. Intuition is regarded by some philosophers as the source of a high spiritual knowledge, achieved by contemplation or by vision. (*Intueri* means "to see into".) A special characteristic of this knowledge is the strong conviction of its truth, apart from any rational proof. Bergson has gone even farther in his estimation of the value of this knowledge, defending the point of view that in it the true nature of reality is immediately understood. In psychology we are required to consider the functions in all their various forms, both deficient and highly differentiated. And the simple forms often give a better idea of the characteristics of a function than its more complicated manifestations. We will, accordingly, try to get a better view of the simple forms of intuition.

Here again, in any attempt to convey the essential quality in intuitive experience, we take, as our point of departure, our own introspective experience, and what is told us by others concerning such experience. Our first question may be whether intuition must be regarded as a separate function. The answer depends on whether it is possible to distinguish the special properties of intuitive experience. In looking for such properties, we are struck first of all by the fact that an intuition refers to matters of a certain complexity. It is impossible to have an intuition of a single object. If we take an object, for example a chair, as the focus of an intuition, we see that it is the relationship in which it stands to other circumstances which is the essential thing. Let us discuss this in connection with some examples.

If we listen to someone speaking in a foreign language, we may clearly understand the words, and even something of the speaker's emotions, so that we should probably be able to give some account of his state of mind. We experience him in our instinctive sphere. But as soon as he changes to a language with which we are familiar, all these sounds suddenly coalesce to an entity. We are no longer concerned with them as sounds, but with their meaning. Or, as another example, we may take a boy faced with a mathematical drawing. At first this looks to him like nothing but a criss-cross of lines; if, however, he works out their mutual relationships, he may suddenly perceive the meaning of the whole.[1] From now on, his contact with the drawing is different from what it was before. In the same way, a man may experience a Beethoven symphony as mere noise, if he is not musical; but it may also happen that a piece of music suddenly begins to become full of meaning. Intuitive insight may also occur in relation to a memory; for example, we hear someone in the course of conversation make use of a certain expression; only later do we realize why this was said, and what its real meaning was. The expression which we heard fits into its place within a larger whole, a totality full of meaning.

This kind of conscious experience is something special, in addition to the instinctive sphere of experience. It possesses the following distinguishing characteristics:

(*a*) Compared with the continuity which is characteristic of happenings in the instinctive sphere, the form assumed by intuitive experience has about it something momentary, more or less sudden and unique. Often it comes like a flash of lightning.

(*b*) In intuitive experience there is spontaneous insight into the relation of a certain group of facts, as a result of which they assume an added significance. This is something quite different from the practical instinctive knowledge which results from emphases in sensation.

(*c*) Intuitive knowledge appears as something new, while instinctive experience is always associated with the effects of earlier experience.

(*d*) This insight has a peculiarly convincing quality. It brings with it conviction of the validity of the revealed relation, in contrast to the empirical adaptation of instinctive experience, where conviction covers no more than can be dealt with in practice. (Later, it is true, criticism may shake conviction; but at the moment there is no element of doubt.)

(*e*) Intuitive experience is more personal than is instinctive

[1] Here thought plays a large part in the origin of the intuition, since it makes it possible to recognize the meaning of the details in the drawing. I shall deal further with this relationship between thought and intuition in the chapter on thought.

experience. It is as if by our insight we were in control of something, as if relationships and possibilities were revealed to us. An intuition is something special, having a certain value for the person concerned. As a result, intuitions may, owing to the personal form in which they take expression, exert persuasive influence on others.

(*f*) A sixth characteristic of intuition is the form it takes in memory. In recalling an instinctive experience, memory may proceed from emphasis to emphasis in sensation, and in this way reproduce the actual experience. This is not possible with intuition. Here a totality, with its distinctive structure, must be recalled. This totality is fixed in the memory in the form of a certain image, which serves to bring the whole experience back to life. This image may be of something incidental—for example, the person who gave us the intuition, or the place where it occurred. It may, however, bear some relation to the whole, and reflect certain of its features. In this case the image becomes a symbol. Word-symbols have been of particular significance in the development of mental life. (In this connection I may point out that the words of primitive languages refer to relationships rather than things.)

Having thus described the characteristics of intuitive experience, I must now discuss an objection which is frequently raised against the admission of intuition as an independent function. Sudden insight is explained as a consequence of unconscious thinking, so that intuition is regarded as a special form of thinking. In some cases it can be demonstrated that conscious reasoning may lead to a certain conclusion, and it is then assumed that the appearance of this conclusion in a spontaneous way is the result of unconscious reasoning. Further, it is somewhat hastily presumed that this explanation will hold good for all forms of sudden insight. Various arguments may be adduced against this attempt to explain away intuition. First of all, we must remember what William James called the "psychologist's fallacy". Psychologists are apt to think that anything which can be thought concerning a psychological fact must have been present in the mind—their own, or that of another—at the moment when it occurred. If there is no trace of this in recollection, then it must be assumed that it was there nevertheless, but unconsciously. But this is not consonant with sound scientific psychology, which must be based on perception and careful description, and not on speculation. For this reason, I propose to try first of all to describe what does occur in consciousness when an intuition appears. A second argument against this explanation by unconscious thinking may be found in the suggestion that it proves somewhat far-fetched when applied to primitive peoples, in whom thought is developed only slightly, if at all; or to cases where there is a gift for intuitive calculation, such as is occasionally found in imbeciles. Thirdly, there are many cases where thought cannot possibly offer any explanation of a particular flash of spontaneous insight. As a rule, psychologists tend to deny facts of this kind; but they exist nevertheless, particularly in women. In many of the cases investigated by the Society for Psychical Research the concept of intuition may be of value in the classification of forms of insight which appear to have no foundation and yet prove to be correct. As a fourth argument, I can refer to my own experience with very intuitive people, that they often find it extremely difficult to understand the rational basis of their intuitions, and indeed (where thought is poorly developed) may sometimes not succeed in doing so at all. It appears to me incorrect to assume that in such cases there is in the unconscious a superior form of thought. I prefer to describe these manifestations without further explanation. And since this description reveals that there are many special features in intuition, it seems to me practical and justifiable to give these phenomena a special name in psychology.

We have now got a clearer idea of the special form of intuitive experience, viz. a spontaneous, occasionally extremely sudden, form of insight into certain relationships in the field of instinctive experience. Some people are very familiar with it, others may find it difficult to differentiate this form from the other contents of their conscious life. This function appears to me to play a very large part in all mental life, and although in some cases it may be very striking, intuition is also often made use of without our being aware of it. We shall see later that this form of conscious experience is very closely bound up with aspects of thinking and feeling, and where this is so, it may be difficult to analyse out the influence of intuition in complex mental structures.

In regard to intuition, as with other forms of conscious experience, there is a tendency to objectify the experience, by assuming that it also occurs in others. Here we also find support in the fact that others describe corresponding experiences to us. Even when this is not possible, we still venture to draw conclusions from their behaviour as to the state of mind which is impelling them. Thus the question arises here also, as to whether there are special forms of behaviour which are more particularly associated with the intuitive form of conscious experience. We may attempt to differentiate such forms, even though we recognize that the special form of expression in words, as used to communicate introspective experience, is the surest guide. In addition to this, we have, however, simple verbal expression, and other kinds of behaviour, as factors to help us in our estimation of other people. As far as the latter is concerned, it may be noted that spontaneous insight effects spontaneous, more or less sudden, changes in action, usually inexplicable by external changes, and thus giving an impression of a certain capriciousness. And if these changes are accompanied by words, it may become evident that there is, as personal motive for the change, a profound conviction in regard to some flash of insight. From this we may conclude that spontaneity is a characteristic of behaviour which is controlled by intuition.

The behaviour of primitive people, and the images in which they give expression to their convictions, impel us to regard intuitive experience as an essential factor in their mental life. We may even go farther and assume that intuitive experience can occur even in the anthropoid apes. A large number of experiments have been made with various animals, with a view to investigating the possibility of learning by experience. If, for example, coloured feeding-buckets are used, and food is always placed in a bucket of the same colour, it is observed that the number of mistakes made in finding the food gradually diminishes, so that the animal finally goes straight to the bucket of the particular colour. Yerkes carried out a similar experiment in a more complicated way with an orang-utang, and found a remarkable difference in this form of learning.[1] For a time the number of mistakes did not greatly diminish; but suddenly a change took place, and no more mistakes were made. It was as if the meaning of the connection suddenly dawned on the ape. This may be compared with similar modes of behaviour in children, described by Bühler as the "Aha!" experience. Similar modes of reaction were also observed by Köhler[2] in corresponding studies of chimpanzees, and these also give one the impression of the development of sudden insight.

Thus we find intuition in the earliest unfolding of human consciousness, and before I pass on to the significance which it may have in the minds of certain people, I must spend a little more time on this aspect of the subject. Intuition seems to me to be of the utmost importance as a source of development in mental life. Before the dawn of intuition animals had but one form of adaptation. After this there exist in the consciousness of primitive man (and perhaps of anthropoid apes) two forms, capable of mutual

[1] Robert M. Yerkes, *The Mental Life of Monkeys and Apes: a Study in Ideational Behaviour*, 1916.
[2] Wolfgang Köhler, *The Mentality of Apes*, 1917 (Eng. Trans., 1923).

inter-action. Both forms are primarily directed towards practical adaptation, and at the beginning these conscious forms are related, both in memory and in actual experience, only to real existing things and relationships. Intuitions may also arise, however, which do not entirely coincide with reality. A relationship or a possibility which has been divined, may prove to be incorrect when compared with the facts, or two intuitions concerning one and the same thing may clash with each other. As a result, the images of intuitive experience are more or less independent of reality. They form in the conscious mind a region which may lead us to ask how much corresponds to reality, and how much is imaginary. Primitive people do not see it as imagination, but ascribe such contents of the mind to spirits, demons, etc. The fact remains, however, that a new form has arisen in consciousness, more or less independent of sensory experience, which is possibly "only psychic". In this way intuition may, although originally directed towards the real world, lead to imagination, and it is still possible to observe this process taking place in intuitive people.

As a second effect of intuitive experience in consciousness, we may regard the increased significance which it gives to the ego. While instinct is guided step by step by sensory experience, keeping in close touch with the material world, intuition reveals the possibility that we can control things by our insight. Since this recognition comes to us in the form of an experience of understanding something in a very personal way, the importance of one's own personality is more keenly felt. In the field of instinctual experience, the overcoming of a difficulty may give a sense of power; but with intuition the experience remains in memory as a picture in which the "I, who did this" is an important figure in the foreground. In this way the ego becomes more and more a central image, an important symbol of power; and "I wish" becomes more and more "I will". "I will" means a conscious reinforcing of the impulse, under the influence of intuition. It seems to me that we may recognize this result of the appearance of intuition in the young child, in the development of narcissism. In intuitive people the latter is also found as a powerful factor, intensifying the personal significance of experience of all kinds.

A third possibility arising out of the existence of intuitive experience is the development of a more or less independent mental life. In the instinctive sphere, inner needs and the inner meaning of life find expression in action and conduct. Intuitions are probably first of all directed towards the external world and practical adjustment to it, and while in this form, they do not arouse any awareness of mental activity. But when once images have been formed of relationships in the world and between man and the world, these images may be employed to reflect a certain aspect of an inner state of mind. A savage may, for instance, say that he felt like a lion being attacked, or a woman may compare a certain situation with the birth of her first child. Such images are often inevitably difficult for the uninitiated to understand, since they cannot possibly be familiar with all the special experiences of these people. Extremely fantastic images may at this stage be the best expression of their first recognition of an inner life. Such recognition cannot at this stage be described as introspection, since this term is usually reserved for a more actively controlled perception. Very significant material is, however, contained in these images, capable of giving a lead to introspective perception. In some people this intuitive mode of expressing inner relationships in a metaphorical way may be much in evidence. The dream seems to me to be a product of intuitive activities of this kind, and the form assumed by many curious symbols in waking life can only be explained in this way.[1]

These general considerations lead us to the conclusion that intuition must be recognized as a function of great significance in psychology. Without this concept, many phenomena can find no place in scientific description. It will also prove full of significance in the explanation of special forms of thought and feeling. The influence of intuitive experience in mental life is particularly striking in certain people, in whom this function predominates over other modes of conscious orientation. Where this is so, spontaneous insight, and the images resulting therefrom, take precedence over simple practical application of facts, and over the established rules and ideas governing thought and feeling. Such people rely on their ability to see the rights of a situation at the moment when this becomes necessary. Hence they make few preparations, and rely much less on sound common sense or on tradition than do others. Since they see every situation as a fresh problem, it is more difficult for them, than for others, to learn by experience. Facts have little significance for them, unless they are seen in some association of meaning and purpose. They approach reality through the images of their imagination. These images may, however, conceal the real facts, instead of revealing them. With intuitive people we find an intensely personal mode of attacking problems, and a strong conviction of the correctness of their insight. Their behaviour may

[1] The reference is here only to the form of the dream and similar symbols. Their contents require a different mode of explanation, which psycho-analysis has worked out.

appear capricious. They may occasionally exert powerful suggestive influence. They do not feel bound to their opinions, however strongly they have expressed them; for intuition demands liberty to see things at any moment in a new connection. They not only avoid the rigidity of facts, preferring images, but they only make use of thought and feeling when these possess a certain flexibility and elasticity, allowing for readjustments under the influence of spontaneous inspiration.

(B) *The Extraverted Intuitive Type*

The vision of the extraverted intuitive individual is directed chiefly on to relationships and circumstances in the external world, which are suddenly seen in a certain context, without his being able to work out how he came to it. This knowledge, and the spontaneous activities in which it is expressed, often prove to be absolutely correct and to the point, when checked by later experience. The extraverted intuitive is also readily able to grasp the views of others. Whereas outwardly directed sensation submits to the guidance of material facts, intuition sees in the external world all manner of connections in an original and personal way, and is charged, as it were, with a mission to realize certain possibilities. These relate particularly to personal development and activity, both for the self and for others, and intuition seeks them everywhere, and has a special flair for finding them. Even in cases in which intuition is not the most important function, it will often provide a solution in circumstances in which none of the other functions can find a way out. Jung writes: [1] "If intuition be the leading function, all ordinary conditions of life seem to be enclosures to which intuition must find a key. It is forever seeking new paths and new possibilities for outward life. For an intuitive person all circumstances soon become a prison, an oppression, and they long for liberation. Things in the outside world seem temporarily to have an exaggerated value, namely, when they can be of use for a solution, or a liberation, or for the discovery of a new possibility. They have, however, scarcely served as steps, or a bridge, when they seem no longer of any value and are cast off as unnecessary ballast. A fact is only valued so long as it opens up new and more important prospects, which in their turn will liberate the individual. Sudden possibilities become compelling motives which the intuitive mind cannot disregard, and for which it may sacrifice everything else."

[1] C. G. Jung, *Psychological Types*, p. 527.

The extraverted intuitive is in many respects the opposite of the introverted instinctive person. Whereas in the latter great passivity and a certain dependence on the environment is found, the extraverted intuitive manifests much spontaneous activity and independence, even to the point of rebelling against any obligation. This may be evident at a very early age. Children of this type are merry and full of the joy of life; but often extremely tiresome. They are always thinking out something fresh, and their imagination continually suggests fresh possibilities. They have a finger in every pie, want to know everything, and at an early age seek to become persons of some influence in their environment. They like to impress others by startling remarks or behaviour, and at an early age want to be something special. Later, also, one finds among these intuitives particularly lively people, active in mind, and expressing themselves with freedom. When they are at the top of their form, there is something radiant and inspiring about them. They are able then to entertain a whole company, and have the art of bringing other people out of themselves. They are fond, also, of making use of this capacity and of being the centre of enthusiasm. They prefer to radiate enthusiasm and to stimulate others, rather than to work something out, or enter on any lasting relationship with anyone. Novelty attracts them, both in people and in things, which makes them extremely changeable. They are often pleasanter with strangers than they are in the home circle. They constantly reveal new facets of their nature, which seem to come to light spontaneously. This was eloquently expressed in the dream of a very intuitive patient. He saw in this dream a large postal delivery van which had met with an accident, and heard the people standing round express their indignation about the reckless driving. It was at the time when these vans had just been introduced. He defended the driver, saying that these chauffeurs had constantly to drive fresh cars, and thus never got to know them properly. Analysis showed that this really represented an excuse for mistakes caused by his own recklessness. He had great difficulty in managing himself, owing to the constant irruption of fresh inspirations and impulses.

Owing to this excessive spontaneity in their nature, extraverted intuitives find it extremely difficult to bind themselves to keep rules or appointments. They cannot always be depended on. Their activity is often very great, but somewhat incalculable. Their whole energy will be concentrated, almost apart from their will, on the opportunity offering at the moment. They like, however, to see quick results, and failing this, their attention is readily distracted to something else. They show more impulsive energy than concentrated will-power. They are stimulated by difficulties, for they are by nature combative. They do not like to admit that they cannot do a thing, and they will discover fresh possibilities where others have failed to get on. Many discoverers and inventors belong to this type, but also the business man, who with great assurance sees new possibilities for extending his business; many lawyers, also, and politicians, even artists who manage to find new modes of expression, possess this mental structure. Among them are found leaders [1] in many fields. In women of this type, intuition plays a part particularly in the establishment of personal relationships and in social contacts. This type of woman is peculiarly successful in initiating and organizing social activities. The pride of these people is that they see possibilities of putting something through which others regard as impossible. They are frequently better at taking the initiative in starting something than at working it out to a finish, while others will be able to profit by their idea.

With intuitive people judgment takes the form of a strong, momentary conviction, which they often express so persuasively that others are influenced by it. Sometimes it is possible to confirm this conviction logically, but not always; and even without such confirmation, such a judgment will for most intuitives be binding. Where the intuitive function is highly developed, it will often be found to be astonishingly correct. But even in such a case, an intuitive may nevertheless be profoundly mistaken, and in the absence of any capacity for rational self-criticism such mistakes will also be made with complete conviction. If he notices his mistake, he is usually very adroit in correcting it or covering it up. For these people are really startlingly clever; they give an impression of making nothing of the difficulties with which others have to struggle; they can get away with anything.

Reason is in intuitive people subordinate to spontaneous inspiration. It is often well developed, but is nevertheless influenced by qualities peculiar to intuition. One of the results of this is a great liveliness and flexibility in reasoning power, and a striving after originality. People of this type are able to converse in a lively way concerning all kinds of problems, and soon come to be regarded in their circle as authorities in any field. Their views often appear original, but they are frequently taken over from other people and cleverly made use of. At the same time they are apt to be ill-considered, and are seldom, if at all, elaborated into useful ideas. Thought is for these people nothing but a means to attain some

[1] Lloyd George is a typical example.

effect; it is never an end in itself, as with the intellectual person who seeks in it some foundation for his life. At school, children of this type are the despair of the teacher, because while they show clear evidence of good reasoning powers, it is difficult to persuade them to make use of them and to develop them, unless they can see some immediate advantage from so doing. If they have promised themselves to fulfil some purpose, or if their competitive interest has been aroused, they may occasionally distinguish themselves in the intellectual sphere; but in thought itself they find only moderate gratification. Many intellectual perceptions seem to come to them, as it were, unbidden; but if this does not happen, they generally fight shy of the trouble which it will cost them to master anything. Hence there is often something fragmentary about their knowledge. They will let contradictions stand side by side unresolved without being troubled by them, and in their theorizing they are apt to be very inconsistent. Their knowledge is not regulated by any objective system, but develops in line with their personal experiences and needs. Thus a certain ego-centricity will be evident. Since they must always allow some scope for inspiration, they will never tie themselves up too closely with formulations and rules. Room must be left for further possibilities. This occasionally gives an impression of insincerity, and may indeed lead to it. But if this characteristic is kept under control, it will imply a wide understanding, and receptivity to the views of others. This quality enables them to contribute a great deal in scientific and practical problems towards the examination of new points of view, and to bringing people of various kinds together. The special qualities in the thinking of such an individual are well illustrated by Count Keyserling.

Feeling, like reason, may play a large or a small part in the lives of intuitives, but it also will be under the influence of their peculiar spontaneity. Here, also, there will be found great liveliness and flexibility in the feelings, which are very individual in their mode of expression. Many clever people belong to this type, and the majority of artists. There is a lively expression of feeling, but it does not last long, the intuitive person being more concerned with expressing himself, and making a strong momentary impression on others, than with the formation of a lasting relationship. To this type, also, belong those people who carry on entire conversations without paying the slightest attention to the replies or remarks of the other person. When they do want to stimulate some response, it is usually with some special intention, and not because they want a closer personal contact. They shrink from intimate relationships, owing to a fear of limiting thereby their freedom to act in accordance with their intuitions. As a rule, they are on friendly terms with a large number of people, and have a wide circle of acquaintances, but no really intimate friends of either sex. Their surface of contact with others is limited, but intense, and at the same time mobile. This mobility makes it appear wider than it is, while hindering any more intimate tie. It is a characteristic which enables them to evade with considerable skill conflicts both within themselves and with others. A joke or a compliment will be made to distract attention from any difficulty or contradiction. The consequences of feeling will always be avoided, if in any way possible. As a result, there is at times with people of this type a tendency to play with feelings: they prefer them in the form of fireworks, rather than as a flame. If they should be caught up in them, it is usually to some extent against their will.

The result of this attitude is the same as where thinking is concerned, a marked ego-centricity in the emotional life. Feeling is not for them a sphere of influence, whose laws they accept, but a playground for their own personal opportunities, and the ego is the determining factor. The weak point in the emotional life of the extraverted intuitive is his vanity. His enthusiasm is usually only aroused by something in which he himself can play an important part. He is thrilled by other people only when they have some value for his personal life, or, more especially, when they appreciate something in him. If his vanity is wounded, he will generally not let it be seen at once. He will answer to a criticism only if directly challenged; otherwise he will prefer to keep out of the way of the critic, or himself will assume a very critical attitude. Here the effect of vanity is in contradiction to that chivalrous generosity which in other circumstances bids him make allowances for mistakes and faults in others.

This tendency to keep at a distance and to avoid conflicts, in the sphere of feeling as in the sphere of thought, is associated with a certain insecurity, concealed behind an appearance of decisiveness. These people are sometimes conscious of this sense of insecurity, but sometimes not. Its source lies in the dependence of intuitive people on images. Adaptation, based on clearly perceived images, seems to them to be safer and more exact than other modes of orientation based more on trial and error; but this is only so long as these images and the connections they express are not questioned. When this happens, the suspicion dawns on them that these images are not the facts themselves, and that things may possibly be other than they appear. The customary assurance of the intuitive individual then forsakes him, and he will be apt to try and escape both facts and arguments based on reason or feeling.

The aspect of life which the intuitive finds it most difficult to accept is that which is most congenial to the instinctive individual. The facts of the external world, and physical and instinctual needs, are likely to be the greatest hindrance to anyone whose constant aim it is to realize fresh possibilities. This is particularly true of the compelling aspect of his instinctual needs; such people often show a compulsive tendency to deny their own bodily and instinctual needs, even to an extreme degree. When consumed with zeal for their work, they will, for example, easily forget to eat or sleep until exhaustion overcomes them. As a rule, too, they take no trouble in the reasonable ordering of their sexual life, with the result that their sexual impulses take them unawares. They find the instinctive side of life somewhat disturbing, and prefer to ignore it.

(C) *The Introverted Intuitive Type*

The introverted intuitive perceives connections and meaning in the internal world, and with as much spontaneity and conviction as the extraverted intuitive sees them in the external world. It is not primarily his own personal inner life that he grasps in this way, but rather inner life in general, the inner nature of things. The aim of intuition here is to perceive the ideal essence of all things—animate and inanimate, and in their inter-relations. The clearest example of the kind of thing is seen in Plato's "ideas", which give a purer representation of the inner being of the world than does reality itself. Jung calls these mental images, supplying meaning and a standard of comparison, "archetypes", and he regards them as a deposit of ancestral experience. Others see in them the immediate expression of a spiritual world. These questions lie outside the realm of psychology, and would lead us to that of metaphysics. Here we must confine ourselves to the statement that intuitions of this kind concerning the inner essence of things do occur in the human mind, and that for a certain type of mind, that of the introverted intuitive, they determine and control the direction and the content of life. Here, also, intuitive knowledge is felt by the person concerned as objective and as having the universal validity of truth. Here we find, in addition to the tangible reality of sensory perception, and the conviction of instinctual impulse, another source of certainty, of great significance for humanity, for from this intuitive knowledge there arises not only religious conviction, but, in fact, all spiritual assurance. Spinoza speaks in this respect of "*scientia intuitiva*". Hence there are found also among intuitive introverts great spiritual leaders, prophets, founders of religions, all those people who, for the sake of some sacred inner conviction, will endure the world's misunderstanding and contempt.

It would be a mistake, however, in studying a function, to consider only its extreme potentialities, in which all that is most profound in the human mind has taken form. For this type assumes also many much less noble forms, and there is peculiar difficulty, where this inner knowledge is concerned, in finding even approximate expression for what is perceived. It is extremely important, therefore, for people of this type to attain through their education a technique of expression, as was the case with two great artists, Rembrandt and Beethoven, both of whom I include in this class.[1] The development of this type is slower and more arduous than that of most other people. In childhood, these people have something about them as spontaneous as have the extraverts of this type; but it is, both in form and expression, more bizarre, and less intelligible, owing to the causes being less explicable from external conditions. Such children are not very amenable to influence from their environment. They may have periods of uncertainty and reserve, after which they suddenly become very determined, and if then they are opposed, they may manifest an astonishing self-will and obstinacy. As a result of the intensely spontaneous activity within, they are frequently moody, occasionally brilliant and original, then again reserved, stubborn and arrogant.

In later life, also, it is a persistent characteristic of people of this type, that while on the one hand they possess great determination, on the other hand they find it very difficult to express what they want. Although they may have only a vague feeling about the way they want to go, and of the meaning of their life, they will nevertheless reject with great stubbornness anything that does not fit in with this. They fear lest external influences or circumstances should drive them in a wrong direction, and they resist on principle. In their mode of life, and in their immediate environment, they seek to regulate everything according to their own ideas, which is apt to make them tyrants within their own small circle. Rather than adapt themselves, they will limit their contact with those who do not fall in with them. The rest of the world matters, in fact, very little to them. In contradiction to this reserve, there is the genuine enthusiasm which they may suddenly display for something. If some individual, or some event, or some object, responds to this sense which they have of the meaning of their life, and reveals to them something of their deeper purposes, then they take up a

[1] As a painter representing the extraverted intuitive type, one may mention Rubens, the master of composition.

different attitude, and become conscious of a more intense, more profound connection in things. The highest form of this function would imply a capacity for perceiving the deeper meaning of everything. The marvellous richness of life would then be revealed. As a rule, however, this only happens at certain moments and in relation to certain persons or things. This contradiction between intimate contact and cold reserve has been very clearly described by the introverted intuitive, Buber, in his account of the "I—you" and the "I—it" relationship.[1] This contradiction also occurs in other people, but not with the same mutual exclusion, nor with such definiteness, as in this type. Where the inner life finds expression, there will be close attachment; but side by side with this there will be a cold aloofness (*Weltfremdheit*). As far as material and instinctual life is concerned, these people feel exceedingly helpless, like people suddenly transplanted from another planet. They feel much more at home in spiritual things. In the realm of the spirit they have far greater assurance than other people. Here they are stimulating; one feels that something peculiar to themselves is operative within them. But its activity often remains indefinite, owing to an inability to find adequate expression for the tension of what they mean. The spiritual side of life can only be approached through symbols; its import can only be understood in mental images, and it is by no means always possible to find this approach. Moreover, a great deal of confusion arises, because it is not understood that this is, in any case, only an approximation. Certainty in regard to the underlying intent is then transferred to the form in which it is expressed, as a result of which formulations become dogmatic and judgment rigid. Incidental and inadequate points in the formulation are then regarded as essential and absolute. The firm conviction of these people may in such cases arouse strong opposition or find blind support. They often lay down the law in regard to what they have perceived, without its even occurring to them that it might be possible to find incorrect as well as correct elements therein. This often makes their influence over others the more effective, but it may prepare the way for great confusion. One is reminded of the influence which a man like Nietzsche has had on our generation.

In the realm of thought we shall to some extent find the same characteristics as we found when extraverted intuition influences reason. Here also the influence of reason is very variable and ego-centric, and knowledge fragmentary. Ideas must come of themselves, and great effort is required if this does not happen.

[1] Martin Buber, *Ich und Du.*

Thought is, however, less flexible than with the extravert of this type, but frequently even more original. Many new ideas, especially in the spiritual realm, have originated with people of this type; but they are often not worked out systematically. Their thought remains aphoristic, and is often expressed in paradoxes. Men like Emerson, Shaw and Chesterton belong to this type. Side by side with ideas expressive of genius, they will occasionally propound with equal conviction mistaken and fantastic views, which they maintain with obstinacy in the face of all criticism. Intuitive conviction stands for more than rational argument, which renders such people occasionally extremely conceited and opinionated.

Where it is a question of feeling with people of this type, it also assumes the peculiar characteristics of intuition. As has already been said, this gives rise to a contact with other people which is changeable and peculiar, according to whether something important is felt to lie in it, or not. As a result, emotional contacts are extremely inconstant; these people are at one moment full of enthusiasm and devotion, at the next utterly cold and stand-offish. It is always necessary, when with them, to be on the look-out for which way the wind is blowing. Spontaneous insight, and the images associated therewith, affect the feelings of the introverted intuitive in a somewhat different way from what we have seen in the case of the extravert of this type. With these extraverts the danger is that feelings are for show, with no development of inner reality. A living relationship with other people and with personal standards is lacking when this is so. With the introverted intuitive, the image of what the feelings should be may easily be substituted for a feeling-relationship. He will then make demands on others, without being prepared to meet the same demands on himself. Egotism, and a desire to dominate, may then make use of these requirements of an ideal relationship, for their own ends. Another peculiarity which may be manifested by feeling, when influenced by introverted intuition, is intense ambivalence, the co-existence of two absolutely opposed emotional attitudes. We have already seen in extraverted intuition how spontaneity favours the loose juxtaposition of opposing manifestations. In the introvert there is less variety in the form assumed by these contradictions, but great inner tension. The introverted intuitive may identify himself alternately with the divine and with the diabolical within himself. Occasionally he is unaware of this himself; when it becomes too intense, however, he feels as if he were being torn in two by conflicting forces within. In this struggle the individual concerned may be thrown hither and thither between the extremes of godlike assurance and diabolical confusion. In extreme cases the result may be a character like Rasputin.

As with extraverted intuition, here, also, contact is least with the facts of the external world, and with instinctual life. Such people live, as it were, alongside their bodies, until these by some disturbance demand their attention. The main thing is, however, that ordinary practical things and the world of facts are far removed for them, and they try to confine their contact with them to that which they can regulate according to their wishes. Everything else appears to them as something disquietingly incalculable, against which they must defend themselves as far as they possibly can.

CHAPTER IV

THINKING AND THE THINKING-TYPES

(A) *Thinking as a Mental Function*

THERE is more agreement concerning the formulated definition of thought than concerning the other functions. Thought is regarded as the mental activity by means of which the material of perceptions and ideas is elaborated into an objective system. To this end, the material is analysed and synthesized to form a coherent whole, without contradictions, and in conformity with experience. Thinking is expressed in judgments containing constant elements. These judgments are combined to make rules and laws, thus building up a system of knowledge whose aim it is to record the constant element in all happening.

This function is not easy to understand in its relation to other modes of conscious orientation, because it is not developed in us step by step, but is taught to us in ready-made forms. As a result, the contents of these forms assume a special authority, as if they were something quite different and of another order, compared with the rest of our mental contents. To understand its psychological relation to other manifestations, we must study the history of mankind, or the development of thought in original thinkers, or the birth of new thoughts in ourselves. In this case, we are less dependent on introspection, since the aim of all thinking is to find forms which are valid for everyone.

If we follow the development of thought in mankind, we shall find good reason to suppose that thought was not always present in our earliest ancestors. The need for judgments of general validity can only develop in communities of some size. Thought develops with social life. We saw how intuition arose at the dawn of human history, and we may regard intuitive knowledge as one of the earliest forms of intellect. It cannot as yet be called thought, however. We have already discussed how the inter-action of instinctual and intuitive experience rendered possible the development of a more independent form, that of mental images. Only later can the question arise as to whether an image is correct or not, when it may even prove to belong to a sphere other than that of reality. Intuition may conflict with sensory experience; two intuitions concerning the same object may even contradict one another. Only at this point does the question of truth arise. From the very beginning truth means a constancy of relationship;[1] and examination of this constancy yields two forms of mental content: the tested sensory fact, which becomes an observation or perception, and the tested content of intuitive knowledge, which becomes an idea. I have already postulated that sensory experience and observation (or perception) are two different modes of awareness. The distinction lies in the fact that by perception (or observation) a certain part of the sensory field is delimited, and is then examined in its constant relation to other contents. In the same way, our ideas differ from our intuitive knowledge in their more definite and more constant content. Only that which proves constant in association is retained. Since investigation of the constancy of such associations involves the comparison of judgments with the totality of our knowledge, thought implies a system in which mental contents, having proved constant, receive their definite place in relation to other judgments. It is clear that analysis and synthesis must work together in the building up of such a system.

The most careful construction of thought-systems is found in the sciences. The system employed in the natural sciences is formed more especially from the inter-action between the sensory aspect of instinctive experience and intuitive insight into relationships. The sphere of instinctive experience may, under the influence of intuitive insight, be differentiated into two parts: one, the more objective sensory aspect, and the other, the more subjective impulsive aspect. In actual instinctual experience there is consciousness only of the more stable objective aspect. It can only appear as distinct from the other after the lightning-flash of intuition has yielded images of certain co-existent associations. Insight into these associations or relationships, and our conception of the world of objects, develop together to a system of correct images of the world. Intuitions relating more especially to the sensory aspect of experience grasp certain associations in it, which are regularly repeated, and as a result yield reliable images. In our sensory experience, we find the world as a coherent whole, in which we are led from point to point through certain emphases in sensation, experience teaching us that any one point always involves the next. The world of the natural sciences is built up in the same way, with the one exception that

[1] This conception of truth is that of pragmatism. But pragmatism does not explain how a truth comes to be established as such, which leads us to the problem of intuition.

in science there is, in addition, an aim, namely, to describe every possible object and process in images. And these images must be such that they can be defined and confirmed. This form of orientation is called explanation of the world by cause and effect. Thinking is orientated not in accordance with emphases in sensation, such as direct our actions in the instinctive sphere, but according to a system in which all that is observable has been in every possible aspect analysed and tested, according to its value for action.[1] And instead of the continuity of the field of sensation, and of happening in the instinctive sphere, there is found in thinking a synthesis of every possible perception, offering explanations, not only of the field of observation at the moment, but of earlier and of subsequent perceptions, and of the connection between them. The continuity of instinctive experience in relation to space and time is thus reconstituted in the synthesis of science, according to the law of cause and effect.

Registering casual relations is not, however, the only aim of science. We can understand intuitively a connection between cause and effect; but our intuition enables us to recognize other forms of relationship as well. Our thinking is developed in connection with our actions, and for the control of this action the structure of the external world is not the only important factor; our own purposes and those of others represent an essential factor in our orientation, and these purposes are also grasped intuitively in the first place. Side by side with the thought-order of cause and effect, there thus arises another order, regulated by purpose, and these teleological definitions and evaluations also form in most sciences an important factor; especially in the mental sciences. Classification of purposive efforts may here give rise to momentous ideologies (e.g. in relation to the state or to religious life).

A third form of systematization by means of thought, in which intuition plays a large part, is developed when, after they have been evolved to a certain point, the categories of thought themselves become the object of insight. Certain rules and norms of thought are then perceived intuitively, and postulated in separate structures. In this way, sciences such as grammar, mathematics and logic are evolved in the human mind.

We are dealing here with an effect of intuition, which is not only possible in connection with classification by thought, but which may also furnish images for the expression of other structural character-

[1] One may compare practical with scientific orientation by taking as an example two men, one of whom can manage his car only from the practical point of view, while the other is familiar with it only in theory.

istics of our life, such as the values of the emotional life, or truths immediately perceptible in the totality of some particular vital experience. This form of intuition spans,[1] as it were, a whole realm of conscious experience, and is able to abstract from it essential factors in their inter-relation. For all abstract and philosophical thinking, this form of intuitive insight is of fundamental value.

It will be clear from what I have said that I regard intuition as being extremely valuable in the development of every kind of thought-form.[2] In ordinary thinking, however, intuition plays, as a rule, practically no part. Its forms were intuitively conceived many years ago, but a few thinkers are still able to discover them afresh (as happens, for example, if one begins to examine the truth of an axiom). Ordinary thinking, however, follows the highway of mental association, without questioning its correctness. The form of thought is a collective creation, even though the purposes which it is used to serve may be personal enough. Indeed, for most people it is to their interest to distinguish their intuitions from their thought-forms. When this does not happen, thought becomes capricious and loses its firm foundations. This may be stimulating in an ordinary conversation, but such thinking will be less appropriate as a guide for conduct.

With some people, however, thinking remains closely bound up with those vital needs from which it arose in the development of mankind, that is to say, with the investigation of the verity of objective and associative images. The consequence is that such persons are at the same time more careful and more enterprising in their thinking. They do not simply accept all the thoughts that present themselves in a generally accepted form, but even here demand some proof. On the other hand, they do not hesitate to combine in fresh ways facts and associations hitherto unrelated. A thought-system is for them a living organism. For them there is always the possibility, that by linking up old truths they may discover a new one. They are accessible to new facts and new views, so long as these can be brought into agreement with the totality of established experience. Hence, for them thought is more closely associated with sensation and intuition. If, however, no connection with the system can be found, mental contents are consigned to the realm of fantasy, and excluded from the structure of truth.

[1] See Translator's note on page 264.

[2] Many philosophers and psychologists identify these forms of intuition with thought. The fact that intuition also occurs apart from thought, and that a great deal of thinking is carried out without any vital contact with intuition, has led me to distinguish between the two concepts.

Nowhere is the dividing line between objective truth and fantasy regarded as of such vital significance as with people of the thinking-type.

The criterion of truth is thus always that a mental content shall prove to be in agreement with the totality of our experience. The presence of this agreement can be shown in four ways: (*a*) such agreement may mean that a certain part of the sensory experience has a constant reference to other perceived facts (*vérité de fait*, Leibnitz); (*b*) or it may be evident that an intuitively divined association is not in opposition to the facts or to the rest of our experience of the context; (*c*) a third form of agreement consists in the adherence of a judgment to a system of truth which has been proved as such (*vérité de raison*); (*d*) also the total structure of a system of truth, or of a field of vital experience, may be envisaged in one moment by means of comprehensive (*überkuppelnde*) intuitions, as a result of which the norms which determine this structure become clear. Even in this latter case, the truth of the insight depends on its agreement with the totality of experience.

Having considered some of the general aspects of thought, we may now proceed to discuss what are the properties of the sphere of thought in our conscious minds. As a general and approximate description, one might say that, in thinking, the conscious contents of the mind possess a definite meaning, which we assume to hold good for others as well. We further assume objective validity for the fixed associations between these and other thought-images. These thought-images are closely associated with those belonging to our sensory and intuitive experience, but are not identical with them. Simply reading the words of a book, without realizing the content, or re-living in memory a previous occurrence, or recalling the impression made on us by someone's personality—all this is not thinking. In none of these situations is there any demand for objectivity. But what about recounting to others something of my own experience? If I make use of words, is my intention not objective, in so far as they are intended to produce, through the images they present, the same effect in the mind of others as they have for mine? Have not, then, all words an objective meaning? Does the use of words always mean thought? And is it possible to say that all thinking takes place in words?

If this were true, it would provide a convenient criterion; but it is not so. In the first place, the speaking and hearing of words is not always related to thought. When I was trying to explain intuition, I adduced as an example the situation of hearing someone speak first in a foreign language, and afterwards in our own. As a result of this change, we are able to hear his utterance as a significant whole. I must now add something to this, to show how far the understanding of his words may be regarded as an intuitive experience, and under what conditions we must allow this understanding a place in the sphere of thought. I can justify the use I made of this example, by pointing out that intuitive experience is always present in such a situation, while the presence of thought depends on certain circumstances, which may occasionally also occur. Supposing the person in the example is reciting poetry (especially very "modern" poetry), or is speaking to amuse his listeners; we should most of us agree that these utterances would not come under the head of thought. Here the most important thing is the expression of something personal. This personal aspect is always present, whether the person concerned is explaining an experiment in physics, or the philosophy of Kant. Through this aspect we receive an impression of the kind of man the speaker is. Words may, just as much as bearing, be a matter of simple expression, and, as such, comprehended in the sphere of intuitive experience (empathy). Occasionally this is the real aim of a verbal contact, but often it is not so. In the latter case, the intuitive, personal aspect of understanding is felt to be subsidiary, and the objective significance of the verbal communication comes to be the most essential thing about it. When an intuition is expressed in words, these words may assume very individual significance. In a joke, its point may be the using of a word in a different sense from that usually ascribed to it. In the explanation of a mathematical theory, both words and numbers, and other signs too, assume a very definite meaning, laid down by definition. In order to understand the discussion, one must be able to fill in the sense of these words with some definite mental content. These contents are often extremely complicated, as, for example, when a theory is indicated by the name of its author. Thus words employed by thought-processes indicate structures possessing general validity for all who are able to understand them. In science, words have recognized and exact meanings. In ordinary thinking—and occasionally, indeed, in science—the meaning of words may be filled out in different ways, without involving necessarily any falsity in thought. Supposing I speak of a tree and a table, it may be that one of my hearers will picture an oak and a four-legged table respectively, while another will have before his mind a fir tree and a one-legged table. Or supposing I am describing the scenery of a foreign country, which I have visited, to people who have never been there; the images in my mind will not be the same as those in their minds. If I induce them to think about this country, the mental structures, associated by them with names and words, will be less objective than mine. Yet, as thinking, their thought is just as genuine as mine. Their minds may, in fact, be working more exclusively in the sphere of thought than mine, since for me it is possible simply to recall my earlier experience, when there will be no need for any names or words or ordering of thought. For them, on the other hand, a certain ordering of thought will be the only means of attaining a more or less correct picture of the country concerned. The words used in thinking require to have their meaning filled out to some extent, but again it must not go too far. Otherwise, thought may be changed into the re-living of earlier experience, or pass over into fantasy or intuitive perception. All of this may take place during a train of thought. Our mind may set out from a certain mental (thought) image, and then wander; in which case we cease to think.[1] Thus thinking means a partial amplification of meaning, only so far as is necessary to lead us to the next concept. All this makes it apparent that abstraction is a distinguishing quality of thought-structures, differentiating this form of conscious experience from both instinctive and intuitive experience.

Thus the essential thing in thought is found to be not the fact that it involves words, but its possession of certain mental structures claiming objective validity. Sometimes the group of people employing these structures will be small, as in the case of the higher mathematics; in other cases, elementary-school education will see to it that the mind of every citizen contains certain of these structures, as a result of which we learn to understand the world and to behave suitably, much sooner than if we had to learn by our own instinctive adaptation or by our own intuition.

It is certainly true that this system of facts and connections is communicated to us by means of words. Is it, then, possible to say that all thinking takes place in words? It has become evident that the relationship between words and mental contents is, in any case, a much closer one where thinking is concerned than is the case with intuitive and instinctive experience, which can be only more or less suggested in words. We saw that the object of the judgment, emanating from the sphere of thought, and expressed in words, was a structure definable by those words. But words are not the only means of suggesting that structure. It may happen that a diagram or a plan or a mathematical formula will come nearer to a satis-

[1] It is true that we may, from the starting-point of a mental image, spin a train of thought of our own, quite independently of that of the person addressing us.

factory representation of the structure concerned. Although it is true that such forms can likewise be described in words, the fact remains that most architects would prefer a drawing, and most mathematicians a formula. Thinking is thus possible apart from words, although even here its essential quality of involving certain mental structures remains. It may indeed happen that certain ideas involving complicated abstract thinking will be absolutely clear to some individual, in spite of the fact that he finds it extraordinarily difficult to express these thoughts in words. In a case such as this we recognize, therefore, that thought, although usually associated with words, may, under certain circumstances, dispense with them.

At this point I will offer what follows as the result of an attempt to state the characteristics of the sphere of thought as experienced introspectively:

(*a*) In comparison with the instinctive and intuitive spheres, thought-forms, both of past and present thinking, appear to us as constant. We pass from the variable experience of the external and the internal world to a region of order and constant connections.

(*b*) This ordered world of thought is not, however, isolated from reality. It reflects the relationships and facts of reality; but since, in doing so, it has regard only to the more essential and constant factors, we obtain a more reliable picture than our total experience provides.

(*c*) This reliability is the consequence of the fact that the structures of the sphere of thought have been built up by humanity in the course of centuries, so that the experience of endless generations is contained within them. The use of these structures is part of our education, and from youth up we are accustomed to regard them as possessing universal validity.

(*d*) The constancy of thought-images is the result of abstraction. Observations and ideas are abstracted from instinctive and intuitive experience, by the isolation of common features from the content of various experiences. According to the stage which this process of abstraction has reached, there may be all kinds of transitional forms between thought-forms and those of intuition or sensation. Starting from certain thought-forms, we may, by filling out these forms with every detail, undo the work of abstraction, and work back to the forms characteristic of sensation and intuition.

(*e*) The definition of the mental structures employed by thought may vary greatly. For ordinary thinking, a certain degree of definition is sufficient, allowing for amplifications of various kinds. For scientific thinking, these structures are more sharply defined.

There are all kinds of transitions between fantasy, in which little regard is paid to factors of reality, and the making of plans, where they must be considered. Speech also fails to make any sharp distinction here; but the more every conceivable factor is weighed, the more truly may one speak of thought. In scientific techniques, action is as far as possible determined by the structures of thought.

(*f*) The fixed structures of thought find expression in us, and are communicated by us, by means of words and other recognized signs. The manner in which we fill out the meaning of what is said, depends not only on the word, but also on its place in the whole train of thought. While words, when used as symbols of intuition, refer to certain personal experiences, when used as tokens of thought they indicate fixed mental structures.

Having established these properties of thinking, from the introspective aspect, we may still ask whether it is possible to distinguish certain characteristics in observable external behaviour, when this is conditioned by the sphere of thought. We are accustomed from childhood to regard thoughts as something common to us all. Thus we count with certainty on being able to find the same mental forms in others as well as ourselves. On the ground of certain peculiarities in the behaviour of others, we assume that they think. This is particularly the case when, from their words and actions, we can deduce the influence of systematic instruction. Also, apart from this, we shall assume the existence of thought in another, the more we see in his words indications of a system, a systematic programme and consistent method. The man who relies upon thought makes use of generally valid arguments, and thus can more or less justify the reason for his action. Hence the surest way to establish how far thought is the basis of certain conduct is to ask the other what are the reasons for his behaviour.

When the function of thought is the predominant one in an individual, this sphere of firmer, more generally valid structures has the most powerful influence on his behaviour and his inner organization. Personal and subjective points of view are then suppressed in favour of the support provided by the sphere of thought. The man of thought is inclined to see everything that happens in himself and around him as mechanisms, interacting in accordance with definite rules and laws. Both nature and the life of the mind are regarded as systems. The individual of this type finds assurance for his actions in principles derived from universally valid points of view.

When in contact with the instinctive sphere, thought directs itself primarily to the sensory aspect, this being the more objective.

Emotion and impulse are apt to be denied, unless this thinking individual sees a way of considering them systematically, and is able in this manner to adopt an objective standpoint in regard to their subjectivity. The domination of thought exerts an inhibiting influence on intuitive experience, by questioning its connection with other points of view. Otherwise the inspirational value of intuition may be admitted; but the flights of intuition are often crippled by ponderous criticism.

Farthest removed from thought is feeling, because here it is just the subjective and personal element which is cultivated to become something of universal validity. There is a polarity between thought and feeling, which will be explained more fully when we discuss feeling. It is for this reason that feeling does not easily attain an independent influence where thinking predominates, remaining, as a rule, in an elementary form.

(B) *The Extravert of Thinking-Type*

The extravert of thinking-type is guided by the structures and laws of thought, as these have been taught to him by his educators. He is able to make good use of these forms as arguments, and in his actions. Every sensuous experience is at once fitted into its appropriate perceptual complex, and to a person of this type it would seem impossible that there could be awareness of the world apart from systematized conceptions. Facts are only thinkable for him as parts of an organized reality. Insight cannot even be regarded simply as intuitive experience, but must have its place in some systematic context. This way of considering things appears to the extraverted thinker as such a natural necessity that it is apt to be taken as absolute.

The objectivity of knowledge finds here its main support in facts and authorities. The system according to which the extraverted thinker arranges his facts is also held to be objective, although it is accepted as based on the prevailing authoritative views, and is subjected to no critical examination from within. He orders his facts critically and with great care, and herein lies the strength of the individual of this type. On the other hand, his chosen system may be a weak point, since it is often accepted as unquestionable, without the person concerned being himself aware of this. In his ordering of ideas and judgments this danger may be greater than where facts of sensory perception are concerned, because in the former case there are more likely to be all kinds of subjective and capricious elements in the material itself. There is no doubt that thought can do creative work in its establishment and classification of facts and judgments. In general, one may say, therefore, that this type possesses great receptivity for facts and opinions, but that the formulae by which he tests these, and according to which he classifies them, are frequently somewhat rigid and limited. It depends also on the circumstances, whether the rigid or the receptive side prevails in the development of the type.

It is possible, even in children of this character, to observe these two sides. They are accessible to anything which their thoughts can classify, and are quick to adopt current systems and in being able to apply them. In addition, they also make use of their knowledge at an early age, so as themselves to be regarded as authorities, setting themselves up, with a certain pedantic precociousness, as superior to others. In later life, also, these peculiarities are found in all kinds of variations in people of this type. Their knowledge usually embraces a wide field, and they are rarely unwilling to add something fresh to it. But there must be no interference with the system or with the principles to which they subscribe, and which for them possess absolute validity. Any such attempt is repulsed as foolish, morbid or mischievous. Convinced of their objectivity, they strongly oppose anyone who would be prepared to consider the validity of other modes of classification or other principles. The advantages of their strong side, and the disadvantages of their weak points, are also frequently evident in another field. The official, doing useful work in all kinds of social conditions by the application of tiresome legal stipulations, may at home allow his rigid principles and his niggling exactitude to destroy all happiness in his family, exerting an inhibiting influence on the development of his children. The advantage of a clear and business-like outlook may, when it is applied in petty ways, degenerate into a tiresome and dreary prosiness. Controlling principles and systems then become strait-jackets. Right and wrong, good and bad, are judged by this thinking-type of person according to whether they conform to his system or not. This has for him absolute validity: it is the purest expression of the law of the universe. This is true for his scientific as for his ethical system. Anything that does not agree therewith appears to him accidental or untrue. He is convinced that such facts will, on closer examination, fit into his system, and that anything in his nature which is contradictory to his ethical conceptions is a chance imperfection which he will ultimately be able to master.

If the standpoint adopted by such people is a broad-minded

one, they may exert a settling and purifying influence, both where it is a matter of profiting by experience and where controlling principles are involved.

Among people of this type are found excellent officials, organizers and scientists, people who distinguish themselves, both in practical and theoretical fields, by their thoroughness and their wide knowledge. Few women belong to this type. These people are always most effective in the external aspect of their sphere of influence, since their adjustment is mainly in an outward direction. Here their aptness for system introduces a new clarity and vision. Where things are already in order, their efforts are limited to the maintenance of the *status quo* and to resistance against disturbing influences. Hence in a narrower sphere they are liable to be somewhat conservative and conventional. In such circumstances they may appear to be quiet, pleasant people; but at the same time somewhat rigid and tyrannical, without much understanding of others' needs.

As far as activity is concerned, there is evident in these people a manifestation which we shall also have occasion to notice in introverted thinkers and in feeling-types, namely, the significant place assumed by the will. I agree with Jung in regarding the will as an expression of consciously organized aspirations.[1] In thinking and feeling there is a definite extension of the conscious mental organization. As a result, instinctual and impulsive forces are canalized in the personality, increasing the amount of free energy which is more or less constantly available. In instinctive and intuitive people, unconscious impulse and spontaneous inspiration play the most important part in stimulating activity. In people of thought and feeling, the will is the more constantly essential factor. The consequence is that, in general, thinking-types manifest a constant, quiet activity. In addition to their feeling for order and their conscientiousness, their persistence is a particularly advantageous quality. Their contact with material things, and with theories and systems, is, however, usually better than it is with people. Their disinclination for introspection often prevents their entering very deeply into psychological problems. These reasoning people manifest also, in general, a certain coldness and aloofness, their systematized thinking standing between themselves and the world. Even in extraverted thinkers this is noticeable in their attitude and approach, in spite of their satisfactory adaptation to circumstances.

[1] With some thinkers there is a tendency to regard all effort as will; but this gives rise to confusion.

Both the instinctive and intuitive aspects of the disposition may assert themselves in thinking-types of this kind, and be subjected to the influence of reason. Reason tends to emphasize the sensory aspect of instinctual experience. Instinctual impulse belongs—as I shall show later—more to the life of feeling, and the thinker tries to keep away from this. He does this by representing it as inessential, and by concentrating his whole attention on more material experience. That part of his feeling-life which is affected by instinct, but does not disturb his principles, may then be allowed to add to his joy in life, in the form of "normal, healthy pleasures". Even our intuitions may appear to us as universally valid knowledge, in which case thought, too, is prepared to recognize their objective value; but only on condition that it is allowed to examine and delimit their validity. Extraverted thinking does this by comparing intuitively conceived views with one another. Even their own intuition is checked up in this way by people of this type. As regards the intuitions of others, one frequently finds in them a peculiar manifestation. If, for example, in a debate, another opinion is opposed to theirs, they will regard this too with great objectivity, simply placing the two judgments side by side, and thus giving the impression that they really have no opinion of their own. In reality, they think of all judgments as facts, so as to be able to include as many as they possibly can in the thought-system they are elaborating.

The mental life of people of this kind is farthest removed from feeling, since this would disturb their liking for objectivity. Their feelings are, accordingly, the least independent part of them, and are required to fall in entirely with their principles. Feelings which will not do this remain unconscious, but may well be obvious to others. While consciously they are governed only by principles, it will, for example, be obvious in a discussión that they are personally offended, from the irritable tone of their voice, or from an involuntary hostility to opponents. In such circumstances, also, they may occasionally, in pursuit of their aims, employ means which could not well be reconciled with their principles. In general they keep matters of feeling at a distance, particularly where love and sex are concerned.

(C) *The Introverted Thinking-Type*

The introvert of thinking-type also takes his systematized experience as his guide; but here the emphasis falls on the inner aspect, thus on the need for objective order and on laws and principles, according to which experience is generally systematized. Abstraction of that part of conscious experience which is revealed as constant and subject to general rules is regarded by the introverted thinker as something of vital significance. He tries to arrange the opinions which he takes over from others in a system of his own. In doing so, he will take up a more critical attitude in regard to the thought-material which he is taught than do extraverted thinkers, and his aim is to follow the guidance of his own opinions and convictions. In consequence, we find a most careful working-over of his own experience, but a tendency to leave out of his reckoning facts and points of view which are not known to him. While the strength of the extraverted thinker lies in his easy application of systematized knowledge, the introverted thinker is particularly good at comparing systems and principles. He feels at home among abstractions, and there are many fine shades of meaning in the world of his ideas. Also, as he is more skilled in introspection, he is better able to examine mental facts than is the extraverted psychologist.

Hence we see here a living contact with ideas, and subtle reflection and consideration, side by side with difficulty in expressing and applying what has been thought out, and a certain aloofness from the world of facts in general. There is thus in these people a contrast between their consciousness of the objectivity of their judgment, and their difficulty, of which they are equally conscious, in defending this judgment and securing its recognition by others. This produces, even in children of the type, a peculiar attitude. They are often reserved, somewhat timid and uncertain, and seem not to feel at home in the world. On the other hand, they will, at the same time, manifest an obstinate, somewhat pedantic decisiveness. They have not the cool logicality of the thinking extravert, but take up a more fanatical stand, which may easily degenerate into dogmatism and extreme pedantry. In general, both children and adults of this type are, as a result of their introversion, difficult to convince that they are mistaken. Their inner, logical reasoning makes them feel that they are right, and they may take up an attitude to the external world also, which might be expressed as follows: "That is my opinion, even if I can't prove it; whether you agree or not, it will not change it to the slightest degree." At an early age they have learned that the fact that they inwardly regard something as true does not in the least mean that others will accept it. As a result, their attitude is, in general, more sceptical in regard to the validity of any truth than is that of a thinking extravert, and they are more inclined to allow for the existence of differing views, even when these do not entirely tally with theirs, or with those of prevailing authorities. At the same time, however, this gives rise to a feeling of aloofness in regard to any generally recognized system of truth, for this often seems to them something quite unattainable. On the other hand, they never cease to be surprised that what seems so obvious to them should not be equally clear to others. Occasionally such people will go to great pains to express themselves as objectively and clearly as possible, but sometimes they give up the attempt and simply present their views in the form in which they arose. In the difficult language of some philosophers we find the effect of both influences—sometimes in strange combination. As a result of this somewhat sceptical and resigned attitude in regard to form, the judgments of introverted thinkers have often about them something cautious, cold or stiff-necked. It is as if they already reckoned on difficulty in convincing others. Jung says of this type: "Even if he goes as far as giving his thoughts to the world, he does not deal with them as a careful mother would with her children, but he exposes them as foundlings, and at the most he will be annoyed if they fail to make their way." [1]

This inner conflict between certainty as regards conviction, and uncertainty as to how to maintain and apply this conviction in the world, intensifies thought concerning personal conflicts and problems. Hence many philosophically disposed persons belong to this type. They aim at having, at least inwardly, a foundation of pure ideals and definite principles for the ordering of their lives. Such people make, as it were, endless preparations for life; they constantly renew their efforts to perfect their equipment, so as to be equal to the fight for existence. This they do, not only in the big problems of life, but also in ordinary practical matters. They like to have a systematic view of the whole situation before entering on any new ground. In order to be able to adapt themselves, they need to have order in their life and work, and they love making programmes. When travelling, they eagerly study maps and guide-books, or they may even try to master the language of a foreign country, before ever they go there. Such people like to be able to foresee all the possible difficulties which may arise in their business or work, so as to be able to take precautions against them in good time. Occasionally this leads to the most elaborate reckoning with every important practical detail. Ford seems to me to be a good example of the potentialities in practical adaptation characteristic of this type, with his elaborate preparations down to the smallest detail, coupled with a theoretical justification of all his ideas. In a mind

[1] C. G. Jung, *Psychological Types.*

less clear and with less insight into what is essential, this preparation may, however, lead to much fussiness and complexity, and in such cases much energy and attention is wasted in warding off imaginary dangers.

These thinking people are also found more especially among the male sex. Great philosophers, such as Kant, belong to them, and also many mathematicians and psychologists. Or they may be found in all kinds of practical and applied sciences, and taking leading rôles as careful organizers, legislators or contractors. On occasion, however, they are unable to get over certain unpractical traits, and will then cause difficulties with their fanatical exactitude in details, or by everlastingly insisting on their pet principles in any discussion or practical undertaking. This makes co-operation with them in any large combine somewhat difficult. Socially, also, they are somewhat surly. Their attitude to others is more or less studied, seldom absolutely spontaneous. Here again, their systematic thinking stands between them and the world. Their words are usually carefully chosen and weighed, and thus are a kind of mask. People of this type are usually aware of this; but they see no possibility of adopting any different attitude. One usually learns to know them better in a smaller circle, where they will be more spontaneous, and even cordial or original; but even so, with a tendency to be awkward as a result of over-sensitiveness or irascibility. It is more easy to see them as they really are in some sphere in which they have begun to master the technique.

As among the extraverted thinkers, here, also, we may find keen concentration of will and constant activity. Since the introvert finds the motives for his aspirations more within himself, he is less dependent on external stimuli. This is counter-balanced, however, by greater susceptibility to inner difficulties, which, accordingly, may damage his working capacity. And while his independence of circumstances gives him great perseverance, even where initially no success is to be looked for, it may also happen that he will squander his best powers on something impossible from the practical point of view, without realizing this in time.

If the instinctive life manages to gain some influence, it will be conducted along definite paths by a controlling reason. As a rule, introverted thought finds support in the perceptual aspect of instinctive experience, since this represents its objective aspect. This type of thinker is, however, in philosophy, natural science and psychology, more inclined than the extravert to speculate on the nature of perception and the object. In addition, he is, as an introvert, more in touch with the subjective side of instinctual life.

He is more conscious of the inner struggle between instinctual drives, and here also he will seek to create order with his reason, in which case it will depend on his principles as to how he will do this. The theorizing idealist, full of his ideal of the purity of love, and despising as filthy anything remotely associated with sex, will, in the inflexibility of his system, be not far removed from those who defend licence on the principle that nature must not be denied. Both attitudes are in point of fact calculated to evade the practical complications of the problem, and to keep it, so to speak, at a distance. The introverted thinker will sometimes have a great deal to say on such subjects; but he is not, for all that, better, or more skilled, in practice.

Intuition may also influence people of this type to a greater or less degree, giving them something original, which is, however, subdued, since it can only be permitted to play any part in their life after it has been carefully tested. Intuition also reveals to them the schemata and principles according to which thought may classify experience. But the immediate results of personal vision, both in regard to the internal and the external world, tend rather to be mistrusted, unless it is obvious that they will fit into the system. These results may, however, give rise to alterations and extensions in the system. Nevertheless, fine inspirations frequently remain unfruitful, owing to the ponderous way in which they are dealt with.

Feeling, again, gives rise to the chief difficulties in people of this type. Anything which conforms to their principles and views is allowed; but even this cannot easily find expression, owing to deficient familiarity with current modes of expression. As a result, people of this type will often display a strict conventionality, or else a childish disregard of these modes. Inwardly, their feelings, moods and impulses cause them much more unpleasantness than they do to the extraverted thinker, the latter being less aware of them. An introverted thinker, when in love, feels awkward, uncertain and ridiculous. He will try and talk himself out of his feelings, or else make endless preparations to give expression to them, which is, naturally, scarcely conducive to spontaneity.

CHAPTER V

FEELING AND THE FEELING-TYPES

(A) *Feeling in Psychology*

FEELING is the function offering the greatest difficulty as regards clear definition. The word is used for many different kinds of mental contents, when these more or less lack definition. For example, one hears it said that someone has a certain "feeling" in his leg, when actually a certain sensation is meant. But although physical sensations may be regarded as an element in feeling, the two must be distinguished. There is a second difficulty in relation to intuition. We say, for example, "I 'feel' that some trouble is brewing", or "I 'feel' that he wanted to say something different". Here the main content of the mental happening is a vague intuition. The greatest difficulty, however, is found in distinguishing between feeling and emotion, concepts which many psychologists regard as equivalent. Some of them identify emotion with feeling, and distinguish sentiment. In my opinion, it does not matter much what names we attach to our concepts, so long as we explain our meaning. I shall use feeling and sentiment as synonyms, and shall try to indicate in what respects they differ from emotion.

In the chapter on instinct, emotional reactions were regarded as an element in instinctual experience, forming part of a totality of conscious experience, just as sensations also are part of the totality of the field of instinct. It is, however, possible, both in ourselves and in others, to distinguish certain kinds of emotion. The way in which we do this in the case of others is clear enough. I have shown how intuition is able to grasp certain manifestations on the part of another individual as a whole, the image of these being later labelled as the concept of a certain emotion (e.g. fear or anger). When these same emotions are experienced in ourselves, they appear quite different. When we feel fear or anger we may not ourselves be aware of the part this is playing in our experience,[1] but it is expressed in that experience and in our actions. We are,

[1] To become aware of an emotion may mean that its activity is intensified or diminished, according to what is happening at the moment in the other spheres of mental activity.

it is true, aware of something, but supposing, when the emotion has passed, someone enquires, "Why were you so cross?", or, "Why were you afraid?", it becomes evident that the emotion as experienced at the time, and the subsequent awareness of it, which enables us to attach a label to it, are two quite different forms of conscious experience. Recognition and classification take place in quite a different mental sphere from that of the experience itself. To describe this experience in concrete terms is extraordinarily difficult, because everything happening in the instinctive sphere is closely associated, and there is often a certain lack of definition in its structure. To get a good description, we must be able to account in a plastic way for both the various sensory elements and for the subjective reactions inseparably bound up with them. Otherwise there will be nothing but an extremely vague abstraction from the experience, in the form of a concept of tension, or of an internal disturbance which carries us away.

Later, I shall try to explain the distinction between emotion and feeling as revealed in their external manifestations. For the moment, let us see wherein lies the distinction between the internal experience of feeling and emotion, and what constitutes the distinguishing marks of feeling. If we compare sexual excitement with being in love, or anger with indignation, we note that in the two latter cases there is a much more definite structure. Sexual excitement and anger may be expressed in very various forms, while love and indignation aim much more at a definite form of expression. Thus feeling is more plastic than emotion.[1]

In the second place, feeling possesses a much closer association with its object. It is possible to vent one's wrath on another person or on an animal, but indignation cannot so easily be displaced; it is also much easier to express sexual excitement in regard to a different person from the one who originally aroused it, than would be the case with love. Feeling seeks a certain plastic relationship with a certain object. Here I whole-heartedly agree with Shand and McDougall, who regard feeling ("sentiment") as "an organized system of emotional tendencies, centred round some object".[2] McDougall seeks to define certain feelings as combinations of emotions, for example, reproach as a fusion of anger and tender

[1] Jung expresses the opinion that emotion is not only less complex than feeling, but also more intense and more physical; but this does not seem to me to be an essential difference. Feeling may be intense, and an emotion weak; and a strong physical expression may, moreover, be found with feeling as well as with emotion.

[2] W. McDougall, *Social Psychology*, 21st Ed., p. 105.

emotion. A feeling may thus be expressed in many kinds of emotion. "When a man has acquired the sentiment of love for a person or other object, he is apt to experience tender emotion in its presence, fear or anxiety when it is in danger, anger when it is threatened, sorrow when it is lost, joy when the object prospers or is restored to him, gratitude towards him who does good to it, and so on."[1] In this connection I may mention a situation in which this plastic attachment of feeling to a person may be clearly seen. Freud has shown how feelings, developed in early childhood towards the parents, may in later life still be of special significance, owing to the fact that in certain circumstances they may be transferred to other persons. In the study of the transference we are struck by the unity and definite structure of feelings of this kind. Anyone who is undergoing analysis will from time to time become forcibly aware of the existence of such fixated forms of feeling.

A third point of distinction between feeling and emotion is the connection with the ego. In an emotional state the ego is passive; we are carried away by an emotional manifestation, but in feeling we take a much more active part. We stated that the influence of the object on feeling was a certain desired relationship; that of the ego is, on the other hand, a certain attitude developing under the influence of feeling. This does not mean that we need be consciously aware, when experiencing a feeling, of that attitude or of that relationship in a discursive way, as separate entities; but it is possible to analyse them from the concrete experience. Awareness of these factors reinforces the attitude of the ego, and in this way an emotional manifestation may be transformed into a feeling. A short example may illustrate this. A boy may, in his rough play, hurt his younger brother in his violence. His mother tells him he is naughty, and points out what he has done. On another occasion when beginning to play in a similar way, he may become aware that this means being "naughty". This implies that he is seeing his behaviour intuitively as a whole, involving a certain kind of behaviour towards his environment; and if in spite of this he persists, he will also become more or less aware of a certain attitude towards this environment. It is possible that this attitude was already there, unconsciously, but the fact of becoming conscious of it makes a great difference, because his ego is now involved. What he does now will no longer be merged in the totality of his instinctual experience, and a certain feeling of responsibility will be the consequence of this development of awareness. Our feelings are much more part of us than are our emotions; one might even say that

[1] A. F. Shand, *The Foundations of Character*.

feelings are the most constant and the most plastic expression of our subjective being.

This brings us to a fourth characteristic of feeling. Feeling expresses something of more or less constant worth to us. From the many forms of contact with the world, our feeling selects those which have a certain personal significance for us, and seeks to guard and elaborate them. Feelings are not only emotional attitudes, but attitudes to which we cling, and which we cultivate. Why do we feel them to be valuable? Might it not be because feelings are able to reduce our divergent emotions to the unity represented by attitudes? Suppose that a young man is hurrying along a busy street, and somebody gets in his way: his first emotional reaction may be that of vexation; but if he perceives that the object of his annoyance is a child, or someone very frail, an instinctual reaction of sympathy may be aroused. These opposing emotions may then fuse to form an attitude of feeling, prompting him to guide the helpless creature before him to a safer place. This attitude of wanting to help and guide may then express itself in action; if not, the inclination may give rise to a fantasy of such an action. Feelings have value for us, because they combine various inclinations in a form which renders it possible to express them, devoid of inner contradiction. The more impulses we can combine in an expression of feeling, the more value shall we attach to the latter. This explains also why we cling to such manifestations, and why we strive to include certain attitudes in the stock of means of expression at our disposal.

Most of our forms of expression have not been achieved by ourselves, but have been taught us through our education. At that time the proper attitude in regard to all kinds of circumstances was shown to us, and we have amplified this teaching by following the example of our elders, although in this way wrong attitudes may also be adopted. Some of these attitudes and forms of contact may be accepted only within a certain group of people (customs, etc.), while others have a more general validity, and may be considered to have universal value (moral values). All these varied possibilities in the way of feeling-expression are, so to speak, models, available for our use in developing emotional expression. It is a characteristic of the life of feeling, that its every expression is subject to the influence of these norms and modes. While emotional expression remains part of the total momentary instinctual experience, a feeling-reaction is capable of detachment from that momentary situation, as something independent, to be brought subsequently, moreover, into association with the life of feeling, taking its place among other forms of expression. These various forms of expression are not stored at random in the sphere of feeling, but are arranged according to certain situations and values. One may speak here of a hierarchy of values. The more the personality is expressed in these forms of contact, and the more they take circumstances and other people into account, the greater is the value attached to them. In this way, norms and ideals of behaviour may be evolved for all kinds of situations, and their influence forms the most essential distinction between the expression of emotion and the expression of feeling. We are prepared to account for our feelings, but not for our emotions; and where we do take responsibility for some emotional reaction, it means that we transfer it to the sphere of feeling, after it has taken place.

What does it mean when we speak of transferring a mental content to the sphere of feeling, and what are the characteristics of the contents of this sphere? Here I must return to my conception of the relationship between the various spheres. As I have already said, I regard the instinctive sphere as the most fundamental form of conscious orientation, characterized by a fusion of sensation and reaction. To this there are added, in the intuitive sphere, certain images of relationships, some of the contents of the instinctive sphere being, as it were, taken out of it, and adopted by the intuitive sphere in a particular form. In this way there arises a world of images, and these are in their turn transferred by thought into its own sphere of constant meaning, and there moulded to become perceptions and conceptions. Since intuition forms images also of emotional expressions and of feelings, these may also be moulded into conceptions of emotions and feelings by the agency of thought. It is possible to get a psychological view of feeling, only by trying to construct these conceptions as well as we possibly can. In doing this, we must bear in mind that we are producing something other than feeling. But the same is true also of thought in regard to instinctual experience and intuition.

Supposing we ask ourselves, what happens in us when a conscious content is adopted by the sphere of feeling. We shall find that our best point of departure is the fact that intuitions select certain contexts from instinctual experience. These cannot, at this stage, be regarded as perceptions or conceptions; they are simply images, having reference to a concrete context. In contrast to the function of thought, feeling sticks to this concrete form, as isolated by intuition. This does not mean, however, that it leaves it unaltered, any more than thought does; but it shapes it in its own way. While thought abstracts the constant element from the world of images, and objectifies it, feeling provides concrete, more or less stable forms for the subjective aspect of its own attitude and for that of others. Imagination, as a mental form, precedes feeling, as it does thought, but its contents are very differently evaluated by the two functions. Feeling is not concerned with constant elements, but lays conscious emphasis on every mental content calculated to further the expression of a plastic attitude, obeying, in doing this, its own rules and ideals.

When an emotional reaction is perceived intuitively in isolation, this development of awareness is likely to make it possible for the reaction to become a feeling, but not necessarily so. The emotion may find expression and disappear; it may be suppressed by the influence of feeling, or it may be considered, without thereby giving rise to any real feeling. Feeling enters into the situation only if this reaction, perceived in isolation, is associated with other forms of expression, such as regulate the relationship with the environment in a more or less constant manner. The effect of the sphere of feeling is to mould the emotional expression to a form consonant with other accepted forms in the expression of feeling. This may happen in several ways. Where the emotional reaction is syntonic with the majority of these forms, it is not only intensified thereby, but it may find expression in a large variety of plastic forms, making free use of every corresponding form. In this way its influence in the sphere of feeling is heightened. Supposing, for example, a man experiences a sexual attraction towards a girl, or a woman, who answers in every way his pre-conceived ideals. Such an instinctual emotion will easily find expression in the sphere of feeling, and be thereby reinforced. Frequently such an emotion will come into conflict with certain ideals of feeling-relationships, and with other personal relationships, although it is in harmony with the man's own feeling-attitudes. For example, the woman concerned may correspond to his ideal of a wife, but the circumstance that she is married brings his inclination to win her into conflict with his moral conceptions. The emotion will be then dealt with in various ways in the sphere of feeling. Feeling may attempt to attribute another significance to his attitude, by seeing in it only friendship; or the emotion may be pushed on one side as unimportant, or his entire interest in the woman may be represented as something so ideal that it is untouched by anything sensual. Or occasionally the consequence may be that the man gets into a state of conflict with himself as to what his correct attitude should be. If the emotional manifestation proves to be opposed to all his accepted norms of feeling, it may be entirely repressed.

Comparison of forms of expression and contact with other forms takes place in two ways. We may test our attitude against the reactions of others, by carefully trying out different modes of expression; or we may take our own feeling-reaction as a standard, experiencing the different modes in fantasy. Many people will never give free course to an emotional reaction, particularly when feeling is doubtful in regard to it, and in such a case they will seek forms in harmony with the environment and with their own ideals, by trying out various modes of expression in turn. People of feeling-type often have a special gift for seeking the right feeling-contact in this way, even in the most complicated circumstances.

Here I must consider a little more closely the rôle of fantasy in the sphere of feeling. I should like to distinguish between the concepts of imagination and fantasy. Imagination I regard as the product of intuition, by means of which the connection which has been perceived is retained in a personal way in a certain image. These images reinforce the plastic expression of emotion. It would not, however, be right to say that intuition is controlled by emotion, although a certain one-sidedness in insight may arise from emotional interests. But intuition remains independent in its vision. Where feeling is concerned, intuition is placed much more in the service of certain aims. Previous intuitions have made it possible to isolate and compare forms of emotional expression. An image having been made of the present emotion, it can be opposed to these other forms of expression. Feeling seeks to make use of the images of other forms of emotional expression, in order to find expression for the present emotion. While thought tends to make the images formed by intuition more abstract and objective, feeling treats them in its own way, by constructing composite forms of expression from them. When imagination is in this way employed for the requirements of feeling, it would be better to give it a separate name, and to speak of fantasy.

The elaboration by fantasy of images which have arisen spontaneously takes place in very different ways, since in the sphere of feeling various wishes and ideals find expression. Fantasy is as capable of developing in plastic form simple ideals relating to sex and ambition as it is of representing moral demands or ideals of holiness and self-denial as the essential factor in our lives. Moreover, the conflict between these different forms of feeling may also be fought out in fantasy. Fantasy is imagination under the control of feeling. When contents from instinctual experience or thoughts stimulate fantasy, they are made into concrete images, and as such made use of by feeling. The transition may be a very gradual one.

The laws which govern these processes in their own sphere continue to operate, it is true; but the whole course of the process comes under the influence of a feeling-attitude, which alters a good deal in it, and sets a limit to its independence. This usually happens without our being clearly aware of what is taking place. If, for example, while writing this book, I let my thoughts wander, and begin to imagine what effect it will have on the readers, whereupon possibilities of contact or of conflict with people whose opinion I esteem present themselves before my mind—my thinking will gradually become more and more dominated by feeling. In a lecture, this kind of thing may induce the speaker to leave out important parts of his lecture, for fear of opposition from his audience. In the same way, our intuitive insight into the intentions of another person may excite fantasies in our minds as to the excellence of our own intentions, whereupon the influence of the sphere of feeling also begins to exercise control over our mental processes. Feeling may leave the mental contents intact, but it makes use of them in its own way.

From the foregoing it will have become clear that the difficulty in getting a satisfactory psychological description of feeling lies mainly in the fact that feelings are concrete, plastic and composite, so that an abstraction from them offers only a pale reflection of the actual thing. It is true that the same difficulty was found in describing instinctual and intuitive experience in terms of thought; but there was the advantage there, that it was possible to demonstrate certain fairly clear-cut processes as illustrations. Where feeling is concerned, there are always other mental processes at work, although their course may have been altered and, as it were, absorbed in the totality of the feeling-process. For this reason, an abstraction offers a much less satisfactory representation of the significance of a feeling than the whole of its concrete expression, or the fantasies to which it gives rise. In such an elaboration of feeling, the resultant feeling-attitude collects all the mental material that fits in with it, and suppresses all that is alien. A feeling accordingly displays, as its most characteristic quality, a definite form of development as a result of the grouping of mental material. The question constantly arises: in what way does this feeling seek to combine in one definite unit of expression every possible kind of mode of expression? Upon the answer to this question depends the significance attached to a feeling, and its influence on the whole of mental life. A tendency to develop along certain lines is not, where feeling is concerned, variable and momentary, as with emotion, but is expressed in more or less stable and individual forms. There are always a large number of feelings, as there are thought-forms, at our disposal, available for use under every kind of circumstance.

The forms of feeling might be compared with vessels of various sizes and shapes, in which mental contents are collected, and more or less moulded to a unit of subjective associative experience. While thought constructs a whole from mental material, by reducing certain experiences to form serviceable building-material, and then putting this together, feeling pours, so to speak, various contents into a common mould, and uses the whole for its expression. Hence we can differentiate feeling-forms only according to the influence which they exert on the contents of experience and expression.

My next attempt will be to characterize the contents of the sphere of feeling from introspective data:

(*a*) In the sphere of feeling, emotional expression and its influence on other mental processes is felt—in contrast to the instinctive sphere—as a separate mental activity. This is made possible by the isolation by intuition of this activity from the totality of the mental experience. Having attained in this way an independent position in our consciousness, it can enter into combination with other forms of emotional expression.

(*b*) By this contact with other possibilities in the way of expression, the expression of feeling is influenced in the direction of a greater plasticity and stability. As a result, a more definite attitude on the part of the ego arises, directed towards a special form of contact and a definite relationship with the object. In this attitude there are combined in one entity various forms of emotional expression.

(*c*) Such forms of feeling may arise spontaneously, particularly where there is awareness of contradictory emotions; most of them are, however, taught to us in our education, or have developed in imitation of others. In all these cases, intuition is an essential factor in the realization of these forms.

(*d*) There are in the sphere of feeling various plastic forms of expression ready for use in bringing our mental experience into definite combination. These forms are arranged in a hierarchical order, according to whether they express more or less of the whole of our being, and according to the breadth of contact which they imply. The value attached to many of these forms is understandable, when one realizes that in them contradictions in our emotions can be resolved. The highest place in the hierarchy of the sphere of feeling is ascribed to ethical values.

(*e*) Feelings cannot be immediately grasped by introspection, either in the moment of experience itself or in recollection. We are only able to recognize them by the influence which they have on our mental and bodily activity. Outwardly, this influence is expressed in certain complex forms of behaviour; inwardly, it is seen more especially in the activities of fantasy.

(*f*) In all feeling there is an effort to find the right mode of behaviour. The transition between emotion and feeling may be very gradual; but emotion becomes feeling according as its form of expression is compared with other modes and norms. In the same way, there is a transition between intuitions of feelings and the feelings themselves. An intuition of this kind means an image of a certain form of contact. This gives rise to an actual feeling, if it is related with other modes of behaviour in ourselves and with the reaction of others.

Having now learned to define feeling from the introspective aspect somewhat more exactly, we may enquire if it is possible to distinguish certain forms of behaviour as determined by feeling. There is a tendency in all of us in this direction, because most feeling-forms are taught to us as something of universal validity, as we saw was the case with thought-forms. We expect to find in others those modes of expression or behaviour which according to generally accepted opinion belong to certain situations. This might lead us to the assumption that feeling provides the inner motive-power in situations where emotional expression is regulated by certain norms. Caution is, however, indicated, for appearances may be deceptive here: behaviour of this kind may be conceived intuitively and made use of, without being related to the whole of the feeling-life. In such cases, the distinction between the intuition of a feeling and the feeling itself is of great importance. In certain situations we may behave according to prevailing conceptions, while our feelings are impelling us to something quite other. Anyone skilled in the use of modes of expression can suggest a wealth of feeling, which is merely borrowed from the picture-book of human relationships; these pictures or images dwell side by side in the intuitive sphere of the person concerned, with no mutual contact, and feeling has had little to do with them. In contrast to this example, there are other people the depth of whose feelings may paralyse any capacity to express them. Is it possible to find external signs by which to judge whether a person is playing a part corresponding to some inner image, or whether he is seeking a living contact of feeling? It is often very difficult to decide; but in outstanding cases it can usually be done, and when this is the case, two factors tend to be particularly helpful. In the first place, the form of contact experienced with the person concerned is essential: where intuition is at work, the aim is the form, and through that form to influence others for some purpose; while for feeling it is not the form, but a satisfactory contact, which is the main thing, and this latter requires a reciprocal expression of feeling from others. A second characteristic is found in the circumstance that feelings imply more or less permanent modes of behaviour, representing a part of an organized whole. By this they are immediately distinguishable from spontaneous, personal modes of expression, and it is this characteristic which finds outward expression in a wider connection with other emotional manifestations, in a certain harmony of form and in a greater stability. Just as we saw introspectively that the transition from intuitive manifestations to feeling was a gradual one, so also, from the external point of view, it is impossible to draw a sharp line of demarcation.

A further difficulty in recognizing feeling as the basis of external behaviour arises when we try to distinguish between a manifestation of feeling and one that is entirely emotional. Someone may be friendly to us, for instance, because the fine weather has put him into a good temper. Were we to take his behaviour as representing a feeling-attitude towards us, implying a certain relationship with us, we might be greatly disappointed the very next day by a complete change in his bearing. His friendliness was nothing more than an emotional manifestation. In the case of many people, whose eyes fill with tears when hearing of the sufferings of other people, there is no question of deep feeling; it is simply emotion. Others, incapable of expressing anything outwardly, may sometimes be deeply sympathetic, this sympathy coming later to expression in a readiness to help. Here, also, it is not easy to make a distinction, owing to the existence of a gradual transition, although there is a wide difference between the extremes. The search for a contact is, for instance, not necessarily the mark of feeling, because emotion may also seek contact with others, but the other characteristics of feeling which have been mentioned hold good here, viz. more widespread connection with other manifestations, more harmony in form and greater stability; and this the more so, in that emotional expression has essentially a simpler structure and is more impersonal. A *nuance* of expression in a few words or in the tone of voice may often express more feeling than a violent emotion.

Owing to the existence of so many shades of transition between emotional expression and expression resulting from intuitive imagery on the one hand, and, on the other hand, the expression of feeling, many psychologists have been led to make no distinction between them. In daily life, however, this distinction is quite often made, and hence it should be accorded a place in psychology. Although a more careful description and differentiation will only be possible with the aid of introspection, nevertheless the study of human behaviour cannot dispense with these concepts, if it is to give a satisfactory account of forms of expression. The history of mankind reveals how these forms have come more and more to represent an independent force. It seems to me that feeling, like logical thinking, has little significance for primitive man. For him there is as yet no appeal to moral law. Mutual relationships are controlled by the instinctual life, and by images of connections grasped intuitively. Only in larger and more established communities are more stable relationships evolved. The priests were the first to become conscious of them, as they were of the earliest recognitions by reason. Subsequently, relationships of feeling between human beings gradually came to be tested by ideal norms. The attitude of princes to their subjects, of the latter towards their ruler, of the faithful towards their priests, of children towards parents, of brothers among themselves, of husband to wife, and of the individual to his God—all these relationships come to be regulated more and more in accordance with conscious conceptions, and their value determined by similar standards. Man learns to account for his conduct, not only by rational considerations, but also by arguments based on feeling in relation to himself and to others. At this point I must again emphasize that the experiencing and testing of these values is very different from their description. In what follows it will be seen that feeling is particularly likely to occur in women as the dominating function, and that in general the moral order plays a larger part in their lives than it does in the lives of men. Its formation in ethical laws is, however, partly the work of reason, and as such is more the work of men. Recognition that there are laws proper to this sphere developed simultaneously with awareness of the laws of thought. The same Socrates who sought the basis of logical judgment was also the first to recognize moral law. And the teaching of Christ, with its deep understanding and revelation of the moral laws of life, has, in many of His followers, developed feeling into a creative and regulating force of extreme significance.

When feeling is the dominating function in an individual, his actions and thoughts will be to a high degree controlled by ideal images of external relationships and inner harmony. For such people, the requirements of the life of feeling are as absolute as are the laws of thought for the individual of thinking-type. Moreover, they constantly seek to apply them in their daily life. A consequence of this is, that in the expression of their feelings they reveal greater stability, plasticity and subtlety than do other people. They see the world as a system of relationships, in which harmony must be found and maintained. They seek, in their actions, the right mode of behaviour and a satisfactory contact. The forms in which their feeling finds expression may in some be influenced more by the community, in others more by an inner ideal; but in either case, contact with the order prevailing in the sphere of feeling remains for persons of this type the foundation on which they construct their lives.

When feeling predominates, the development of the other functions is influenced to a marked degree thereby. In regard to instinctual experience, this is expressed by the subordination of all instinctual needs and emotional manifestations to accepted ideals. Simple, uncontrolled manifestations are suppressed, since everything must be in harmony with the standards of the sphere of feeling. Feeling will seek to find expression for as many emotions as possible in forms having reference to relationships, but it will reject and repress anything that is in opposition to its ideals.

Intuition may also be subordinated to the requirements of feeling. Whereas thought removes the personal element from intuition, this is intensified by feeling; on the other hand, its objective element is more likely to disappear under the influence of feeling. Any inspiration calculated to further expression of a feeling-relationship is accepted forthwith, without investigation of its correctness. This makes intuition, when under the influence of feeling, and in process of becoming fantasy, extremely unreliable. It frequently involves, however, considerable charm of personality, the warmth that is characteristic of feeling irradiating the vitality of intuition.

Where feeling predominates, thinking is least independent, since the objective and material are incompatible with the elaboration of a personal attitude. Where thought adapts itself to feeling, it is accepted. Thought collects data and possibilities, and sets them side by side, while feeling combines them in a subjective way. Feeling can make use of the products of thought, in that it finds in these a choice of material for its own combinations. In this case, it regards the classification made by thought as a kind of preliminary preparation of material for feeling to work on. The man of feeling-type is at the same time often quite unaware that he is prepared to accept the classifications of thought only in so far as these conform with feeling, and that he is excluding anything that does not do so.

(B) *The Extravert of Feeling-Type*

The extravert of feeling-type lives entirely for contacts of feeling with other people. His feeling-attitudes assume a form which is generally approved in the community. As a rule, the life of the individual of feeling-type is not dominated by violent emotion or overwhelming moods: at the same time, in this particular type it is the influence of less differentiated kinds of feeling which tends to find expression. All the actions, thoughts and observations of people of this type are, however, governed by the effort to establish relationships of feeling with other people. In this, feeling constantly seeks expression, and tries accordingly to arouse corresponding feelings in others. People of this type often show extraordinary skill in drawing out feelings in others, sometimes by means of almost imperceptible manifestations on their own part. The fine shading of their own emotional life enables them, moreover, to read the feelings of others from the smallest indications. In this case, their insight is not always consciously employed, but is more likely to be revealed in an adjustment of their own reactions to such feelings on the part of other people. As a result of this swift understanding of the attitude of others, and of the immediate adjustment of their own reaction, extraverted feeling is extraordinarily valuable in social intercourse.

Human relationships form the element in which the individual of feeling-type is most at home. He knows exactly how things ought to be among the people among whom he has grown up. As an extravert, he derives his sense of security from the forms current in the external world. In his experience, feeling-attitudes are things of objective value, and he finds support for this conception in the fact that others also possess these feelings, and that the life of the community is itself based on them. In such people there is a vital need to find corresponding feelings in others. They are exceedingly unhappy when out of touch with their environment, and must always seek to re-establish contact. If they meet with no sympathy, they will prefer strife to indifference, and since in this case also they know how to get at the feelings of others, they may be extremely unpleasant and harsh to those whom, as opponents and disturbers of their harmony, they would like to get rid of. They are first-class members of a community, seeking for themselves modes of life which others will approve. People and things to which their feelings are attached are particularly esteemed by them, such objects being singled out from the rest of the world.[1] In their judgment of others this may easily lead to exaggeration, their tendency to idealization making them ready to overlook faults. For a woman of this type her husband is an exceptional being, and her children are regarded in the same way. This characteristic is likely to be found to some extent in everyone, where feeling is in question, but nowhere is it so marked as in people of feeling-type, because with them all relationships are conceived in somewhat ideal form. This means that anything which fits in with their feeling-life is strongly emphasized, and anything which does not do so is ignored. As a result, repression has much greater influence in these people than in representatives of any other type. Everything is repudiated, both in the loved one and in themselves, which might disturb the harmony which is necessary to them. If, as a result, they manage to conceal from themselves certain marked characteristics, it may happen that even so these are to some extent apparent, and this gives an impression of something artificial in their harmony, and something a bit unreal in their idealism.

In children of this type, it is often possible to observe these traits at quite an early age. They are more taken up with their parents, or with others who attract them, than are other children. They idealize their parents, for instance, to a marked degree, and refuse to hear anything against them. They also try to live up to an ideal themselves. They like to be praised, and show a certain over-sensitivity if others do not meet them in this. They have a great need for love, and want constant demonstrations from older people of their affection for them. At the same time, they very soon find out the soft spots in the feelings of the persons in their environment. While extraverted intuitive children want, as a general rule, to make an impression, with young people of this feeling-type this is more a means to establishing emotional contacts with others. Probably most children long to be their mother's or father's favourite, but nowhere is this felt to be such a vital question as with children of this type. They are apt, in their enthusiasm, to see in their ideal a combination of all that they value, and to fall into profound despair when they are unsuccessful

[1] Jung sees the essence of feeling in the assignment of values to everything. Although this happens to a very marked extent in the sphere of feeling, it nevertheless does not appear to me to be an actual characteristic, since values are assigned by the other functions as well.

in establishing the relationship they desire. At a later age, also, the happiness of these people usually depends on some feeling-relationship with another person, or with several others. This type is particularly found among women, and family life certainly offers a woman opportunities of developing the happiest side of feeling. In the daily life of a woman of this type, the striking thing is not so much an intense expression of feeling as the remarkably appropriate and fine shading of this expression. Such a woman will never do or say anything to disturb the harmony of her environment, but, on the contrary, will create and reinforce it in all kinds of small ways. But, as a rule, she is also well able to wound if she feels so inclined. If harmony is not attained, she feels it much more than would others, and her life may appear to be quite broken up as a result. Where idealization is remote from reality, exaggerated expectations are often followed by great disappointment, and the individual of feeling-type will take this terribly to heart, so that it fills his whole horizon. "*Himmelhoch jauchzend, zum Tode betrübt*"[1] is a particularly appropriate description of the state of mind of this type of person.

When anything happens which touches on feeling, an individual of this kind finds it impossible to be a simple onlooker: he helps to create the atmosphere by the way in which he gives himself up to every impression. Extraverts of this type often possess a peculiar gift, amounting to genius, for giving expression to what everyone is feeling at the time, for they are able to express the most varied shades of any feeling in such a plastic way that they readily arouse response in others. Hence there are found among the representatives of this type many famous preachers and priests, great orators, and gifted actors and actresses. Even their outward appearance expresses the attitude of feeling which is most prevalent with them. This is true not only of the well-bred woman or girl, or of the clergy, but just as much of the *demi-mondaine* or of the gentleman come down in the world who may belong to the type.

Not only feelings, but thoughts also are usually expressed in very plastic form by extraverts of feeling-type, which often makes them very gifted in instructing others. It is obvious that in such work contact with pupils is an essential factor. They think in a dramatic way, as if they were before an audience. Their thoughts take shape while being expressed. The effect of this on people whose thoughts are abstract and swift is one of unnecessary circumlocution, for the individual of feeling-type not only conveys his

[1] "Rejoicing to heaven, grieved unto death."

thoughts, he develops them before his audience. For a teacher or orator this may have great advantages, for his listeners are more able to experience what they hear. But it is difficult for a person of this type to make a brief and matter-of-fact communication. The domination of feeling in their thinking has as a consequence that the contents of their thought are not always very clearly or distinctly worked out, although they are conveyed in beautiful images and in well-sounding words, calculated to reach the fantasy and the heart of their listeners.

When there is good adjustment by means of extraverted feeling, these people feel at home in every kind of milieu, and extract enormous satisfaction from experiencing their skill in adaptation in ever-fresh settings. They like to have a large circle of friends and acquaintances, and take an enthusiastic part in the life of the community. They like to have a constant series of appointments, and are always ready to make fresh contacts. Since intercourse with people offers more opportunities for adaptation by feeling than do relationships with inanimate objects, with animals or with nature, they prefer to share all their pleasures with others; they dislike being alone. They will, for example, always choose those forms of sport in which they can join in with others.

An individual of this type really only sees himself and his own life as reflected in his relationships with other people and in their opinions of himself. Hence he is very susceptible to praise and criticism. Encouragement will very quickly intensify and extend a reaction of feeling, while a comment or an objection which cannot be refuted may exert an exceedingly depressing influence on his spirits. Especially where some uncertainty might exist in regard to agreement between his own views and those generally current does he feel it absolutely necessary to prove to the world that his own feelings are right. When under the influence of powerful feeling, such people are able to exert great influence in their environment, particularly if they find support for their feelings in followers and onlookers. With most people of this type, however, feelings are expressed less in impressive actions than in the creation of a harmonious atmosphere. In their relationship with those around them they do their best to insist on friendliness and fair play, and they are usually conscientious and orderly even in small matters. Since they make similar demands on others, they frequently come into conflict with others, who do not always see the same necessity. Their punctiliousness may degenerate into pettiness, and occasionally such people may become very tiresome and pernickety about details. They will "go on" endlessly about something they feel to be wrong, and since they attach universal validity to the judgments of their feeling, they cannot stop trying to convince others. As a result, they may be tiring to those around them, in spite of their kindness and friendliness. In their persistence we see again the significance of the will for this type. They may give themselves up with extraordinary self-sacrifice and devotion to those whom they love, and to the purpose which they have set themselves.

Since the way in which these people live is for them the most immediate expression of the meaning of their lives, they are acutely affected by external things. This may give others an impression of formality and conventionality. Prevailing forms are, however, for them a much more important expression of life than they are for people who make use of them without conviction. This does not exclude the danger that even for people of feeling-type such external forms may lead to pretence, although they are themselves less aware of this risk. Thus they make use of various forms, all of which possess a certain worth, but are nevertheless essentially incompatible, and in consequence introduce an inner contradiction into their lives. For a person of this type, it is, for example, quite possible to be an outspoken socialist or communist, and at the same time to live in luxury and idleness.

Where feeling predominates, its influence on the instinctual life consists in the organizing of instinctual impulses into a moral structure, and the subordination of the impulses to this. If in this way the whole of the instinctual life is able to assume harmonious forms, the finest aspect of feeling is revealed. But this happens very rarely, because the demand for harmony may at the same time give rise to repression and dishonesty. Thus the results of the influence of feeling on the instinctual life are often seen in a splitting of the latter into two parts, one of which is incorporated into the manifestations of feeling and is thereby ennobled, while the other is repressed as being inferior and ineducable, and is thus condemned to remain fixated in elementary forms. If it is the sexual life which is regarded as worthless, people of feeling-type will be particularly affected in their personality by the results of this cleavage; but other primitive tendencies, such as the urge for power, may in theory have the same effect. This tendency towards repression is also expressed externally, in the sense that only those people who mean something to their feelings seem to have any existence for them, all others being disregarded.

Where extraverted feeling predominates, it will leave its mark on intuition. Intuitions come to be primarily valued when what is perceived is in harmony with feeling. Sometimes they make possible the expression of fine shades of feeling, and when this is so, there may be great charm in the behaviour of such people. Spontaneous insight which does not accord with their feeling-attitudes or relationships tends, however, to be repressed. Their ability to sympathize with the intuitions of others also depends very much on the relationship. If it is one of sympathy, then even the most fantastic inspirations are accepted with enthusiasm, whereas great difficulty is found in sharing the feelings of anyone with whom they are not in sympathy.

There is no independence in the rational judgment of persons of feeling-type. It is not always easy to recognize this, because they often make good use of their reason; and, moreover, they are quite unaware themselves that in thinking they pick and choose entirely according to what fits in with their sentiments. It is usually not easy to make them see that the objectivity and criticism of thought is something quite different from moral judgment. In practical matters they can generally make good use of reason to work out and defend what they consider to be right, but they admit only those arguments which accord with their feeling-attitude. This is probably the case with most people in questions of feeling; but nowhere is this effect of feeling so strong, and so many-sided, as in extraverts of feeling-type. For example, even in scientific problems they will take sides in a violently personal way.

(C) *The Introvert of Feeling-Type*

The introvert of feeling-type finds support and guidance by shaping the subjective aspect of his own feeling-attitudes in accordance with an inner ideal of general validity. Here the activities of feeling are hidden, and from the outside there is, as a rule, little to tell us that we are dealing with a person of feeling-type. Feeling aims more especially at an inner harmony, trying to discover what under various circumstances should be the right relationships between people if life is to be beautiful and well balanced. Reality, however, reveals in most cases that this ideal is not attained, and introverted feeling is particularly vulnerable in regard to such experiences. This vulnerability, which may become as intense as that of the sensitive plant, is one of the most characteristic peculiarities of this type. Just as with the introvert of thinking-type, we find here, too, a marked contrast between inner security and uncertainty in external behaviour. But whereas with the introverted thinker this opposition gives rise to thought concerning the problems of life, with the individual of feeling-type it leads to deep feeling, and to a strange mixture of inner tenderness and passionate conviction. These people are absolutely certain as to the soundness of their ideals, but this is accompanied by a helpless feeling that it will never be possible to realize them in this world. They do not, however, reject the world, for feeling means the making of ties and is directed towards social contacts. In spite of ever-repeated collisions with the world and with other people, they can never give up their wish to love them both. They conceal their sensitiveness behind a mask, which may be childish, or simple, or again conventional, remote, or it may be friendly. But behind this mask the search goes on for someone who will understand, and for a community which will embody their ideals. However disappointed they are, they still in their innermost being believe implicitly in what their feelings tell them. Even if they are not able to express it clearly in words, they are inwardly quite certain as to what accords with them and what does not. Outwardly, their feelings are not very obvious, for when these are affected, these people tend to withdraw into themselves, and if they do express anything, it will only be much later, after they have had time to work it all over within themselves. In ordinary life their mask conceals what they really are. But there is, nevertheless, something very individual about them, sometimes remarkably so, which will come to expression particularly in certain moments, in relation to certain people. This happens more especially in two situations: when they achieve real contact with another person, and when, in a state of high emotional excitement, they stand up for a threatened ideal. In the first case, a very profound relationship of mutual understanding may suddenly come into being, all the wealth of their minds being unlocked to the confidant; sometimes this contact will later be broken off just as suddenly and unexpectedly, in defence of their own vulnerability. And where his feelings are aroused, the person who appeared to be so impersonal, remote and somewhat insignificant may suddenly burst out with a personal point of view, expressed with such conviction and such force of feeling that it compels respect. Such people may also resist with extreme obstinacy anything that does not accord with their sentiments. This resistance may be justified, in so far as it is based on a motive of fine feeling; but the means used to give it emphatic expression is ill-suited to the external world, and in this respect incorrect. The consequence is that they are nearly always misunderstood, and they tend more or less to resign themselves to this situation.

This contrast between a clear intention, directed towards harmony, and uncertain modes of expression, giving rise to misunderstandings, is found again and again in the lives of these people. In childhood they are gentle and dreamy, and somewhat reserved, but with occasional violent outbursts of emotion. In familiar surroundings they can be unrestrainedly gay; but more often they are liable to violent resentment if circumstances do not correspond to their feelings, and it then seems to them that harshness and indifference prevail in the world. As a result, they seem to show signs of disappointment at a very early age, and a certain distrust of life. Owing to their inability to express themselves clearly, and to realize their ideals themselves, there may arise a feeling of impotence and inferiority. They are apt to seek the fault in themselves, and may suffer much from a sense of guilt on this account. Here, also, feelings have a tendency to extend their influence, with the result that their whole being may be plunged into depths of unhappiness; but at other times a genuine emotional contact with someone will once more fill them with a quiet and enormous delight. Now they will look at the world again with new eyes, and a feeling that is almost religious will embrace both nature and man. Later, also, the happiness of these people will depend on the emotional attachments which they are able to make, though they find it less necessary than do extraverts of this type to be in immediate touch with other people. The expression of other people's feelings in poetry and music, and the realization, through the reading of stories and biographies, of the depths of their spiritual experience, may have the effect on these people of making them feel more at home in the world. In this way, there develops in them a life of the spirit, which is carefully concealed from strangers, and which may be expressed, for instance, in a secret piety, or in poetical forms, which are revealed only with great unwillingness.

This feeling-type is also particularly found among women. Whereas the woman of extraverted feeling-type has it in her to create an atmosphere of harmony around herself, in the introverted woman of this type all the riches of her mind will be developed into a love which is inwardly directed towards the highest ideals of harmony. Without saying or doing much, such a woman will emanate a feeling of rest and security. It is difficult to describe an influence of this kind, expressed as it is in such indefinite forms, which it employs merely as an indication. But on the immediate environment it may be very effective. A mother of this type may have an even greater influence on her children than the devoted and radiant mother of extraverted feeling-type. These women are often able to implant and foster something of their own ideals in their children, exercising in this way a quiet force which helps to keep a respect for moral authority alive in the world. All the modes of expression for the deeper impulses of the spirit in religion and art find great support in such people. Whether they are artists or scientists, they are still primarily attracted by problems of the emotional life. They express themselves in such occupations with great care and precision. Here again the persistence and devotion of the individual of feeling-type become evident. When they do give form to their inner feeling—in a poem, for example—they will carefully weigh every expression; at the same time, they will often neglect generally accepted social forms, which for them have no significance, or they will employ conventional and simple forms as a mask, from behind which a more genuine and finer feeling will occasionally come quite unexpectedly to light.

Although in these cases the will, under the direction of strong moral conviction, represents an important factor in the psyche, it is less evident than in the other rational types, owing to the fact that the controlling activity is directed more inwards, and feeling is expressed more indirectly. It is most evident in the strong sense of duty characteristic of these people, and in their faithful discharge of their duties. Their activity frequently suffers as a result of moods of discouragement. When this is so, they lose themselves in pessimistic feelings, giving up their efforts to make themselves better understood, or to alter things in their environment. After a time they recover from such moods, since they tend, as a rule, to regard them as a fault in themselves. This contact with their own moral judgment represents an essential factor in the lives of feeling-introverts. They are not bound by the judgments of others —as is the feeling-extravert—for the standard by which they judge their own behaviour is an inner moral law, intuitively felt to be binding. While the extravert of feeling-type will repress, for the sake of harmony, things both in himself and in the external world which do not accord with his ideal, the feeling-introvert will remain more aware of such conflicts. In him, however, the limiting and excluding activity of the demand for harmony may be detrimental in a different way, everything not consonant with that harmony being regarded from a negative point of view, as opposed to what is ideal and good. It is impossible for these people to see the world or themselves objectively, and their continual comparison of things with ideal requirements gives them an exaggeratedly critical point of view. Since this also applies to their own lives, there is an undermining of their own self-confidence, as well as of their confidence in the world, which may seriously affect their happiness in life. It is necessary for these people to recognize that things which do not exactly accord with their ideals may yet have a value which may be developed.

In these cases, also, the instinctual life is to a very large extent subordinated to the regulating force of feeling. Since the relationship between moral conviction and instinctual impulse is here worked out more within the mind, there is less danger of pretence for the sake of the external world than with extraverts. Instinctual feelings are subordinated to the ideal. At the same time, there may be a too forcible suppression of the instinctual life, in which case it will lead not so much to a split in the emotional life as to a certain joylessness, and to the feeling that life is passing without bringing any true fulfilment. There is too often a need to associate all pleasures and joys with some moral value, and to condemn them if this higher satisfaction is not obviously found in them.

Intuition is also subjected to the authority of introverted feeling. Intuitions here bear more on the inner aspect of feeling than on its expression in other people. They may give form to the laws of feeling, but in images rather than in concepts. Where intuition is developed, it is of great assistance in finding expression for introverted feeling, both in practical life and in art. Intuition may also provide a link with religious life, which, in this case, will be specially developed in its feeling-aspect: inner moral unity with God and with his fellow-man has greater significance for the man of feeling-type than ecstatic experiences or philosophical problems. The domination of feeling is revealed in the constant search for a harmonious relation and in the weight given to views on morality, love and justice.

Thought is, as a rule, not very essential in the lives of these people. They accept the thought-forms as taught to them, and make conscientious use of them; but this is not vital to them, as the judgment of feeling is. In their thought-processes, they argue from preconceived attitudes of feeling, and frequently do not embark on any logical thinking at all, leaving the realm of reason to others to deal with.

CHAPTER VI

COMPLICATIONS

Having offered a general description of the types, I should now like to mention various factors which may in practice complicate the typical picture. It will only be possible to discuss these factors in their general aspect, as it would take up too much space to go more thoroughly into their influence on each of the types.

A first point of difference between people of the same type is found in the stage of development which they have reached. In every type there is a simple form, in which the differentiation of the prevailing function has only just begun, and its modes of adaptation are still being tentatively tried out, although a clear preference for typical forms of adaptation can already be observed. At a later stage the dominating function has found its forms, controlling these with great assurance. Anything which is not in accord is, at this stage, suppressed. With a few people there follows a still further stage, in which the other functions are permitted more development, to compensate for any one-sidedness, and the pronounced typical picture is again modified to some extent by the unfolding of a fuller and richer expression of human nature.

A second complication consists in the development to a certain degree of independence of a second function, in addition to the dominating one, which may take place either before or after the full development of the latter. As a rule, there is, as we have seen, one function more particularly opposed to the typical function, and this one is accordingly least able to develop; but either of the remaining two functions is more easily able to assert itself. In an instinctive individual, for instance, intuition will find it very difficult to attain any independence; reason or feeling, however, may be developed in such a way as to supplement his personality, so that it is possible to distinguish between an instinctive-type with well-developed reason and one in whom feeling offers subsidiary forms. Similarly, with a person of feeling-type, reason is least able to attain any independence, but instinct and intuition are capable of a more free development; so that it is possible to find people of feeling-type in close contact with either the instinctive or the intuitive side of their natures. The same type of complication is possible also with people of intuitive and rational orientation. But in all such cases the second function is less developed, and, moreover, subserves the dominating function. Since, in the foregoing chapters, I have described this effect of the dominant function on the remaining functions in each case, these subsidiary forms may easily be deduced from these descriptions. I may add, however, that the subsidiary function frequently tends to control adaptation in the direction towards which the dominant function is not orientated. For example, an introvert of thinking-type will employ his instinct or his intuition particularly for purposes of external adjustment. Or an extraverted intuitive will seek contact with the inner world through thought or feeling.

A third complication results in yet another variation of the type. It may happen that an individual has little contact with a subsidiary function, but that the polar, or opposite, function stands in a relation of peculiar inter-action with the dominant function. This inter-action is different from that arising from the existence of a subsidiary function, in that the dominant function is less able to maintain its authority in this case, and suffers more frustration as a result. Consequently, these people have something contradictory in their conscious personality. They might be called people with polar activity. I will illustrate this briefly.

The majority of instinctive people are orientated towards the instinctive side of life, and are completely satisfied with this orientation. At the most, they will seek to supplement their lives through reason or feeling. But side by side with these people we find others of the same type, who are continuously dissatisfied with themselves, and who cherish a particular admiration for intuitive people, trying to find a further fulfilment of their lives in spiritual things. Since the instinctive individual finds it difficult to create his own personal forms in this sphere, there will exist in such a case a very strong dependence on traditional forms and authority in the spiritual realm. Anything which is adopted in this way, e.g. in politics or religion, will then be more intensely valued, and more fanatically clung to, than the more familiar forms actually belonging to his own type. Besides these traditional forms, certain archaic intuitions of his own may become prominent in a person of this type, which may then lead to superstition and a kind of cheap mysticism, expressing itself in materialistic forms.

In the intuitive, the effect of the polar function may be to awaken interests normally opposed to those of intuitive people: an enthusiasm for nature, for the high value of the instinctual life, and for personal hobbies and amusements in which contact with concrete things is sought (e.g. sport, collections). Simple, instinctual tendencies also play a larger part in the lives of such people than they do in the case of other intuitives.

The man of thinking-type, affected by the influence of his polar function, will himself recognize the limitation and one-sidedness of reason, and will feel the need of an expression for feeling, both in art and in contact with other people. Since his own forms for expression of feeling are developed with difficulty, he particularly admires people in whom these are well developed, and tries to copy them. His awkwardness in applying them, and his own more primitive expressions of feeling, may sometimes be a cause of considerable difficulty to him. People in whom the polar function is effective tend in general to fall into the danger of being taken advantage of by the people whom they admire.

The individual of feeling-type who is affected in this way will set a lower value on feeling than on reason, and will look upon science and philosophy with great admiration. His own thoughts, sometimes of a childish or primitive kind, will also be regarded with great interest. Such people are apt to take over the thoughts of others ready-made, when they will defend them with fervour and in a very dogmatic way.

There may also be an effect of polarity between extraversion and introversion. In this case, the extraverted individual will condemn his own marked inclination to extraversion, and will admire people who are self-contained. They will try also to make something of significance out of what goes on within their own minds. In a similar situation, the introvert will try to get away from himself and to make a better adjustment to the world, which may lead him to attach himself too quickly or too intensely to people or to accepted forms, and to be too much swayed by his own primitive forms of extraversion. Finally, I should like to point out that although these effects of polarity in conscious orientation are more potent in some people than in others, they may nevertheless develop in anyone under the influence of circumstances, and for a time dominate his life.

A fourth complication, which may be a cause of differences among people of one and the same type, arises from the existence of fixed mechanisms (psychisms: see footnote on p. 118) and complexes. The life of the mind is presented to us as a continuous stream of consciousness (William James). But besides this movement and change in all the spheres of conscious experience, we find in them all more or less constant and established forms, which offer us guidance and enable us to fix events in our memory. In the sphere of instinctive experience these are the patterns (Gestalten) and emphases which determine action and habit. Intuitive experience is fixed in images and symbols. In thought and feeling, the aim is the development of fixed mental structures: percepts, concepts, rules and laws in the one case, and conventions, social forms, feeling-relationships and morals in the other, offer a wealth of fixed, reliable mental contents. These contents are associated according to certain rules, making it possible to study them. In the natural sciences, certain facts are singled out, and an attempt is made to establish the mechanisms which determine alterations in them. In psychology we attempt to differentiate mechanisms (psychisms) linking together more or less fixed contents of mental life. Each of the functions has its own forms and mechanisms, dependent on education and experience. The instinctive forms of the farmer are different from those of the sailor; feeling-attitudes differ according to nation and social class. A man's knowledge, together with his mode of thought and speech, reveals the kind of education he has had. Differences like these enable us to establish distinctions, in which we may take as criterion, not only predominant mental contents, but also a certain style of life. Such differences cannot be explained by the type of conscious orientation, but are the product of factors operating during the evolution of the personality.

Sometimes certain influences give rise to a greater rigidity in the mental mechanisms than they usually possess. As a rule, mental forms and mechanisms are never quite fixed. Having been formed as a result of certain experiences, they may undergo change through later events. This liability to alteration diminishes with age. There are, however, other factors which may lead to rigidity in certain definite directions, namely, repression and fixation. Repression is a product of the activity of feeling. It was first described by Freud as an essential factor in neurosis, but later it was shown by him and by his pupils to be present also in normal people. Under the influence of a certain attitude of feeling, the contents of consciousness are rearranged, and as a result, certain contents which do not fit in with the whole may be entirely repressed from conscious experience. In other cases, the association between one content and other contents may be severed, whereby the whole assumes a more innocent appearance. Some contents are, as it were, fenced off. This influence may operate in any of the mental spheres: but its point of departure is, in my opinion, the sphere of feeling.

Wrong habits, developed in the instinctive sphere, may, for

example, be fixated by a feeling-attitude of obstinacy, or through the influence of a spoiling mother. Intuitive insight, made use of, leads to further insight; but an attitude of conceit may hold up the development of further insight, by finding sufficient satisfaction in admiration of that already achieved. Or insight may be repressed because it would lead to painful conclusions in regard to a beloved person. Knowledge and principles may likewise become rigid if they come under the influence of a feeling-attitude. And feelings themselves are particularly apt to be influenced by other feelings, so that certain of them, if in contradiction to accepted attitudes, are denied, or at any rate very definitely limited in their activity.

Psycho-analysis has shown how attitudes of this kind, particularly when arising in early childhood, may exert a dominating influence on behaviour, and how not only disturbances, but also certain character-traits, may be explained thereby. Many psycho-analysts have a tendency to explain all mental activity by two causes: namely, inborn characteristics in the instinctive sphere, and fixation of affective reactions, arising under the influence of the environment. This point of view seems to me to be too limited.[1] It is not possible to explain in this way the whole structure of a character. But although I cannot accept infantile fixations as the basis for a general classification of character, I willingly admit that this factor is indispensable in the explanation of certain character-traits. This prompts the question as to whether it is possible to find any connection between the types of conscious orientation which I have described and certain forms of fixation. What peculiarities of a character may be described as the consequence of a certain inborn mental structure, and what are to be explained by inborn emphases, not necessarily connected with such a structure, or by chance influences, operating during development?

In studying my patients and other people, I have repeatedly asked myself this question, and although I cannot adduce here the material upon which my conclusion is based, I wish to state this conclusion. The types of conscious orientation which I have described seem to me to be congenital; I cannot possibly see the

[1] The attempt to explain character in this way was begun by Freud, in an essay on the "anal-erotic character," in which the sense of order, obstinacy and thrift were associated with disturbances in the anal function in the first years of life. Abraham and Jones have developed this conception, and the former distinguished three forms of character, according to whether fixations took place in the oral, anal or genital phase in early development (Abraham, *Selected Papers*). The totality cannot, however, be entirely explained by a summation of mental forms and mechanisms, even though one admits that their influence may be of the utmost importance.

origin of this congenital structure in inborn emphases in the instinctive sphere. This will probably be obvious to the reader who has understood my description of the functions. The congenital character of the types I can only state as an impression gained from my experience, which needs confirmation by further research. Here I can only say that I have often been able to establish the presence of these types of conscious orientation in quite young children. Sometimes the parents and the other children belonged to quite a different type, while the child concerned possessed the type of orientation of one of the grandparents, whom it had never seen. The influence of an identification with an older person is in such cases scarcely probable. The influence of instinctual emphases and of circumstances giving rise to complexes is not sufficient to explain the totality of a character, since these influences may assert themselves in a similar way in people of very different type, as far as conscious orientation is concerned. Certain forms of father- or mother-fixation, or of auto-erotic manifestations, etc., occur in persons of different types.

Does this imply that there is no connection between character-traits dependent on complexes and the character-structure as a whole? There may surely be a connection, although not a very simple one. We might formulate it in this way: that the significance of certain complexes may be increased by the characteristics of a certain type of conscious orientation. The latter may offer a soil in which certain fixated mental mechanisms flourish more readily. I will try and indicate how this happens in the case of the various functions.

Instinctive people take their instinctual reactions for granted, and as a rule are right in doing so, because these reactions are well adjusted. If, as a result of circumstances, wrong modes of expression (for example, various forms of auto-erotism) have been developed and fixated in consequence of some emotional situation, such manifestations (bad habits, perverse activities, and compulsive defensive reactions against these) may still be taken for granted as are other instinctual reactions. They are, accordingly, more readily incorporated in the total structure of behaviour, in the form of character-traits or persistent symptoms, than would be the case with people of another type, where they would exist in less close relationship with the organized personality. Wrong thoughts and maladjusted feeling-attitudes will, with such people, be more likely to cause an attempt to effect some change in the personality than manifestations in the instinctive sphere.[1]

[1] This problem will be more fully discussed in the psychiatric section of this book.

In intuitive people, insight, arising in a spontaneous personal form, is the most important influence in mental life. This insight may be controlled by objective criticism or by comparison with ideals or with facts, but where this control is lacking, there will still be no uncertainty in the mind of an intuitive. This ability to dispense with such control may be strengthened by feeling-attitudes, and in this respect narcissism seems to me to be a danger to which an intuitive is particularly liable, because this intensifies the personal quality of intuitions, without his being aware of the fact. As a result, all kinds of influences emanating from fixations, and making insight extremely one-sided, are given free course, since they are subjected to no correction.

People of feeling-type will be less able to modify fixations in the sphere of feeling than in other functions. In other spheres also, in my opinion, fixations are the result of the influence of feeling; but this type of person feels less master of the situation in the other spheres and is, accordingly, more ready to accept criticism. Certain events and situations in the sphere of feeling may, however, also give rise to fixation, and the fact that all feelings are accepted as right, once they are incorporated in the totality of feelings, prevents a person of feeling-type from recognizing that a certain feeling-attitude, e.g. towards the parents, has become fixated and is transferred to others, where it does not at all meet the situation. Fixations of this kind, revealed more especially in the transference, have even greater rigidity in persons of feeling-type than in others.

Thought may also be influenced by feeling-attitudes and consequently become fixated to a greater or less extent. An individual of thinking-type, while rendered insecure by emotional influences which he meets in more or less direct form, may occasionally adopt them without noticing the fact, if they make their appearance in a purely rational form. The moment principles and theories are formulated in an abstract and theoretical way, they become part of the sphere of objective truth. When this happens, fixations caused by feeling will not easily suffer correction, because they appear to be just as well founded as other contents in the sphere of thought. Hence the rationization of unconscious complexes is the special danger of people of thinking-type.

Summarizing the foregoing, we reach the conclusion that no single fixation is specific, and that any kind of complex may occur in any type. The modification of a fixation may, however, offer peculiar difficulties in that sphere whose contents are most easily incorporated and permanently adopted by the type of individual concerned. Thus, while I accept Freud's explanation of complexes, I see the possibility of further complications in the inborn character-structure, which at the same time offer a better explanation of the peculiar position to which complexes may sometimes attain.

As a fifth complication, we must discuss those manifestations of the unconscious which cannot be described by the term complex, because they are not fixated as a result of emotional influences. Yet they do not belong to the structure of conscious orientation; they represent a more adventitious part of the total personality, which under certain conditions may become an essential factor in the explanation of a person's behaviour.

In characters affected by polarity of function, these factors are sometimes more conscious in their activity, and when this is so, they make the structure of the character more complicated and more contradictory. In most cases, the influence of a mental foundation, too broad to be fully dealt with in conscious life, acts more indirectly. In the latter case, there are no conscious conflicts; but other people may be aware of inconsistencies in conduct. I touched briefly on this problem in the first chapter, when showing that the distinguishing characteristic of Jung's typology consists in its view of the types as an extract from the unconscious psyche. We saw there that it is possible to observe in the behaviour of outstandingly extraverted people, whose motives are entirely derived from their environment, certain manifestations which can only be explained from inner, personal interests and desires. Similarly, it is possible to discover in outstandingly introverted people, who consciously cling exclusively to their own point of view, an extraordinary susceptibility, in certain matters, to public opinion. This kind of behaviour, opposed to the attitude which prevails in consciousness, may be found in all types of conscious orientation, making the concrete form very much more complicated. I will endeavour to describe briefly the different forms in which this may occur.

In the first place, there may be an irruption from the unconscious into the ordinary picture, expressed in simple or archaic forms. The individual of thinking-type, with his desire to see everything objectively and from without, will become passionate or irascible, or will allow himself, in despite of all his principles, to be carried away by simple feeling. The usual excuse in such circumstances will be that he was not himself at the time. Or the person of feeling-type will seek to attain his ends in a coldly calculating way, without regard for his ideal of a good relationship with others. Later he may perhaps say: "Yes, that was horrid of me." An intuitive person, who in ordinary life will do anything to realize his visions, grudging the time demanded for food and sleep, will occasionally get an uncontrollable craving for certain simple pleasures, or will devote peculiar attention to his food or to creature comforts. Or the instinctive person, usually interested only in what is tangible and matter-of-fact, will become superstitious and attach great significance to all kinds of omens and good and evil influences.

A second form of this influence from the unconscious is less elementary; but it still remains more or less isolated from the rest of conscious orientation, as a very personal peculiarity, for which the owner himself is unable to account. In this case, a person of feeling-type will, for example, become an ardent Christian Scientist, adopting a doctrine which definitely sets out to restrain too great sensitiveness towards oneself and towards others, or he will stand up vigorously for war. Or an individual of thinking-type will throw himself into some form of philanthropy. An intuitive may be stirred by the sufferings of animals and take up "prevention of cruelty" work, while the more instinctual side of life otherwise leaves him somewhat cold. An instinctive person may join some religious movement. In all these cases, the exceptional activity has little influence on the rest of the life. It is a speciality, a hobby-horse, which is really out of touch with the rest and which must be explained as an influence from the unconscious, unrelated to the typical structure.

A third form of unconscious activity is seen in a certain fanatical adherence to conventional views which are actually not consistent with the conscious attitude. One meets thinkers who go in a great deal for social forms, in spite of the fact that these have no logical basis; or people of feeling-type with an enormous enthusiasm for pure science. There are intuitives who stand up for the maintenance of tradition and custom, while they themselves are, as a rule, most averse to being bound. And instinctive people will occasionally adhere ardently to certain religious dogmas, although otherwise indifferent to abstractions. There is in all this a contrast between these more conventional forms and the usual pattern of life.

A fourth manifestation of unconscious activity, of a compensating kind, is the strong power of attraction which people of an entirely different type may sometimes exert over us. It is understandable that we should feel indifferent towards people who are quite different from ourselves, or that they should tend to alienate us by their—to us—essential strangeness. But that they should be able to arouse particular sympathy in us is much more surprising. Sometimes, however, it is just these opposite types who seek one another out.

It is in such cases as if that which is undeveloped in ourselves is attracted by the fully developed forms revealed by another. In discussing the relationship between the types in the following chapter I shall deal more fully with this point. Here it will be enough to regard this effect as a kind of attempt at compensation from the unconscious.

Finally, there is a fifth form in which the compensatory activity of the unconscious may be expressed. This consists in the disturbance which the prevailing function may experience in certain points or at certain moments, as a result of activities in the unconscious. People of very pronounced type have a tendency to apply their dominant function where it is not suitable; a thinker, for example, in decisions in affairs of feeling; an intuitive, with a view to regulating material affairs by means of inspirations, and so on. If they go too far in this way, it may happen that their habitual assurance suddenly deserts them, and another aspect of things, an aspect usually ignored by them, forces itself upon them, thereby upsetting their equilibrium to a greater or less extent. The thinker will then begin to doubt his logically constructed conceptions, and be hampered by unpleasant feelings. The intuitive will suddenly fail to see any more connections and possibilities; the endless actuality of things will seem to crowd in on him as a chaotic mass, with which he has no idea how to deal. The instinctive person will no longer be able to accept things calmly, as is his usual way, but will feel he must be doing or attempting something, without knowing what. And the individual of feeling-type comes to mistrust his own feeling, and to look for something steadier and more objective.

On considering the inner state of mind when such disturbances as these are being evolved, we may occasionally be led to quite remarkable observations. Let us take as an example a thinker who has thought out a plan, based on excellently rational motives, but which may injure very good friends of his in an extremely unpleasant way. The result may be that at the moment when he is about to execute his plan he becomes uncertain and is overwhelmed by depression of spirits. Or an intuitive desires to realize something which is beyond his powers, or which would demand the application of too much of his attention for a considerable time in one direction only. Again unexpected uncertainty and confusion may arise. The form taken by such disturbances is capable of many variations. Those little disturbances in daily life, first described by Freud, may depend on compensatory activity of this kind. In many pathological manifestations, also, it is possible to demonstrate a conflict between the unconscious and the conscious form of typical orientation.

It is not possible to go into all this thoroughly; but I should like to discuss briefly the question as to what the relationship is between compensatory influences from the unconscious and the effect of complexes as described by Freud, which I have dealt with as a fourth complication.

Most of Freud's followers regard all disturbances originating in the unconscious psyche as determined by complexes. In my opinion, only some of them are susceptible to this explanation, complexes being only a special form of unconscious activity. Since the conscious personality is developed as an extract from the totality of the psyche, it is possible to regard less conscious or unconscious activities as complementary to the conscious personality. The majority of the forms assumed by compensatory activity do not necessarily lead to the development of complexes. It is true that they are also not incorporated and elaborated within the conscious personality; but they appear unimportant and subsidiary. Some of these manifestations may, however, come into conflict with the ideals of feeling, which to a certain degree are in control of the conscious life; and if these manifestations are then repressed, the impulses expressed therein being particularly powerful, the result may be the organization of a complex.

A powerful sexual emotion, arising for the first time in the life of a child, may be regarded as an extension of his conscious life, as so far developed. Since the form taken by the emotion is ill-defined or primitive, it does not accord with the totality of conscious life, and this the more where education has succeeded in evolving an attitude of feeling in the child which requires the condemnation of such emotions as bad. There then arises an opposition between the conscious personality and the unconscious psyche. The manifestation of the unconscious now never occurs without a great deal of attention being paid to it, but at the same time it is, from now on, forbidden. The impulse, which might have been gradually developed into a better form, now tends to be rejected forthwith. The opposition then becomes even greater, owing to the lack of any further development in this particular form, and also because the tension involved, finding no outlet, may bring about regression to even more primitive forms. Such forms as these, excluded from the development of the personality, are then fixated, together with certain measures adopted for their suppression. Hence there is, for these forms, no longer any possibility of effecting compensation for the one-sidedness of conscious orientation. Only after the removal of repression are they able to regain their mobility and thus become once more available for use.

Hence we see that complexes are to be regarded as a special form of unconscious activity, while other peculiarities and disturbances, arising from the unconscious, may also occur in a more general, less well-defined form. These more general forms may more easily lead to compensations and corrections in conscious attitudes than is the case with complexes.

A sixth and last complication is provided by the various temperaments, which may likewise have an effect on the structure of the character. Temperament is dependent on a tension which is always present in mental life, on the sense of intensity, on a certain *tempo* and feeling of vitality, factors which vary very considerably in different people (Ewald's *biotonus*). One person will possess powerful inner tension, enabling him to withstand fatigue and to be ready to assert himself at any moment; another is weak and easily exhausted; while yet another may show evidence of great tension at certain times, while in between-times feeling very flat. Temperament stands in close relation to the physical state, and may be studied in physical reactions, which gives rise to the danger of introducing biological speculations into psychology. Some psychiatrists attempt to explain normal and pathological characters by reference to temperamental differences in various manifestations. In my opinion, temperament may explain certain alterations and differences in tension, but not the totality of the character-structure. Temperament is essential in the clarifying of certain peculiarities in the character. In an individual possessing great force of will, a temperament marked by great tension will explain the driving power of the will, but this will be of little use unless it is directed towards an aim (this aim having been first consciously conceived by intuition), and unless there is some persistence in the organization of this inner concentration within the totality of the conscious personality (through thought and feeling).

As a rule, explanation by temperamental differences has made psychologists blind to other mental differences. It is most desirable that the inter-action of this factor with the structure of the psyche, and with complexes, should be investigated, but this lies outside the bounds of this present study.

We have now recognized six complications which make it possible to describe the personality of an individual in a more concrete way. Although this may still not yield up the last secret of personality, our understanding of another person nevertheless increases, the more we are able to distinguish these factors. I will now summarize these factors once more, arranging them in relation to mental contents and structures, and to the distinction between inborn and acquired characteristics:

I. Inborn factors:

A. Factors relating to mental material:

(1) Temperament.

(2) Instinctual emphases (impulses).

(3) Variable, little organized manifestations of the unconscious.[1]

B. Factors relating to the structure of the conscious personality:

(1) The type of conscious orientation.

(2) The secondary function, or polarity.

(3) The ratio between organized personality and unconscious drives (capacity for sublimation).[2]

II. Factors dependent on circumstances:

A. Factors relating to mental material:

(1) Mental mechanisms (psychisms) resulting from environment and education.

(2) Complexes (also dependent on I *A* (2) and I *B* (3)).

B. Factors relating to the structure of the conscious personality:

(1) The stage of development in typical conscious orientation.

(2) Character-traits (dependent on I *B* (1) and II *A* (2).

This differentiation of types of conscious orientation can, in my experience, explain many peculiarities in the motivation of behaviour and in conduct. I admit, however, that the type of conscious orientation is not always the most pronounced factor in such explanation, in which case manifestations may be better explained

[1] Had we been studying personality-types instead of types of conscious orientation, we should have had to add to these factors qualities of disposition, such as talents, capacities and gifts dependent on organic development. These have, however, little to do with a person's motivation, or with his conscious attitude to the world and himself, and I have accordingly omitted them from consideration here.

[2] This ratio is also dependent on circumstances and education ; but there is also an inborn factor. Some people have much greater capacity than others for finding conscious forms for impulses and needs. This is acknowledged in psycho-analysis by the assumption of a certain capacity for sublimation as an inborn factor.

by reference to unconscious drives and to their organization in complexes. With many patients, complexes are more important to our understanding of them than the type of conscious orientation.

As a rule, the description of a character is necessarily very complicated, if it is to cover all the facts. Many people prefer simple schemata, and present-day psychology offers plenty of them to satisfy their needs. For my part, it would surprise me if a simple system proved adequate to explain the many differences that exist between people.

CHAPTER VII

THE INTER-RELATION OF THE TYPES

THE happy relationship of people among themselves is very frequently disturbed by misunderstandings, and it is the task of psychology to clear these up as far as possible. Freud has made a notable contribution in this direction, by focussing attention on important problems of the emotional life and shedding new light on them. Freud's views are of special help to us in understanding the difficulties, failures and mistakes of others. They need, however, some amplification as regards the psychology of normal people and those who have made a success of life, and Jung has led the way here in his classification of typical forms of adaptation. This classification has made it easier for us to understand others in their success, even when their attitude towards life is very different from our own. Moreover, the elaboration of this conception of types has enlightened us as to the causes of those typical misunderstandings and conflicts which so frequently stand in the way of co-operation and sympathy. I shall proceed to discuss briefly some of these conflicts.

In very clear-cut cases, there is an impassable gulf between introverted and extraverted people. The extraverted individual strikes the introvert as superficial, taking life at its face-value, changeable and unreliable. He may occasionally admire the easy sociability of an extravert; but, on the whole, an attitude of criticism prevails. The introverted individual, for his part, finds it difficult to understand the difference between his own conventional adjustment to his environment and the personal and differentiated adaptation of the extravert. The extravert, on the other hand, sees in the other an opinionated, eccentric and unaccountable person, even though he may occasionally admire his independence. As a general rule, however, he believes him to be dominated by some kind of peculiar emotion or egotistic motive such as perhaps once in a while he has been aware of in himself.

No less defined is the difference in standpoint between the two groups described by Jung as rational and non-rational. In the mental life of instinctive and intuitive people, what happens is seen as fact or as the consequence of other facts, while those of feeling-

and thinking-type are impelled to weld such events into a hierarchy of values or into some objective system. Objective happening may be logical, or it may be fortuitous; that is to say, we call it logical when it corresponds with our rational view of things or with our emotional attitude, while we designate as fortuitous anything that does not correspond with these. In so far as it is logical it can be accepted by reason, but where this is not so, it cannot be dealt with in this way. Non-rational people pay little, or at least less, attention to this aspect of events, and they are thus more readily able to deal with fortuitous happenings than are people of the feeling- or thinking-type. It is not so much that they do not reason, as that they are, to a high degree, prepared to accept anything that comes. The reason in things is for them of subordinate importance. This dependence on chance circumstance gives to the man who brings reason to bear on everything an impression of opportunism and lack of character, even though his admiration is aroused by the capacity of the non-rational individual to enjoy life and to profit by circumstances. On the other hand, the non-rational individual finds it impossible to understand how anyone can attach more significance to ideals and rational principles than to living reality. In so far as he is able to make any kind of picture of such an individual, he regards him as an unpractical enthusiast or a theoretical fanatic, whose first concern is to insist on principles and to exercise power, thus more suited to be a professor or a minister of religion than for ordinary life.

Quite other is the conflict between a man of feeling- and one of thinking-type. And here, again, we see clearly how one can judge another only by taking oneself as the object of comparison. The consequence is that an individual of exclusively thinking-type conceives of the feelings of a person of feeling-type as being just as undeveloped and inferior, or as conventional, as his own. A man of feeling-type will, on the other hand, belittle the thoughts and principles of one of thinking-type, because he assumes that these will be as little worth serious attention as are his own. Regarded from the hard-and-fast standpoint of reason, the man of feeling-type may indeed appear a pleasant person, but quite as unreliable in his ways and as swayed by circumstances as one of instinctive- or intuitive-type, and this makes him appear incredibly subjective in his general attitude. A man who is governed by reason, however, seems, to an individual of feeling-type, to be, with all his ability, making use of circumstances in a cold, hard and cunning manner, and this to an even greater degree than do, in his opinion, people of intuitive and instinctive type.

Even the instinctive and intuitive types show a contrast. The calm acceptance of circumstances and adjustment to these and to inner instinctual needs, the inclination to make the best possible use of all that happens—characteristics that prevail in persons of instinctive type—do not accord at all well with the active, restless seeking for opportunities and the expression of personal views which characterize the second type. Again it is a case of judging the dominating function in another by one's own corresponding undeveloped function. The intuitions of an individual of instinctive type interfere with some of the enjoyments for which he strives, although, if the conflict in himself is not too great, they may offer him occasionally a pleasant change and something that he feels to be special and peculiar. He therefore tends to see in one of intuitive type a domineering, capricious and restless person, who, on account of his vanity and capricious notions, misses opportunities of enjoying life. On the other hand, he sees in the originality of the other a valuable intensification of the sensations offered by life. The individual of intuitive type is occasionally restricted in his freedom by external facts or by internal states of mind, and he is aware of a similar lack of freedom in the individual of instinctive type, even though, on the other hand, the latter gives him an impression of calm and solidity.

The contrasts to which I have just called attention may be the cause of still further complications. For instance, an introverted individual of thinking-type will find it doubly difficult to understand an extraverted individual of feeling-type, and in a quite different way he will be bewildered by an extraverted person of intuitive type or by an instinctive individual. When one reflects on all these possibilities for mutual misunderstanding, one may wonder that, in spite of it all, there do exist so many satisfactory relationships between people. Various factors are responsible for this. In the first instance, it is to be remembered that only part of us is expressed in our conscious personality, and that the unconscious part of our being is in much closer agreement with that of others, so that in simple matters we are more alike in our feelings and behaviour. Moreover, when we estimate the more complicated manifestations of another personality according to the characteristics of our own, the result may be not only that a more highly developed function in the other is judged by our own corresponding less well-developed function, but that we may attribute to the inferior function of the other the same significance which attaches to the prevailing function in ourselves. A good thinker will often over-estimate the capacity for comprehension in others, and, since his mistake is not always disclosed by subsequent events, there may arise an illusion of a deeper mutual understanding than actually exists. By this means, the contrasts between the types may be responsible, not only for unjust de-valuation and rejection, but also for valuation and attraction on insufficient grounds.

Attractions of this kind may also arise from the operations of the unconscious. A conscious agreement in matters concerning judgments of reason or feeling (in the case of rational types), or those concerning circumstances and aims (in the case of non-rational types), may bring people a sense of conscious contact, in spite of themselves. "Like to like," as the proverb says, and it is often very true. The unconscious may, however, also be responsible for contacts. These may be of a simple nature, an undeveloped instinct in one person being attracted by the elementary characteristics of the same instinct in another, in whom they are less repressed and exhibited more freely. For example, a girl who has been brought up in exaggeratedly moral principles, and who has had to renounce everything to do with sex, may feel a strong attraction to an idle philanderer, or an honest business-man may, under a similar attraction, fall into the hands of a trickster. In such instances, there need be no opposition of types. But sometimes the distinctive behaviour of an entirely different type may exercise a magical attraction, which is frequently mutual. The bond which is then formed may be partly explained by the fact that such people, in practice, act as complements to one another, so that they become very necessary to one another. One frequently sees something of this kind in marriage or between friends. This, however, does not explain how such relationships arise, and moreover persist, without giving any practical advantage. In such cases, one may assume that the presence of an unconscious undeveloped function brings to the one a vague awareness that in the other there are differentiated and developed capacities which may be of very great value for his own development. We saw in the case of people who had an influence of polarity upon one another that this attraction may be a fully conscious one. For the most part, however, such a relationship could not stand conscious investigation, since this would emphasize the contrasts and lead to mutual disparagement; for the very quality which gives a superiority to the one personality is the weak point in that of the other, and *vice versa.*

Although there may be an unconscious desire to escape from that which is undeveloped in oneself, in practice it is usually obvious, for example in a marriage, that the union of two such opposite types of people will not simply increase the one-sidedness of their characters. As long as they stand back to back, as Jung has put it, to defend themselves against life's difficulties, their incompleteness will be mutually made good, often to an astonishing degree. If, however, they have time and opportunity to occupy themselves with those characteristics in the other which do not correspond with their own, then it will become clear how consciously inhibited they are in regard to other values and other modes of conscious orientation. They cannot understand one another. They seek each to undermine the convictions of the other, and finally they entrench themselves in their own point of view. For normal people, there is probably no field where a science of character of general validity is so sorely needed as in modern marriage. In bygone times it was in practice the custom for man and wife to stand, as it were, back to back, each surveying his or her own province; but a modern marriage demands much more contact between the partners. Development of individual personality and a reciprocal relationship play in these days a much bigger part than in the past. Anyone who deals with psychogenic disturbances must realize again and again how intimately difficulties in personal equilibrium and in personal development are bound up with the marriage relationship. The psycho-analyst, in elucidating a personality to himself, has indeed often to add to his task that of acting as interpreter, explaining the mode of expression of two different people one to the other.

Experiences of this kind tell us a great deal about the significance of character-types, at the same time revealing the great value of such a recognition of types. In my opinion, the influence of this knowledge may be of great consequence in many spheres of human relationships. Although it is true that mutual understanding is of paramount importance where contact is most constant and the bond the closest, as in the family, between husband and wife, and between parents and children, yet in the social sphere there also occur many unnecessary misunderstandings and irritations which might be cleared up. Religious and political—even scientific—views are determined not only by other factors, such as complexes, but also by the type of conscious orientation.

Recognition of these types should make a man more objective in his judgments of others; but it may also help him in his own development. We have already gone some way when we become aware of the fact that we are all one-sided. And if we try to give other people their true value, this will mean that we shall have to learn more about the organs with which we do this, especially our own undeveloped functions. In this way, our own human development and an understanding contact with others unfold themselves side by side. As we advance in the former respect, so we come to understand that no single function in our adjustment to life is of greater value than the other, so long as they are all given the fullest possible outlet in their own spheres; and that the fullest development of humanity is seen only when all the functions work in proper co-operation. While this division into types shows up clearly the differences between people, it does not imply impassable divisions, because the foundation of our being is common to us all, and our emotional development brings us still closer to one another.

Finally, I should like to point out that the value of this classification and its correctness can only be fully understood by going deeply into it and finding out by practical experience whether its essentials are revealed in the psychological study of one's own personality and that of others. This theory of types has arisen out of medical practice, and it must be tested by the practical experience of others. In the following section I propose to expound further its practical value in the field of psychiatry.

PART II

PSYCHIATRY AND THE TYPES OF CONSCIOUS ORIENTATION

CHAPTER I

TYPE AND COMPLEX IN PSYCHOPATHOLOGY

MANY difficulties and misunderstandings in psychopathology could be avoided if psychologists would pay more attention to certain fundamental distinctions. For this reason, I will begin by clarifying an important distinction in the sphere of scientific description. This distinction is valid for all sciences, but it has been particularly the source of misunderstanding in psychology.

In science, as in ordinary life, an abstract explanation does not always mean the same thing; for instance, a father sitting in a train with his son may explain to the child, as they cross over the river on a bridge, that this river is the Rhine, and may remind him of a map on which it is obvious that one must cross the Rhine if one travels in this particular direction. Shortly afterwards, they see a dam on one of the banks, and the father may now explain to his son that this dam was placed there some years ago, because floods constantly took place at this point.

Another example illustrating the same thing is the following: a medical student learns that it is possible to feel the pulse at different spots in the body where the artery passes over a hard surface. A further explanation is unnecessary on this occasion. But he also learns that an unusual thickening in one of the bones must have an unusual cause, which he then proceeds to find; e.g. in a former inflammation or in a fracture. Similarly, short bones may in one case be regarded as a racial peculiarity, while in another they must be attributed to disease.

It is not always realized that we are dealing here with two quite distinct forms of thought. In the first case, the explanation always refers to a certain structure into which a fact is fitted. In the second case, attention is drawn to certain causes or factors which have operated upon one another at a certain time and under certain circumstances. This latter form, causal explanation, is by some investigators incorrectly regarded as the only scientific form of thought. Description of structures has, however, always played an important part in science. In some sciences, such as geography, anatomy or morphology, it is, in fact, the dominating factor. Other objects of study, such as physics, economics, physiology and others, deal principally with causal relations. It is nevertheless important to realize that it may be as important to explain a fact through its connection with structure, as through the causes which have brought it about; and in so doing, it is possible to distinguish between static and dynamic explanation.

Both these types of explanation are applicable in psychology. An observer may note from the way in which someone expresses himself that this mode of expression is characteristic of one particular family, or nationality, or character-type. This mode of expression is thus seen as part of a definite mental structure, and as such labelled, for example, as inborn. One can, however, also imagine a situation in which a man is anxious, because at some earlier period he has been in a similar situation and has had an unpleasant experience, or he may be at the moment undergoing some trying experience. Here also it is a matter of two different forms of thought. In the description of a typical form of conscious orientation, such as I gave above, the static explanation of structure is most prominent. In psychopathology the dynamic explanation of phenomena is of great importance, and hence it is necessary to study further this type of explanation, and to try to shed some light on the interaction of both forms.

At the end of the last century, scientific interest, under the influence of Darwin, was concentrated on the explanation of definite structures. Mental disorders and peculiarities of behaviour were explained primarily by the characteristics of the disposition. Man's destiny appeared to be chiefly determined by his inheritance. As a result, medical psychology laboured under the influence of biology. But, in addition, an attempt began to be made to study individual mental phenomena in their inter-relation with one another in the same way as it is done in the natural sciences, in dealing with objects formerly considered more or less isolated. The school of psychology known as Association Psychology sought to explain mental events causally, as the product of influences which regulated the operation of individual conceptions upon one another. It has become more and more obvious that this view was much too simple to account for things as they are. Established forms, as they exist in consciousness, come into being through a process of continuous modification, which has been defined by William James as an unbroken progressive stream. These established forms, which we find alongside variable and much vaguer contents, have a special kind of existence. They come into being at a certain moment, under certain influences, and they may be changed by other influences. Ideas are, however, not the only established forms in our consciousness: in the sphere of instinctual experience, we find patterns (*Gestalten*) and habits; in the intuitive sphere, significant flashes of insight, held in images or symbols; in the sphere of thought, perceptions and conceptions; and in that of feeling, attitudes and ideal norms for relationships. The close connections which exist between these forms may be designated and described as mental mechanisms.[1] Since the period of Association Psychology, dynamic psychological explanation has developed in various directions.

Although the study of the emotional life remained at the outset in the background during this process, and even now plays a relatively insignificant rôle in academic psychology, this side of life has recently been investigated with great success, particularly by certain psychiatrists. It became clear that certain definite disorders must be regarded as stereotyped expressions of feeling, and this discovery in itself led the investigator to study the dynamics of emotional expression. Janet regarded all kinds of phenomena in hysteria as mental automatisms, to which he gave the dynamic explanation, that they arose from certain traumatic events. The fixation of the effects of these, as a result of which they are later repeated automatically, was ascribed by Janet to general predisposition, thus to the structure of the whole. In Germany, this repetition of the reaction was explained by several psychiatrists as being a matter of emotional expression. Such expression is characterized, as a rule, by being always the same in certain emotional situations. Freud went farther in showing that there was in certain cases a special reason why these expressions of emotion appeared so rigid and unalterable; it is a result of repression. The flexibility which normal emotional expression always has to some degree is here restricted, because a painful conflict is involved. The proper expression of the emotions is, as a result, restrained, and only indistinct and indirect forms of it are revealed. There is a fear of permitting any alteration, because under such circumstances the original conflict might arise again. These effects of emotional experience are not only responsible for the repression of certain feelings or memories of certain events, but also conscious behaviour in situations connected with them assumes a diminished mobility and tends to follow a fixed course. As a result of anxiety lest thoughts and feelings be permitted free outlet in certain situations, mental processes are, more than is usually the case, conducted along certain established routes. Such groups of ideas or emotional manifestations, fixed in rigid form by an emotional conflict, are

[1] See Translator's Note on following page (118).

called a complex. The effects of complexes are found in every sphere of mental life. In this way, certain instinctual modes of expression, products of intuitive insight, thought-sequences and feeling-attitudes, become inaccessible to alteration through experience. For example, a man who has evolved a theory may easily find it difficult, as a result of emotional influences, to make changes in this theory unless these originate within himself.

The problem of dynamic explanation, as to when and why a certain mental content has arisen, may in some cases be further extended into a similarly dynamic investigation into the reasons why unconscious emotional influences have produced a special kind of rigidity in the expression of this content. Our insight into the origin of complexes enables us to explain much more clearly many of the manifestations of both pathological and healthy mental life, and we become aware of powerful emotional influences in our own life-story. Novelists and biographers have already in their work shown insight into this historical connection, but it is Freud who first brought scientific clarity to this insight. The great importance of early childhood in the development of fundamental modes of reaction may now be assumed as generally accepted. In this way, dynamic explanation is possible not only of simple limited reactions, but also of very complicated modes of behaviour, and these not only in psychopathology but also in normal mental life.

Dynamic psychology has, like bio-chemistry, a certain tendency to neglect problems of structure, and to regard as explanation only that which describes causal relationships. In biology, Driesch has instituted a reaction against this point of view. He has shown that a living form has in itself its own particular influence, and that this cannot be deduced from causes determined in space and time. This influence of the totality can only be determined scientifically by means of a description of structure. In processes such as growth, restoration after injury, and adaptation, this influence dominates the whole process. Also in mental life there are phenomena which are to a high degree dominated by the totality, while other phenomena may be more easily dealt with as separate mechanisms (or psychisms).[1] In these days more attention is being given, both in psychotherapy (Jung, Maeder) and also in general psychology, to

[1] In German the word *psychism* (French, *psychisme*) is used to express the structural *product* of mental mechanisms (e.g. a neurotic "psychism"). I have translated it as "mechanism", although the latter word is also used to express the mental *process*, because this word is familiar in psychoanalytical writings in both senses. The phrase "mental mechanisms" on the previous page (117) is used to translate the German "*psychische Mechanismen*" and has not the same reference.—TRANSLATOR'S NOTE.

problems of structure. Kretschmer's researches, showing the connection between bodily and mental structure, have stimulated interest in these problems. His psychological differentiations are quite different from those of Jung. With Kretschmer, temperamental differences, as expressed in the psycho-somatic field, play a large part, and in this respect his work approaches that of investigators such as Ewald or Hoffmann. With Jung, it is a question of another kind of division, namely, in regard to the emphasis in conscious orientation. I have tried to clarify these structural divisions phenomenologically, and to show their practical significance for normal people.

I now propose to consider the significance which these different types of conscious orientation may have in psychopathology, and this brings me to the problem of the relationship, in practice, between dynamic explanation by means of complexes, and static explanation with specific reference to these personality-structures. Let us first look at this problem from a general point of view.

In ordinary life, as also in reaction to certain pathological disturbances, we all behave on occasions dynamically and causally, and on other occasions statically and according to our structure. If you see someone regularly manifesting in a certain situation unusual uncertainty or anxiety, you will be right in looking here for a definite cause, even though it may not be easy to discover one immediately. When, however, a mental condition appears to be simply an exaggeration of the ordinary peculiarities of the personality, for example, when you get a manic condition in an individual of hypomanic character, then it seems natural to apply an explanation from the structure of the personality. This does not mean that another way of regarding the situation must be totally excluded. In the case of a definite fear, the character of the patient will help to determine how the fear is met: whether, for example, he seeks support from others, or whether he relies on his own stoical attitude to life. And the occurrence of a hypomanic condition will also be influenced, as a rule, by certain definite circumstances and susceptibilities. But in clear-cut cases the one factor will be recognized as dominating and the other as subsidiary.

It is, accordingly, possible to classify pathological mental manifestations in various categories, according to their connection with the total structure of the personality. When such manifestations show a peculiar organization, existing more or less apart from the structure of the personality, it seems natural to consider them as mechanisms (psychisms), and when there is fixation by emotional influences, as complexes. When, however, these particular manifestations stand in close connection with structural peculiarities of the personality, then it seems to me that we are obliged to regard them in relation to their place in the structure concerned.

This structural consideration may be followed up in various ways, since the mental as well as the bodily structure of people may be studied from various points of view. In the mental field one may, for instance, estimate a man according to his temperament or according to his mode of conscious orientation. In what follows I shall limit myself to the significance which the mode of conscious orientation may have in certain disorders. And we shall see that there are various possibilities in the explanation of the origin of such disorders.

An individual's conscious orientation becomes more obvious when his external and internal adjustment comes up against difficulties, and in such an event a solution of the difficulty will be sought through conscious activity. In this process, the various emphases in this orientation will become more clearly visible. One kind of difficulty, however, requires a different mode of attack from another. A man whose car has sprung a defect will not improve matters by sitting down and reflecting that he ought to have followed his principles and have taken a course in running repairs before he bought a car. A man who falls into a state of internal conflict concerning the expression of feelings which contradict his ideals may seek a solution by throwing himself into philanthropic work in order to quieten the conflict, instead of facing his inner conflict and solving it in a more direct manner. Thus in any internal or external difficulty we may proceed to act in a correct or a mistaken manner. Sometimes the mode of dealing with the problem comes spontaneously, but on other occasions we may seek consciously for the right way of dealing with the problem in hand. This right method of attack is usually sought in the sphere in which the individual feels most at home, because it corresponds with his own type of conscious orientation. This confidence may, however, give a feeling of assurance for which there is no proper basis. It may result in the overlooking of points of view arising naturally from less fully developed functions, and these functions are, in fact, apt to be less dependable. An intuitive individual, for instance, may be so capable of sound thinking and feeling as to be able to make good use of these functions in certain situations; at the same time, he is aware that thought and feeling have no absolute validity, and may be tainted with human weakness in others as in himself, and as soon as he suspects such a taint in these functions in himself, he prefers to trust to his own spontaneous vision of the whole. In this way he may reject perfectly sound points of view arising from the thinking or feeling part of his mind, and rely entirely on inspiration. A man will not readily admit that his conscious orientation in his most highly developed function is mistaken, because he knows from experience that many possibilities are open to him as far as this function is concerned, if only he persists in his conscious search. This is true in the case of the preponderance of one of the four functions, as well as in the case of introversion and extraversion. An extravert will always look for the disturbance outside himself, while the introvert looks within, but this does not always mean that the chief difficulty is to be found in either place.

If the problem whose solution has been sought in conscious orientation fails to be solved in this way, conscious activity is intensified, and this may happen in two different ways. Active search for a solution usually assumes the form of the dominating function. This is, accordingly, stimulated to activity of a somewhat compulsive kind. At the same time, other quite involuntary contents may appear in consciousness, illuminating the problem in one way or another, for example, ideas, fantasies, intuitions, impulsive moods, violent emotions or superstitious notions. These mental forms will be frequently less differentiated than those of the prevailing function, and may belong to spheres of conscious orientation in which the subject is less at home. Such forms are particularly hampering when they represent fixations, and thus assume an obsessive character.

Such neurotic forms arise in connection with problems that are chronic, unresolved and repressed. As a result of the tension investing unresolved problems in consciousness, varying less neurotic, fixated mental forms may also occur, and likewise become insistent and cause disquiet. While the active form of search for a solution will show typical peculiarities in accordance with the type concerned, these forms that I have just described, which arise involuntarily, are not specific for the type. A healthy individual of feeling-type will be less primitive in the expression of his feelings than one of any other type; but superstitious intuitions or superficial opinions may take in him the same forms as they would in an individual, say, of instinctive-type. Let us consider a few examples.

A woman of extraverted feeling-type knows how to maintain a friendly, affectionate atmosphere in the family, but she cannot follow her husband in his intense absorption in his work, and finds it difficult to understand the problems of her children. As a result, her husband and children withdraw more and more into their own interests, and this makes her uneasy. She will now be likely to redouble her expression of feeling; but she will probably not get what she wants in this way, because the cause of the trouble lies elsewhere. In such a situation, the woman may now develop ideas in regard to her children's education, or plans for her husband, or her anxiety for the physical welfare of her husband and children will drive her to take constant practical measures; these exertions, however, are the product of less well-adjusted functions, and will thus frequently appear deficient and capricious. Her disquiet is not reduced, and she now turns back to her former, more accustomed attitude, and seeks support and security in feeling-relationships. These become, accordingly, exaggerated. She will be inclined to make emotional demonstrations in regard to her husband and children, or to cause scenes when she is not able in this way to bring about the contact she desires. She will also begin more and more to discuss these problems with others, and thus to endanger still further her good relationship with her own family, with the result that she now begins constantly to seek new friendships in order to be able to express her feelings, until finally her whole relationship with others becomes restless and tense.

A man of introverted thinking-type will try to solve the problems of life through objective contemplation, seeking his support in definite rational principles. As a conscientious scientific worker he will bring the problems with which he has to deal to the test of that system which he has learned to use in his own self-development. The time will come when he finds himself faced with a scientific problem which cannot be solved by means of his familiar system, so that he has to assemble his facts in a different way. Intuition might bring the solution here. It may further happen that one of his children acts in a way that is in direct opposition to his father's principles, and that the latter is not able, with all his representations, to persuade the child into the direction he desires. Here affectionate guidance, appealing to the feelings of the child, might have attained much more. This thinking-type of man, however, is, in his scientific work, likely to be very ready to dismiss as unscientific vague intuitions arising in his mind, and, in bringing up his children, to reject his own affectionate impulses as sentimentality. These intuitions and feelings may, however, disturb him, so that he clings more and more to his theories and principles, handling them with increased precision. In this way, a certain compulsive quality infects his thinking, making it dogmatic and rigid, so that he becomes more and more inclined to deny facts which do not correspond with his point of view. He then tries to force facts to accord with his theories, and may thus in the bringing up of his children become the tyrant of the home.

An extraverted woman of intuitive type finds security and purpose in the tasks and opportunities which she meets by the way. For example, she becomes interested in social problems and art, and is successful in setting all kinds of things going and in establishing relationships with interesting people, because of her capacity for identifying herself with the situations and mental outlook of others. In all this, however, her concern for simple duties and for her own health may very well be neglected. Moreover, as regards her family, she assumes as a matter of course that their simple needs are not particularly important. Should a disturbance arise in this world of regular daily needs and established ties of feeling, as a result of illness or of difficulties in her sexual life, she will at first expect to find help in these problems too from direct inspirations. When, however, her sudden ideas and spontaneous expressions of feeling do not alter the situation, she will again seek distraction from her disquiet and insecurity outside her home, in all manner of new relationships and undertakings. As a result of her nervous unrest, the operations of her intuitive faculty may now be interfered with, because she pays less attention than formerly to the realization of opportunities, with the result that a certain superficiality becomes apparent. Such a woman, persistently led hither and thither by her intuitions, begins to dissipate her power and health in worthless problems and intrigues, while her family suffers through her restlessness and instability.

Similar examples might be taken of the other types, but these that I have described will have shown sufficiently clearly that through the one-sided exaggeration of one form of conscious orientation, a situation may arise which is felt to be wrong both by the subject himself and by his environment. Since there is a gradual transition between the usual forms of adjustment and these exaggerated manifestations, the nature of the disturbance is usually not very easy to identify.

It is important to point out here that this explanation of disturbance is not incompatible with the view that many such disturbances arise from false reactions fixated by means of complexes. In the disturbances I have described, a part may be played by such reactions. The woman of extraverted feeling-type may, for example, in her longing to produce a state of emotional harmony in her family, be governed by memories or fantasies which were of importance in her childhood. The introverted man of thinking-type may, in his attitude towards his son, be hampered by vague homosexual inhibitions, connected with his own adolescent experiences. The extraverted woman of intuitive type may be inhibited in the fulfilment of her duties as wife and mother by an inner protest against her femininity, arising out of her own personal development. Occasionally, moreover, it may be the fact that the situation is so dominated by a complex that the latter must be considered of prime importance in its explanation. In such a case, the psycho-analytical point of view is of the greatest importance. At the same time, there are also cases in which the difficulties and complexes play only a variable and subordinate rôle, while the conscious one-sided orientation of the personality dominates the picture. Where a complex is the dominating factor, it will determine the direction in which flight will be made from one particular outstanding problem. Where the type dominates, there will be, as a result of the conscious one-sidedness of the personality, a correspondingly one-sided reaction to every kind of problem.

In addition to these two forms of pathological reaction: (*a*) vague, misunderstood and upsetting manifestations of the less well-developed functions, and (*b*) exaggerated and impulsive manifestations of the dominating function, yet another typical form of disturbance may arise, namely, a crippling of the most important function. As a rule, the development of this situation is preceded by a period of nervous tension, when the two kinds of reaction which I have described dominate the picture. If the main function, after being employed in this compulsive manner, suffers damage, then there develops a state of great insecurity—in fact, frequently of helplessness and despair. There is a great similarity in this state in all the different types, whereas the condition which preceded it, the type of problem, and the manner in which a solution is sought, are often very different. A few examples may make this clear.

A young extraverted girl of intuitive type had shortly after puberty to take on the responsibility of her family in the place of her mother, who had died. She managed to adjust herself to the circumstances with some skill, but her emotional life remained held up in old fixations, as a result of which several opportunities for marriage came to nothing. She failed to cater for the needs of her emotional life, but through a vague sense of unrest was driven to philanthropic and religious activity, each time taken up with enthusiasm for new people and fresh opportunities. She gradually became more and more restless and impulsive, until finally at a given moment her dominating form of adjustment completely deserted her. She lost her faith, could no longer find satisfaction and support in her duties, and fell into a condition of helpless uncertainty.

In the case of a young girl of extraverted instinctive type we find a similar state of affairs, but as a result of different reactions. She also had the care of her family on her shoulders from an early age, and in consequence remained arrested in her emotional development. Consequently, she was inclined to seek the solution of every problem along purely conventional lines. As soon as she met a tolerably suitable man she became engaged to him, and then, becoming restless and anxious, she tried to solve the difficulty by entering into sexual relations with him. The result of this was that she got into a state of great insecurity and anxiety, and no longer dared to tackle her everyday duties, which previously she had managed perfectly well.

Another case concerned a man of extraverted thinking-type, a scholar who suddenly lost all confidence in his power of thinking. Such a condition is usually regarded as the consequence of overwork. But a closer investigation will reveal that the compulsive work which preceded this condition was more its consequence than its cause, and that the difficulties in his work which floored him could only have been solved by intuitive insight into his general attitude towards the world.

As a last example, I will mention a woman of introverted feeling-type who was never able to establish in her marriage a satisfactory relationship with her husband and children, although she persistently sought for the right attitude in herself and fulfilled her duties conscientiously. The more dissatisfied she felt, the greater became her care for her husband and the house. She became more and more quiet and depressed, until finally she lost her entire confidence in life and felt a violent resistance against all her duties and her whole manner of life.

In such cases of mental disablement, the presence of serious complexes may always be assumed, and, as a rule, it is necessary to work through them to establish a cure. The picture of the condition itself, however, both before and during the period of disablement, may not reveal much of these complexes, so that it may be preferably described as a compulsive one-sided orientation with subsequent crippling of the main function. For the proper understanding of such a state, the complexes are not alone of importance, but also the reaction of the whole conscious personality. Moreover, in the therapy of such cases, an understanding of the conscious attitude, and of the compensations involved which may increase its one-sidedness, is extremely useful, because such an understanding helps to establish contact with the patient and thus to make the complexes more accessible.

Thus we see that type and complex provide two points of view from which any pathological condition may be studied. These two ways of studying the problem, however, cannot usually be separated, but overlap at certain points. There may, for instance, be an interplay between certain complexes and certain forms of conscious orientation. Let us now consider the general significance of this interplay.

Fixed forms of expression may arise in any sphere of conscious orientation. Their origin in any particular sphere depends on circumstances in the patient's life-history. Their conscious elaboration depends, however, very largely on the position which these fixed mental structures hold in the field of consciousness, whether this is a part which is usually well illuminated and where distinct differentiated forms exist, or whether they belong to a dimmer part of the field of consciousness, to which, for the most part, less attention is given.

When a mental content or structure exists in a certain part of the field of consciousness with which the subject is very familiar, we find, as a rule, not only a more distinct form in the content or structure, but also a more vivid association among the other contents and structures in the same sphere. Such forms will be more clear-cut and fixed, but if, for any reason they do not harmonize with other forms, an increasing flexibility will be developed, until these conscious forms are brought into harmony again. In the case of less well-developed functions, this does not happen to anything like the same degree.

The fixating effect of complexes may be seen in the contents of the most highly developed function as well as in those of vaguer fields of conscious orientation. In the latter case, the fixation will tend to be more circumscribed in its effect. The fixated form, a fear, for instance, or a certain superstition, may be tiresome in itself, but the conscious personality finds it less difficult to get rid of a content from this sphere, and it is easier to deny it, than in the case of fixed forms in his habitual sphere of conscious orientation. In this latter case, forms arising from fixations will, to begin with, be regarded in the same way as other forms; for the person concerned is not aware that the persistence of a particular form is the result of a complex. We do not ourselves know when we are governed in our relationships with other people, with friend, wife or children, by rigid attitudes originating in childhood. Neither are we conscious that certain principles which we maintain, or a preference for a certain sphere of thought, or certain emphases in our thinking, are determined by fixated emotional motives. An intuition looks like objective insight, even when it is being made use of by unconscious emotional drives, which render it false or one-sided. Instinctual reactions and habits retain that characteristic sense of inevitability even when they are determined by complexes. We notice the diminished mobility and flexibility characteristic of mental life in all spheres where there are unresolved unconscious problems only when a collision takes place between these mental contents and the rest of our mental life. The nature of these collisions tends, however, to be different according to whether the complex is in the prevailing function or in other mental spheres. These other spheres may be more easily excluded if they disturb the whole, and in such a case it is often more convenient to deny the whole sphere, instead of considering more closely the particular content which is in collision, with a view to ending the disturbance. Such a method of evading the problem is not so easy when there is a collision in the sphere of the prevailing function. In such a case, there is increased activity with a view to re-establishing harmony. Such conscious activity does not usually reach the unconscious sources of the disturbance. It cannot remove the trouble, but it establishes a compromise, a pact or a rationalization. This artificial equilibrium is, however, often felt as not quite satisfactory, and the resulting insecurity may have further consequences in conscious orientation. There is a need for unity in the main function far more than in the other functions. We insist with something of fanaticism that there must be no disturbance, that everything is normal and healthy, and that the causes of our difficulties lie not in inner conflicts, but in the outer world. Manifestations of fixed conflicts in the prevailing function become much more part of the personality; it is more difficult to recognize them as disturbances, and more difficult to give them up, because in so doing there would appear to be a reflection on the value of the subject's conscious orientation.

From this it is clear that, while in an individual of one type a disturbance may have profound effect, in another of different type similar profound effects may be caused by another kind of disturbance. I indicated the inter-relation between complexes and the various types of conscious orientation in regard to their general influence on character-traits in the chapter on complications, and I propose in the chapter which follows to go farther into this inter-relationship as it affects certain neurotic disorders. At this point, however, I should like to consider a little more closely the general significance of this inter-relationship. The influence of the type of conscious orientation works in two ways. In the first place, the effect of a complex in the dominating sphere of consciousness is not readily recognized as abnormal or inappropriate, even though contents from other spheres may come into conflict with it. Consequently, it is less likely to be modified. In the second place, a very profound influence is exerted on the conscious personality when the effects of the complex conflict with forms governing order and orientation in the dominating sphere. I will illustrate this with a few examples.

A man of instinctive type has, in general, great confidence in his "natural" reaction to men and affairs. When, as a result of complexes, these reactions begin to develop peculiarities (for example, he takes a strong dislike to certain foods or to certain physical peculiarities in the opposite sex), he will nevertheless consider this attitude normal, and will not permit himself to be swayed by either reasonable arguments in regard to the excellence of the food which he finds unpleasant, or arguments appealing to his feelings concerning the good qualities of the women whom he finds antipathetic. Even in the face of continued mocking criticism by his friends concerning his dietetic peculiarities, or when the happiness of his marriage is jeopardized by sexual inhibition, owing to his susceptibility to some physical characteristic of his wife having driven him to seek satisfaction with other women, such an instinctive man will not feel that he is ill. When the disturbance threatens his feeling of physical health, however, vomiting or diarrhoea becoming associated with his disinclination toward certain articles of food, or his sexual function showing general signs of a more serious disturbance, then there may develop a severe reaction of anxiety and disquiet, causing him to go in for all kinds of remedies to change the situation.

A strongly intuitive woman is guided in most of her decisions by her spontaneous insight. In certain difficulties she will seek this insight in the form of religious meditation or prayer. The intuitions which come to her in this way may occasionally be correct, but in some cases they may be controlled by complexes without her being aware of this. For example, she will try to force a solution of problems in her relationship with her husband and children, or of practical problems such as measures to be taken in the care of her own health or that of others, by using such intuitions as if they were of magical value. The emotional reactions of others, who are irritated by this, or rational criticisms of her intuitions, will not easily influence her to adopt other views, because her intuition, as a rule, serves her as a good judge, and is thus for her a very useful means of adjustment. If, however, there arises a conflict between two points of view, both of them received in this inspirational manner—supposing, for example, she feels herself called upon to accomplish successfully some difficult social task, while, on the other hand, other intuitions tell her that her child is in need of her, or that she is vain—then the certainty of her intuitive function is shaken, and a condition of doubt may arise which she herself feels to be pathological. The consequence of this will probably be that she will seek a solution in fresh intuitions, and her praying and religious ceremonies will be pursued still more compulsively, taking up more and more of her time and energy. Superstitious forms and magical conceptions may then become the expression of her compulsive striving for intuitive certainty. I shall come back to this when discussing obsessional neurosis.

An extraverted woman of feeling-type may also in her emotional relationships with her environment, the chief force in her life, come under the influence of fixations. A woman of this type was, for example, governed in her love for a man by a situation in her childhood. In her youth, the emotional interest of her parents was completely absorbed by the long-drawn-out illness of her only brother. This made her feel inferior and she sought to combine her hopelessness and her rage in a fantasy of her own complete failure and ruin. Behind this fantasy was the secret wish that her father or another man would, because of his love, rescue her from this danger. A family situation of this kind is not a rare one, but a girl of another type would have been able to deal with it more easily. In most cases, such an attitude will in practice be ultimately given up, because of its unpleasant practical consequences, either in the reaction of men to a girl who is ready to abandon herself, or in the restrictive measures of her parents. In an individual of feeling-type, however, these counter-acting influences are less influential, and insight into other possibilities is not sufficient to prevent this attitude from governing conduct with extraordinary stubbornness. Occasionally an individual with no obvious neurotic symptoms will constantly throughout his life land himself in the same difficult emotional situation.[1] Here, also, a feeling of disturbance and of being ill, and the possibility of alteration, will be likely to occur when a different attitude in another, for example, the man she loves, comes into conflict with her own attitude. In the case which I have in mind in this example, a dangerous urge to abandon herself was given up when

[1] Helene Deutsch has described this as a hysterical fate-neurosis in her *The Psycho-analysis of the Neuroses*, Eng. Trans., 1932.

a man whom she loved showed that he had confidence in her character.

In the sphere of thought, also, one finds this same peculiarity, rigidities and disturbances which have arisen from emotional fixations not being readily recognized as errors, even when definite facts and beliefs have to be overlooked, or personal relationships jeopardized because of them, If, however, an insoluble conflict arises in the actual order of thought, through making it impossible to fit ideas any longer into a logical system, or through proving principles to be incompatible, the certainty of the thought-process is threatened and a state of morbid doubt may arise, causing severe reactions in the personality, and possibly changing the direction of the whole character.

I hope I have made it clear that the effect of a complex in the most habitual sphere of conscious orientation is more persistent and more constant than in other spheres of conscious orientation. The question may arise here, as to what are the circumstances which determine whether a complex has its effects in one particular sphere or another. Does this depend on the kind of complex, that is to say, does it arise out of circumstances in early development, that certain manifestations are particularly associated with a certain form of orientation? Or is a certain type of conscious orientation predisposed to suffer certain disturbances? In Jung we find the opinion expressed that hysteria is the neurosis of extraverts, and obsessional neurosis that of introverts. This seems to me to be a much too limited view of the connection between personality-type and neurosis. It is, in fact, a characteristic of neurotic manifestations that they have little connection with the rest of the mental life, and Freud's dynamic view seems to me to offer the most appropriate explanation in this discussion. In practice, moreover, one finds the same kind of neurotic manifestations in individuals of very different personality-type. Hysterical manifestations are by no means found exclusively in extraverted persons, and severe forms of obsessional neurosis can be found in extraverts as well as in introverts. At the same time, Jung's statement is not entirely without justification, for it is certainly true that acute hysteria is mostly to be met with in extraverts and severe obsessional neurosis in introverts. In my opinion, his observation has more bearing on the extent to which a neurotic manifestation permeates the whole character than on the significance of the manifestation itself.

This permeation can be explained in much the same way as the more potent effects which complexes have within the dominating function. In comparison with other neurotic manifestations, the hysterical reaction is distinguished by the fact that it appears to overwhelm the person concerned, as if it were something coming from his own body or from the external world. This is true both for introverted and extraverted patients. But the cause of these manifestations lies in the emotional life of the patients, and is indeed to some degree accessible to them, for example through their own fantasy life, and through their emotional conflicts with others, both of which are likely to express the conflicts which have led to the hysterical manifestation. The hysterical patient himself, however, is in no way conscious of the connection, and will, moreover, make no effort to change these manifestations by changing his inner emotional attitude. An introverted patient, however, will be more likely to become aware of such conflicts, because in any disturbance he is inclined to seek the cause within himself. The extravert, in any difficulty, looks outward first, and tries either to run away from or to alter the difficulties which have led to the disturbance. In so doing, he wanders, as it were, farther and farther away from the cause of his trouble. This, however, would merely explain why extraverted hysterics find it so difficult to gain insight, and why, in their attempt to get rid of their trouble, they manifest increased extraversion. The extent to which hysterical manifestations may permeate the character of extraverted individuals has another source. These manifestations are connected with the emotional life, and frequently express in disguised form emotions which are not compatible with the patients' normal feelings. Occasionally it is fairly clear to others that a woman, for example, will upset the plans of her husband by a sudden illness. In hysterical attacks, also, violent feelings may be expressed which in ordinary life are suppressed. The result is that others react to feelings in regard to which the patient has no insight. The introvert finds it easier than the extravert to ignore more or less such reactions from the environment. He is quite used to recognizing a connection between his behaviour and his intentions. The extravert only becomes aware of his intentions when they take form in some mode of expression. In conflicts with his environment arising out of some hysterical manifestation, the introvert will break off the contact, and thus reduce the difficulty of the external situation. The extravert, on the other hand, will try either to justify his hysterical manifestation, or to make it acceptable to his environment by a declaration of physical illness (when the emphasis will be on the fact that he is ill) or through a fully justified reaction to the attitude of others. In this way, fresh effects, determined by the influence of the complex, are produced on the environment, and these produce fresh reactions on the part of others, so that there is an extension of unrest. Under the influence of extraversion, the whole character may in this way be temporarily or lastingly modified. In the following chapter I will discuss this influence more thoroughly, and will try to show how, in my opinion, moreover, feeling, as the dominant function, may from hysterical manifestations evolve a hysterical character. At this point I am dealing merely with the general point of view, and this I will proceed to illustrate by considering the influence of introversion on obsessional neurotic manifestations.

Obsessional neurosis is characterized by inner defence against feelings which are in opposition to one another. This may be manifested in doubt, or in exaggerated control over personal activities, or in a constant awareness of dangerous inclinations, or in symbolic acts, e.g. ablutions, penalties, reassurances, etc. The solution of problems is sought primarily in an inner change, which never reaches the desired goal, because true insight into the conflicting emotions is lacking. Manifestations such as these are found in introverts as well as in extraverts, and in both cases they are determined by the same mechanisms, the products of certain difficulties in emotional development, such as have been indicated by Freud. At the same time, it is easy to understand that these defence-forms are likely to be more prominent in the conscious orientation of the introvert than in that of the extravert. The former is accustomed from the beginning to elaborate consciously his inner experiences and to conduct himself accordingly. Uncertainties and oppositions give him no rest, while the extravert is more able to overlook them by directing his attention outwards. The consequence is that obsessional neurotic manifestations in an introvert are more likely to influence his whole character. Any modification of such manifestations will in his case be made more difficult because he is less perceptive of the effect of his own feelings on others, and as a result is much less capable of objective control. An introvert finds it more difficult to rid himself of his obsessions. He is under a compulsion to explain them or justify them to himself, and in this way, characteristics such as doubt, self-control and a tendency to seek a solution of his problems by means of symbols become more and more ingrained in his character. Besides this influence of introversion, there are also reinforcing influences from the dominating function. I will later expound how, according to my opinion, it is possible to distinguish two types of obsessional neurotic character, according to whether thought, as the dominating function, intensifies doubt, or whether intuition puts the emphasis on symbols and magical acts.

I hope I have succeeded in showing that the effects of complexes in people of different types are felt in definite spheres of conscious activity, but that they exert a stronger and more lasting influence on conscious orientation when their effects operate in the most highly differentiated sphere. It is, therefore, impossible to say that a certain neurotic disorder will occur only in persons of a certain type. In many cases there will be no need in the analysis of such a disorder to refer to the influence of the type in order to explain the manifestations. In other cases, however, where the character has been markedly influenced and modified by complexes, the type of conscious orientation may explain matters which could not have been fully understood if regarded as an effect of the complex. But we still have not stated the whole truth in this matter of the influence of conscious orientation in the development of disturbances. In my opinion, the type of conscious orientation should also be regarded as one of the factors determining what sort of difficulties in childhood will exert the profoundest influence, and where fixations will most readily take place. Here we are dealing with what Freud calls the "option of neurosis". He holds that the form of neurosis is governed by two factors: by events or circumstances which present certain problems in the child's emotional life, and by the emotional pre-disposition of the child himself, as a result of which he reacts in a specially intense manner to certain situations. In the one case, the circumstances will offer many difficulties, while the pre-disposition will be of little significance; in other cases, however, circumstances will be of no particular interest, but other manifestations in the child's reactions or hereditary influences will compel us to attribute considerable influence to the pre-disposition. It is definitely a very great advance in the conception of the neuroses that Freud has made, in clarifying the inter-relationship between these two factors. But his account of the influence of the pre-disposition seems to me to be too simple. This latter manifests from the outset not only the form and the strength of the instinctual drives, but also it is possible from early childhood to observe that one child will seek the solution of inner and outer problems, and will consciously orientate itself, quite differently from another child. There is, *a priori*, just as little justification for attributing these different types of conscious reaction to emphases in the emotional pre-disposition, as for considering certain attitudes to be determined by peculiarities in the instinctual drives. So long as the psychoanalyst cannot clearly prove as a fact that such types of conscious reaction are derived from definite emphases in the pre-disposition, or from definite external influences, or from both, I consider that a description of differentiated types of conscious orientation has more scientific justification than a speculatively causal explanation from complexes. From my general experience of the occurrence of certain forms of conscious orientation, and also of the distribution of talents in families, I think it is very probable that these are part of the inherited structure. In the last resort, this question can only be answered by researches into the problems of heredity, and at this point I will recommend this problem to the workers in this field for their study.

If we accept that emphases in conscious orientation are determined by inheritance, we may ask if, and in what way, these emphases tend to produce certain disturbances. In seeking an answer to this question, it is best to start from the knowledge which Freud and his followers have given us concerning the sources of neurotic disorder. Freud has clearly shown that the form taken by neurotic manifestations is not determined by the actual difficulties met with, although these may be responsible for the emotions and tensions involved. The form is determined rather by susceptibilities and false reactions arising during the actual situation, for which the way has been prepared in earlier life. Long ago a wrong attitude will have been taken up in dealing with difficulties, and this is repeated again and again in regard to certain problems. As a result of repression, the nature of these difficulties is not clearly in consciousness, and so these unresolved conflicts between undesirable forms of expression and the ideal standards which determine repression persist indefinitely. Psycho-analysis has also taught us that the wrong attitude, which led to the concealment of certain emotional difficulties and to fixated undesirable manifestations, often originates in early youth in the period between birth and the seventh year of life. This important early period of development was studied by Freud, and it was seen that during this period different phases could be demonstrated, which are determined by different modes of expression and by various difficulties in adaptation. The tiny child's modes of expression, and his relation to his environment, are to a large extent under the influence of feelings connected with sensations, stimulating the child to seek for pleasure along certain lines. This seeking for pleasure in sensation is displaced during early development from one organ to another. First the mouth is the most important organ, in so far as it is used for sucking and biting; then there follows a phase in which the sensations connected with the control of defaecation play an important part, and at the same time the child's aggression and control of this by pain or punishment are of very great importance. These two early phases are called the oral and the anal phase respectively. Following this, there is a narcissistic phase, in which there is special gratification in the ego and its accomplishments, while finally, in the genital phase, interest is, *via* the genital organ, directed on to the difference between the sexes, on to the opposite sex, and on to the relationship between the sexes.

In each one of these developmental phases the child finds himself faced for the first time with certain problems of life, and the manner in which he deals with these problems frequently determines the development of a plan of reaction to similar situations in later life. In the oral phase, the child meets for the first time with the difficulty of having to give up a satisfaction in order to accept another in its place, as when the mother's breast and the activity of sucking have to be given up in favour of another way of feeding. In the anal phase, the child learns for the first time that it has to accommodate itself to certain forms of cleanliness and routine, and also that it has a certain capacity to resist these demands. As a result, he meets with the problem of the conflict between resistance and obstinacy in regard to authority, or its acceptance. The narcissistic phase brings for the first time further problems before the child, namely, the need to conform to an ideal, thereby experiencing a feeling of security and personal value, but at the same time discovering the possibility of getting this satisfaction in appearance only, or by means of imaginary magical expressions. Finally, the genital phase brings the possibility of conscious, inwardly determined, and firmly held feeling-relationships with other people, with all the difficulties involved: intense desire for love, great susceptibility to disappointment, a tendency towards idealization, jealousy, and hatred towards rivals.

In this way, psycho-analysis has made it possible to classify, according to their structure, many problems of later life in a definite scheme, which has reference to fundamental failures in the first attempt to solve certain problems of adaptation. Psycho-analysis recognizes the possibility that these first difficulties are caused by violent emotions; that, for example, the way is prepared for them where there are marked aggressiveness or intense sensations in connection with the anal function, or where exaggerated emotional situations have arisen out of conflicts concerning this function. The question before us is whether we can show that these early problems may be accentuated by the influence of the type of conscious orientation. We saw, for example, that in the oral phase the child meets with a challenge to renounce something. Now it seems very likely that an extraverted child will be more easily attracted and distracted by new sensations than an introverted one. We find, moreover, that instinctive types may, at a very early age, show strong attachments to pleasant sensations. Hence one may assume the possibility that, in addition to other factors, a fixation in the fields of sensation in a child of introverted instinctive type will take a deeper hold. This would also be true for anal fixations, the anal phase forming, with the oral phase, the auto-erotic stage of development. It is certainly true that for every child in its first years of life experience in the sphere of the instincts is most important; but, in my opinion, it is nevertheless probable that fixations of instinctual manifestations will more readily occur in children of instinctive type. Intuition probably comes later in the mental development of the child, and I am of the opinion that there is a connection between intuition and narcissistic feelings, since intuition first makes it possible to imitate others, and thus concentrates attention on the personal experience of the ego in different attitudes and in relation to others. This effect of intuition provides the first possibility for narcissistic feelings. Their strength and their liability to fixation depend on various circumstances. It is probable, also, that introversion will intensify both narcissistic satisfactions and disappointments, by perpetuating them in fantasy. In children of intuitive type it is often possible to observe at a very early age a tendency to make themselves felt and to exert influence. The gratification of the sense of one's own worth is important here, and susceptibilities and imaginary satisfactions in this connection may have more stubborn and enduring effect than in children of another type.

In the genital phase we come to the first development of consciously sought feeling-relationships. Without a doubt, these are influenced by special conditions or by intense precocious erotic desires. At the same time, it is also obvious that in the case of children in whom there is a conscious emphasis on the feeling-life certain problems and conflicts in this phase of development will be taken more hardly than they would be by other children. Disappointments and conflicts in the sphere of feeling will be more likely to have traumatic effects and to stimulate repression. Children of other types will no doubt suffer from fixations in the genital phase, but in those of feeling-type one is likely to find a very much more intense effect on the fantasy-life. In such cases, these fantasies may form the foundation for later hysterical reactions. As a result of the stronger tendency found in people of feeling-type to seek a harmonious solution for their emotional problems, their problems are, as a rule, more thoroughly dealt with, but if this fails, there may easily arise a traumatic effect. Naturally, this is more likely to be the case in children, because their feelings are not able to cope with the difficulties of life, and these difficulties are often most pronounced in the genital phase.

As far as the function of thought is concerned, it is also possible to indicate a definite phase in early development in which this function is of particular importance. In the child, the development of thought begins in a gradual way at a very early age, and it may be stimulated, for example, by narcissistic satisfaction in personal achievements in this direction. If this is the case, the child's thought will from the beginning manifest the peculiarity, also found in the development of mankind, of aiming at the exertion of magical power. Thought in the form of systematic arrangement and logical reason, giving the capacity to make use of human knowledge, is developed more particularly during a somewhat later period, called "the latency period". This period falls between that of infantile sexuality and puberty (between about the sixth and twelfth year). The earliest emotional problems have by this time found temporary solution, and school life carries adaptation farther by means of thought. It may happen, however, that unresolved problems from earlier periods still disturb the child during this phase, in which case they will exert a peculiar effect on the function of thought. The latter will then be used, not only in the learning of all manner of new forms of adaptation, but also as a defence against insecurity and certain susceptibilities. During this period, certain false uses of thought may be fixated. This may happen in children of all types, but here again we shall find that the effects of these erroneous thought-forms will not be equally great in all. Where thinking is the dominant function, this kind of defence against difficulties will colour the situation much more than in the case of other children who are able to find other ways of escape. The intensity of a fixation may thus, without any doubt, be dependent on the type of conscious orientation.

In the following chapter I propose to consider in greater detail the connection which may exist between neurosis and the type of conscious orientation. In this chapter my purpose has been simply to indicate how it is possible to explain from the inter-action between type and complex why certain consequences of complexes are more easily worked into the character of individuals of certain types, while others are not, and also why we get severe complexes in one child under circumstances which are readily dealt with by another.

The most useful approach to the study of neurosis is by way of dynamic explanation, through fixated complexes, and this is true even when the neurosis is expressed in the structure of the character, producing the typical neurotic character. There are, however, mental abnormalities where the dynamic mode of explanation is of secondary importance, the main interest lying in a static description of structure. This is especially the case with psychopathic personalities. These resemble the neurotic character, in so far as the disturbance, being closely bound up with habitual reactions, manifests itself throughout the whole personality. There may, in fact, be cases in which it is not possible to decide definitely whether we are dealing with a neurotic or with a psychopathic character. This is particularly the case when both fixated complexes and an abnormal mental structure are clearly present. It then depends on the investigator as to which point of view he considers the more important. Sometimes the study of a certain personality will of itself show which point of view is most appropriately emphasized. For example, there may prove to be potent factors at work during development, or it may be possible to recognize from the outset certain abnormalities in the mode of reaction, and to demonstrate these in other members of the family. In the case of the neuroses, one always finds a division within the personality between the normal healthy part and that which is governed by complexes. In the case of psychopaths, the whole mental structure shows abnormalities, which make certain adaptations particularly difficult, or impossible. Scientific description comes up here against the difficulty of having to determine what is to be accepted as the norm in order to test what is abnormal. This difficulty has already arisen in connection with the physical description of individuals, for example in racial differences. In the realm of mental description it is doubtless equally impossible to determine a fixed normal structure which shall be valid for everyone. Moreover, we find in practice that in one country certain personalities will be regarded as abnormal who are counted as normal in another country. Besides this, mental structure has been very variously conceived and described. Religious and metaphysical ideas and evaluations still exert strong influence upon scientific thought in this respect. Any attempt to establish certain typical differences may also contribute to the better understanding of pathological structures, since the exaggeration of a one-sided mode of conscious orientation may lead to caricature-like structures and to disturbances in adaptation. Recently there have been attempts from different quarters to get a better understanding and classification of the psychopathic character. It seems to me that a differentiation of types of conscious orientation will widen our view of the various forms of abnormal structure. I hasten to add, however, that I do not presume to consider this method of approach as the only possible one in the establishment of structural peculiarities, for I recognize that other peculiarities, for example temperamental ones, are of significance. I shall discuss the connection between conscious orientation and psychopathy in a separate chapter. But we must first consider in more detail the possible inter-action between neurosis and the mode of conscious orientation.

CHAPTER II

CONSCIOUS ORIENTATION AND NEUROSIS

THE conception of neurosis has been gradually altered and expanded during the last fifty years. At first it was dominated by the fact that no organic cause could be found for these physical and mental disorders. From a diagnostic point of view, the conception is a negative one, the cause being sought for in a morbid disposition. The first exact descriptions and analysis of symptoms were stimulated by the French workers, Charcot and Janet. German workers (Möbius, Hoche, Gaupp, Kraepelin, Freud) have since then shown more and more clearly that neurotic disorders are connected with the affective life. Freud has extended this conception the farthest. By means of his detailed analyses, he has convinced many of us that neuroses are to be regarded as the expression of repressed emotional difficulties. Through the discovery of infantile sexuality and the relationship between the emotional difficulties of later and earlier life, it has been possible to give a scientific explanation of many hitherto quite incomprehensible neurotic symptoms. Repressed, unresolved and fixated emotional difficulties are now considered by many workers to be the most essential cause of neurosis. Disposition certainly remains a significant factor in many cases, but is of secondary importance in explanation.

Since, with this conception, it is a question of more or less isolated mental processes, repressed from consciousness, it is reasonable to study these processes as something separate from the personality, conscious orientation having probably but a slight influence on them. Neurotic manifestations appear always in opposition to the normal personality, which is not the case with the psychoses, where the whole conscious personality is dominated by their influence. The dynamic point of view, in its attempt to explain certain definite manifestations from definite causes, is thus particularly appropriate for the neuroses. Static explanation from the disposition had brought us no nearer to the understanding of the neuroses, but Freud has made it possible for us to investigate the causes of certain symptoms, and the results of this hard-won understanding have gradually built up the present-day psychology of the neuroses.

Investigation of the causes of neurotic manifestations is directed chiefly towards the unconscious, where the after-effects of earlier experience are still active. Although I recognize this as right, it seems to me possible to indicate two points where neurosis is influenced by conscious orientation. The first point concerns the origin of the fixation of erroneous solutions of emotional problems in childhood. Certain difficulties are associated with the various phases of early development, but in addition to this, the development of certain mental functions is of particular significance for certain phases (for example, the development of intuition for the narcissistic phase). The domination of a certain function in the disposition is probably perceptible at a very early stage, and the result may be that difficulties in adaptation in certain early phases may be particularly marked. If this is so, conscious orientation will be one of the factors determining fixation, and with this the choice of neurosis.[1] The way in which difficulties are dealt with consciously may be better explained by reference to certain forms of mental orientation. When by means of complexes certain forms of defence in the dominant function are fixated in infantile form, this may from the outset pre-dispose to the formation of a neurotic character. The prevailing function then serves not only the usual purposes of adaptation, but also fulfils the task of warding off certain difficulties. In this way, curious rigidities and compulsive exaggerations arise in the use of this function. Thus the foundations of a neurotic character may be laid at a very early age.

Occasionally, however, we come across another process, leading us to the second point in which a neurosis may be influenced by conscious orientation. It frequently happens that a neurosis appears without there having been any clear evidence of neurotic traits in the behaviour of the individual before the illness. The experienced analyst, in investigating the weak spots in emotional development, will certainly find evidence in certain early manifestations and in peculiarities of character which points to a liability to neurosis, but these indications may lie outside the bounds of the neurosis. Probably everyone has fixated weak places in his

[1] Ferenczi, in his article on "Stages in the Development of the Sense of Reality" (*Contributions to Psycho-Analysis*, 1916), has referred to this problem as follows: "We assume that the wish-content of the neurosis, i.e. the erotic activities and goals which are represented as fulfilled by the symptoms, is dependent on the phase of libido-development at which fixation took place, while the stage of ego-development which the individual had reached when he met with the critically inhibiting experience probably determines the mechanisms of the neurosis." It may be, however, that it is not only the phase of ego-development, but also certain peculiarities of ego-structure which help to determine the way in which neurotic difficulties are dealt with.

development, which, owing to successful repression, are entirely ineffective or are at most revealed in insignificant ways (in dreams or slips). But in spite of this, it may happen that external circumstances (particularly circumstances involving frustration in the love-life) may succeed in upsetting mental equilibrium. Freud has shown that the process may be understood in the following way: as a result of tension caused by frustration, there is a regression. Old wishes are revived, but are now even less appropriate to the patient's manner of life than they were in the past. In opposition to these wishes, repression is intensified, and what had been previously a matter of automatic regulation now becomes an inner conflict. This conflict is expressed physically or mentally in neurotic manifestations. These are seen in various spheres, but may influence the dominant function. The latter is then used not only for ordinary adaptation but also for the displacement of, and defence against, certain external and internal situations; the result being certain susceptibilities, peculiar emphases, and a compulsive mode of reaction. This makes a great difference, if the neurotic manifestations have a strong influence on the main function. In the subsidiary functions, manifestations remain more or less isolated, but the main function is a pivot of the character, and hence there is a greater possibility that it will undergo gradual alteration in a neurotic direction. Such an alteration corresponds in its nature to the character-change, which may take place in a child as a result of the failure to solve very early difficulties, and many of the actual manifestations are similar, since the neurotic character developing in later life shows evidence of regression to infantile characteristics. Some of the manifestations are, however, very different, because the normal part of the personality, with its healthy development, stands in opposition to the neurosis, and is well able to do this, with the result that a more complicated situation arises than in the case of a small child.

The influence of conscious orientation on neurotic manifestations is particularly seen in those cases where the symptoms are less isolated, and where they have led, either from the very beginning or with the first appearance of the neurosis, to strong reactions on the part of the whole personality. I shall now try to explain how and why certain neurotic mechanisms are reinforced by certain conscious structures. Such a point of view certainly needs the confirmation of several workers, and is only offered here provisionally. The structure of certain neuroses has certainly become clearer during the last century, but this work has also raised fresh problems, so that it is impossible to speak at the present stage of any unified conception. Moreover, neurotic forms are very various. I have developed my views concerning the relationships between conscious orientation and neurosis from the study of about 180 patients. They should, of course, be tested on much more extensive material. But in amplification of my description of types of conscious orientation, I should like to give here an outline of how I envisage the relationship of these types to neurotic disorders in the case of hysteria, anxiety-hysteria, obsessional neurosis, mild ideas of reference, masochistic reactions, and in organ-neuroses.

Hysteria and Conscious Orientation

Since Charcot stated the differential diagnosis of hysterical manifestations, hysteria has become a recognized field of medicine. Opinions as to the causes of these manifestations still vary, however. Charcot himself assumed as cause a definite degeneration in the central nervous system. The idea of degeneration is a vague one, and its postulation has thus become a convenient means of explaining anything that is not understood. Liébault and Bernheim indicated the importance of suggestion in hysteria, and Janet followed by defining the conception of degeneration to mean the development of a weakness in the capacity to unify various ideas in a single conception (*la perception personnelle*). Babinski also considered suggestibility to be a sign of hysterical degeneration.

In Germany, a change in the conception of hysteria soon took place. Möbius expressed the opinion that the emotions played an essential part in a hysterical reaction, and Hoche maintained that anyone may, under certain conditions, produce hysterical manifestations as an expression of emotion. The form of such emotions was described by Gaupp and Kraepelin as being primitive in nature, and of a kind likely to arise where there is inferior mental development. Kretschmer, in his study of hysteria, agrees with this view. Primitive and abnormal forms of expression arise where there has been no normal expression (sexual impressions in childhood, severe war experiences). Freud has made an important contribution here, in his conception of the repression of more normal forms of expression, under the influence of anxiety or of moral condemnation. The hysterical form of expression is then fixated, because in it instinctual emotional tension finds at least some expression (and occasionally also because of the secondary gain through illness). This hysterical form of expression may then become the regular mode of expressing emotions under certain conditions. The significance of these symptoms becomes clear when the patient's history is taken, but the patient himself remains unconscious of it. A long analysis is usually necessary to reveal the connections to him. Such an analysis will then show clearly why hysteria finds its expression in such remarkable manifestations.

This dynamic conception of the hysterical mechanism has for most psycho-analysts not entirely excluded the significance of congenital pre-disposition. Freud regards it as a manifestation of the effect of disposition if a child or an adult reacts with peculiar intensity to certain simple stimuli. Hysterical manifestations may indeed arise through the effect of traumatic situations, without there being any special pre-disposition. When they appear in massive form or following insignificant causes, or when the whole character is under their influence, then one may assume that pre-disposition is an important factor. The French conception then comes into its own again. The question next arises: does pre-disposition consist only in a certain instinctive susceptibility (for example, in an intense reaction to sexual stimuli), or does the whole mental structure (in psycho-analytical terms, the ego-structure) in such a case provide a favourable soil for the development of hysterical mechanisms?

A number of workers have more or less denied the dynamic psycho-analytical point of view, while attempting to explain hysteria by means of a simple static characterological conception. It has been pointed out that the hysterical character is found without any actual hysterical symptoms, while several (for example, Kahn) maintain that, on the other hand, hysterical manifestations are found in the absence of the corresponding character. As concerns what is to be regarded as the hysterical character, opinions are somewhat various. Manifestations such as the "flight into illness", which have been regarded as pathognomonic, are also found in other types of neurosis. Jaspers has described the essence of the hysterical character as follows: [1] "Instead of accepting the circumstances and opportunities which life offers him, the hysterical character feels a need to appear more to himself and to others than he is, and to experience more than he is capable of." One finds this need in other types of neurotic character, and what is more typical of the hysterical character is the manner in which this aim is pursued, rather than the tendency itself. Bumke [2] has in addition drawn attention to the increased suggestibility, liability and lack

[1] Jaspers, *Allgemeine Psychopathologie*, 2nd Ed., p. 314. (No English translation.)

[2] Bumke, *Lehrbuch der Geisteskrankheiten*, 3rd Ed., 1929, p. 260. (No English translation.)

of balance in the feelings, to the luxuriance of fantasy, lack of truthfulness, capriciousness and egotism; in the background he finds, as the most essential of all, a feeling of incapacity, which the patient seeks to conceal from himself. Kurt Schneider thinks that the need to be valued is the most essential mark of the hysterical character. Kahn[1] finds a relative or absolute weakness in the instinctual drives and uncertainty in sexual adjustment, leading to a deep dissatisfaction with physical and instinctual endowment, and with this, as a characterological reaction, an extreme insistence on the value of the ego: ego-emphasis arising out of ego-weakness and lack of self-confidence. While Kretschmer[2] seeks to find the main characteristic in the instinctual disposition, Kahn emphasizes in addition the special kind of defence and reassurance mechanisms which may develop in quite early childhood, thus approaching the psycho-analytical conception.

The question arises here, as to how far certain developmental difficulties, and how far a certain reaction-type, may be regarded as specific for hysteria. In psycho-analysis the main emphasis falls on the first point: a certain developmental disturbance in the "genital phase" (the phase during which the first love-relationships appear) which is usually bound up with the conception of the Oedipus complex. With the other group of workers, characterological reactions stand in the foreground. But as regards what is specific there is much less agreement. While Kehrer attributes to the hysteric a wealth of modes of expression, and Bumke and Babinski emphasize his suggestibility, Rümke[3] contests with energy both these points of view. He finds, rather, a certain poverty in the power of expressing himself, especially as regards the finer shades of meaning, rendering him unadapted for work on the stage. Moreover, in his view the hysteric is only very slightly suggestible. To him the central factor in the hysterical character is its insincerity: "The hysterical character is a fraud. Among them we find all the typical frauds: the 'good mother', the 'splendid father', the 'serene and charming woman', the 'understanding fellow', the 'strong, silent man', not to mention the man or woman 'who never complains'. One might even say that an hysterical rogue is never a genuine rogue; not even this honour can be ascribed to him."

[1] Kahn, " Die psychopathischen Persönlichkeiten ", *Handbuch der Geisteskrankheiten*, vol. 5, part 2. (No English translation.)

[2] Kretschmer, *Über Hysterie*, 2nd Ed., 1927. (Trans.: *On Hysteria*, New York, 1916.)

[3] Rümke, " Allgemeine psychologische und psychoanalytische Auffassungen über Hysterie ", *Psych. en neur. Bladen*, 1935. (No English translation.)

The choice of the character to be assumed depends upon identifications, defences, a compulsive ego-ideal, and probably also on the inborn character. For Rümke, a disturbance in the power of expression is the specific factor in hysteria.

Even if we agree that there is something characteristic in this kind of insincerity—and it is certainly constantly met with—I do not think we can regard this as the centre of disturbance. If a man conceals himself behind a mask, he usually has a reason for doing so, and because this reason is not obvious in cases of hysteria, we are not thereby released from the obligation to discover it. Hence it seems to me that the psycho-analytical point of view, in its investigation of the history of affective reactions, is a much more valuable one than the merely characterological. The problem will certainly still remain as to why in one case hysterical manifestations remain fairly isolated, while in other cases they affect the whole behaviour of the patient. It seems to me that this question can only be answered by taking into account the operation on neurotic manifestations of conscious orientation.[1]

One should point out, first of all, that there are cases where the character exerts no appreciable influence. This is true both for cases manifesting a relatively simple hysterical structure, standing isolated from the rest of the personality, and for fairly primitive character-types in which emotional expression more readily assumes hysterical forms, which are, however, not very different from the habitual mode of expression. But if a fairly large section of the instinctual life has been repressed, giving rise to much tension, hysterical manifestations will occur in various fields of conscious experience; and if this conscious experience has a fairly elaborate organization, reactions to morbid manifestations will be likely to be of greater significance in the structure of conscious life. Hence it depends on the dominating forms in conscious orientation whether the pathological forms will attain any great significance, and, if so, what this will be.

To the psycho-analysts, hysterical mechanisms represent a pathological method of dealing with a certain group of problems, whose content relates to love-relationships and the influence of sexuality upon these. It is not indeed always obvious that hysterical manifestations are connected with such feelings, but in many cases a violent maladjusted emotion will manifest itself in a fairly undisguised form (attacks, scenes). In such an event, individuals of

[1] I first described the reciprocal action of these two factors at the Congress for Psychotherapy at Bad Nauheim in 1929, and later in a paper entitled "Psychology and Hysteria," *Archives of Neurology and Psychiatry*, 1930.

a certain type of conscious orientation will feel the need to deal with the situation in some way, while in the case of conversion symptoms there is less challenge to do so. We may expect that there will be in one particular type of conscious orientation a tendency to ascribe importance to such hysterical emotional manifestations. It is, in fact, an essential characteristic of feeling that there is a need to subject every kind of emotional manifestation to the influence of definite norms. We may expect, therefore, that where hysterical manifestations are found in the realm of emotional life, there will develop in feeling-types a more energetic striving to deal in some way with them. Individuals of other types will be more able to dispense with such activity in the sphere of feeling, for they do not recognize its claims. Even where it is a matter of conversion symptoms we shall find, in the case of an individual of feeling-type, some more definite emotional attitude in, for instance, an exaggerated emphasis on the fact of being ill, or in the wish to be sympathized with and spoilt.

What form will the elaboration of the hysterical symptoms by the function of feeling take, when this is undertaken purposively? We must bear in mind here that we are dealing, in these manifestations, with repressed emotions, that is to say, with emotions that are not in agreement with the conscious ideal of the feeling-life, so that their actual significance is concealed from consciousness. If, in spite of this, they break through, a real adjustment is impossible. As a result, there is a threat of a split in conscious orientation. In order to maintain unity in the emotional outlook, recourse is had to two sources of help. The more important of these is the appearance of harmony. The position will be taken up, and maintained with compulsive conviction, that there is no inconsistency. This attitude is not at all convincing to others, who then speak of dishonesty and insincerity. At this point the characterological development of hysteria begins. The second method of dealing with the situation is less apparent. The individual of feeling-type tends to find a reconciliation for his emotional problems not only in his outward behaviour but also in fantasy. A tendency arises thereby to withdraw into fantasy. The opposing attitudes, which in this way are maintained to a certain extent in isolation, give rise, because of their irreconcilable nature, to a pathological state of tension, and this is a source of severe discomfort.

These two modes of dealing with hysterical manifestations will probably be found in individuals of all types of conscious orientation, but in the case of the individual of feeling-type they have a profound effect on the character. There is a considerable difference here between introverted and extraverted feeling-types. In the first case, the inner effect, the consciousness of oppositions in fantasy, is the strongest factor, while in the second case, the simulation of harmony is more obvious. This latter case has been described in the literature as specifically the hysterical character, but the first form appears to me to be of clinical importance, and I will now proceed to give some account of its operations.

In the introverted feeling-type, harmony in the inner life of feeling is the controlling motive. When hysterical symptoms occur, which cannot be simply explained as manifestations of organic illness, there arises, on the one hand, a tendency to pre-occupation with the emotional problems involved, while, on the other hand, a tendency to repression will be perceptible. Inward harmony with the self, and confidence in the dominant function, then suffer a disturbance. The state of uncertainty which now arises bears a certain resemblance to the obsessional neurosis. Doubt and a sense of guilt are also occasionally seen, but the main emphasis is on the affective side. These people are introverted, but repression does not enable them to reach a situation of real inner equilibrium. A state of severe depression and despair may follow, frequently associated with marked physical ill-health. At the same time, confused fantasies may arise in strong contradiction to the normal inner life, although consciously there is often little awareness of their content. But a severe inner tension is the result, which expresses itself occasionally in physical symptoms, or in irritability and restlessness, insomnia and suicidal tendencies. If feelings of guilt arise, the condition may pass over into that of an obsessional neurotic character, while where there is special emphasis on physical illness a hypochondriacal character may develop. A tendency to mild persecutory ideas may even occur, but I will deal with this when discussing this type of illness later. The pathological character which may thus develop from hysterical manifestations is seen in a shy, reserved and depressed attitude, with very sensitive reactions in small affairs, sometimes very difficult to understand, while within there is severe emotional tension, either not expressed at all, or only very confusedly, in fantasy. As a rule, there is a strong feeling of inhibition and difficulty in adjustment to the environment.

In the hysterical character-development of an individual of introverted feeling-type, it may occasionally happen that for a time there is an attempt to maintain a certain appearance towards the outer world, which strikes others as to some extent insincere. This manifestation is here, however, more or less incidental, while in the case of an extravert of feeling-type it dominates the whole characterological picture. It is the habit of the extravert of feeling-type to work out his emotional problems in his relationships with other people. For him, the essence of right living lies in harmony with the environment, in identity of ideals with others, and in the demonstration of this ideal attitude. If hysterical manifestations (hate and impermissible sexual wishes) threaten the relationship with other people, an extravert of feeling-type will make a stronger effort than would another type to re-establish harmony in the relationship. As a result of repression, these efforts will not succeed, and, moreover, since emotional problems cannot be ignored by people of this kind, they have to maintain at least an appearance of solution, or to prove that the fault lies with others. This means, for the extravert, a compulsion to convince others, but these others are usually only partly or only temporarily convinced. It is easier for them than for the patient himself to recognize simulation and pose. The latter is aware of this attitude on the part of others, and reacts to it with renewed attempts to maintain the appearance he is aiming at. As a result, his behaviour is exaggerated, affected and even theatrical. He compensates for his insecurity by a need to assert himself, and this insecurity may then lead to uncontrolled outbreaks or scenes, wrecking his relationships with other people. In the face of such destruction, the patient may lose his confidence in feeling, and a pathological kind of introversion arises, differing from the introversion of the introvert of feeling-type, in that there is much less capacity to recognize it as part of himself. He becomes the prey of fantasies and dream-states which he is unable to master. This introversion, in which all sense of contact is lost, is a very dangerous state of affairs for an individual whose development has depended, to a very large degree, on his relationship with others. His world of fantasy does not help him in his orientation, as it does in the case of the introvert, but in this flight into introversion tends to become a kind of enchanted garden in which to lose himself. In this way, the patient's life becomes more and more remote from reality, since reality for him means, first and foremost, life with his fellow-men. As a rule, this state of introversion alternates with violent attempts to convince others by means of emotional outbreaks. If both these forms, under the influence of complexes, come to exert an ever-increasing control over the patient's life, the hysterical character may ultimately become an hysterical degeneration. The original type may even then remain recognizable in ever-recurring attempts to exert influence on others by means of feelings, thus spreading unrest and intrigue all around. Such people are the doctor's bugbear, both in private practice and in hospital.

These most striking manifestations illustrate the fact, emphasized by Jung, that marked introversion may exert an intensifying influence on hysterical manifestations. This influence seems to me to be understandable, since introversion tends to the repression of internal connections. An extravert looks for the causes of his hysterical reactions in the external world or in his own body. When he meets with difficulties in adaptation, he directs his attention outwards and attempts to alter something there. The circumstances which led to his reaction have to be avoided or changed, and everything must be explained in such a way that there is no reference to his inner problems. This influence of extraversion is seen not only in those of extraverted feeling-type but also in the other types of extraverts. In such cases, there is a characterological reaction to hysterical manifestations which has, in common with the original character, a considerable degree of flexibility. The structure of the mechanisms is, however, stronger, as a rule, than where conscious orientation is less well developed; but a greater skill in the evasion of difficult situations, and in explaining away conflicts, is evident. Since the sphere of feeling can be more readily avoided, the result is less pathological than in extraverts of feeling-type.

Anxiety-Hysteria and Conscious Orientation

Anxiety-hysteria may be given a place between hysteria and obsessional neurosis. The problems are the same as in hysteria, and relate to disturbances in the satisfactions of love. The reaction to the problem is, however, different, and is more like that of the obsessional neurotic. This is the reason for Janet's inclusion of both conditions under the heading *psychasthenia*. In a phobia, the conscious attitude resembles more that of an obsessional neurosis. Here, also, the patient feels himself in danger in certain situations and uses anxiety as a defence. The fear of fear which results then drives the patient to impose ever-increasing limitation on his freedom of movement. Psycho-analysis has revealed that this anxiety is ultimately a fear of one's own instinctual drives and of the danger-situations which they may create. This internal danger is then projected outwards on to animals, storms, illness, closed spaces, etc. The feeling of anxiety is a warning, given whenever there is a threat of any kind of danger from instinct. This phenomenon of a warning signal of anxiety is fairly universal in early childhood. Anxiety of this kind may indeed be regarded as the simplest form of neurosis, and in this primitive form may set the pattern for a later anxiety-hysteria.

But even psycho-analysis has not been able to determine finally why similar problems will lead in one case to conversion-hysteria or to hysterical attacks, and in another case to anxiety-hysteria. Helene Deutsch[1] says: ". . . in contrast to hysterical conversion-symptoms the phobia is characterized by a stronger regressive tendency in the sense of sadistic-aggressive impulses. Hence the super-ego behaves more severely and brings the ego into those dangerous situations which can be projected in the phobia and thus take on the character of an external danger and so be avoided." There is certainly a more conscious awareness of the control of the super-ego than in the case of hysteria. This may partly depend on the circumstances which originally determined the symptom, but the conscious attitude seems to me also to be of importance in determining subsequent development. Jung maintains that psychasthenia is the disease of the introvert, but phobias and obsessional symptoms occur also in extraverts. It is nevertheless reasonable to suppose that there will be a more conscious defence against internal impulses in the case of introverts, even when the actual problems involved remain repressed. I should also like to indicate a second factor, which may intensify the psychasthenic character of the symptoms, namely, a marked polarity in the conscious attitude. Persons in whom opposing functions are often equally operative, thus upsetting habitual orientation, have in consequence less unity in themselves, and so are forced to make more numerous inner adjustments than other people. This conscious lack of unity does not, in my opinion, in itself spell psychasthenia, but if psychasthenic symptoms develop in a conscious setting of this kind, they bring about a more severe disturbance than where the conscious structures are simpler.

Introversion and polarity in conscious orientation are thus factors likely to intensify any psychasthenic manifestation, and certain types of psychasthenia are, moreover, closely linked in their structure with certain functions. This is especially true of the more complicated forms of obsessional neurosis, from which the obsessional neurotic character develops. Defence against anxiety is so universal that it can hardly be regarded as forming a special type, and, as far as I know, there has been no description of an anxiety-hysterical character. Yet there are doubtless people who manifest in general an anxious disposition, and in whom one might predict the evolution of certain character-traits from certain phobias. But, on the whole, this type of reaction is less likely to produce a

[1] Helene Deutsch, *The Psycho-analysis of the Neuroses*, 1932.

distinctive character-type than are the more complicated forms of hysteria and obsessional neurosis.

Obsessional Neurosis and Conscious Orientation

As in the case of hysteria, it is possible in obsessional neurosis to define a certain type of character as the obsessional neurotic character. Here, also, the character may be found in the absence of obvious obsessional symptoms, and, on the other hand, obsessional neurotic manifestations may exert no obvious influence on the character. Here the question arises again, as to why in some cases these manifestations involve the conscious personality. To answer this question, we must investigate the structure of obsessional neurosis a little more thoroughly.

In hysteria, the symptoms are chiefly explicable as the abnormal expression of emotional, and particularly sexual, tensions. In the obsessional neurosis, an abnormal defence against emotional tension is more conspicuous. This defence may take roughly two forms, as Stekel has correctly pointed out: compulsion and doubt. Conscious control of wishes and impulses assumes in these cases exaggerated and occasionally completely incomprehensible forms. Psychoanalysis has revealed the deep sources of these forms of defence. Their origin is connected with the anal-sadistic phase of infantile development, in which the child realizes for the first time, as a conscious problem, the control of his impulses; and also with the latency-period, in which this control is consolidated. The developmental problems at the bottom of obsessional neurotic manifestations belong to a different sphere from that involved in the problems of hysteria and anxiety-hysteria. Feeling-relationships with other people are here of only secondary importance and are under the influence of those other problems, which were the most significant in the phases of early development preceding the genital phase. These are the problems concerning the control of bodily processes and emotional impulses and those concerning submission to authority, or its defiance and rejection. They originally concerned the control of excretory processes and the suppression of impulses of hate and rage. For this reason, this phase in the child's development has been called the anal-sadistic phase. The opposition between the child's own will and that of his parents, the question "May I be bad, or must I be good?" (Fenichel), and the fear of punishment with the guilt-feelings involved, lay the foundation for many further problems of internal and external adjustment. Many later modes of adaptation are affected by successful and unsuccessful solutions belonging to this early period. At this stage, love and hate have not been developed into real personal relationships, and are readily interchangeable in regard to the same person. Sex-difference has so far no great significance, and sensuality is chiefly bound up with undifferentiated physical sensations. Freud has shown (in collaboration with Jones and Abraham) that obsessional neurotic structures represent attempts to avoid the repressed unsolved problems of this anal-sadistic phase, and their successors in later life. As a result, the conflict with the environment is, in obsessional neurotics, to a very large extent internalized; the authority of the parents is represented by the super-ego, which is often very much more severe than were those people responsible for training. Self-seeking and hostile tendencies contend with the super-ego, and, in the obsessional neurotic, these opposing forces vie with one another, now one, now the other, being expressed, and this expression being displaced very frequently on to things of apparently insignificant importance, but having some reference to the conflict. The latter may use up the greater part of the patient's energy and render impossible the solution of the problems of life, particularly those of the love-life. Freud has shown that in this he is repeating a failure in his early development, when he failed to cope with the Oedipus situation. As a result of this, problems concerning love receive too little attention, while those concerning order and control are over-emphasized. This over-emphasis is expressed in many manifestations in the field of consciousness, and conscious activity is therefore always much more affected by an obsessional neurosis than by hysteria. Long ago Freud [1] pointed out that certain character-traits occur with fair regularity in cases of obsessional neurosis, and from this has developed the psycho-analytical conception of the obsessional neurotic and anal-erotic character.

In Freud's earliest description of the anal character he showed how certain neurotics exhibited three character-traits in a very marked degree: a love of order, frequently passing over into pedantry; thrift, readily becoming avarice; and obstinacy, increasing to intense defiance. Primitive pleasure in defaecation and its products is often, with these people, sublimated later in pleasure in painting, modelling and similar activities, or there may be a reaction-formation in the way of a particular compulsion towards cleanliness. Interest in faeces may be displaced, moreover, on to money. In addition to these anal-erotic character-traits, the obsessional neurotic character also manifests distinct reaction-formations,

[1] Freud, "Character and Anal Erotism", 1924: *Collected Papers*, vol. ii.

particularly to feelings of hate. Jones [1] and Abraham [2] have given a full description of these character-traits, and have shown how many peculiarities of later behaviour are connected with the fixation of certain attitudes in this early phase of development. I do not propose to go into details here, but I should like to emphasize one point which is, in my opinion, of importance. It seems to me that these authors have set the limits of the obsessional neurotic character far too wide, so that they are in danger of including in their description a complete picture of the introvert. When Jung declares that obsessional neurosis is the expression of the introvert, he is incorrect, because of his one-sided view. But when Freud, Abraham and Jones set out to explain introversion as anal-eroticism and obsessional neurosis, I must equally object. There are certainly characters which may be pretty completely explained by reference to obsessional neurotic and anal-erotic reaction-formations. But one may also find, though more isolated, similar character-traits in persons whose characters are not under the control of these types of reaction. The extent to which such traits may pervade a character depends, in my opinion, on whether there is an inter-action between these mental structures and the type of conscious orientation. At the same time, there are also well-marked introverted character-types which are only very slightly determined by these disturbances in infantile development, and whose kind of behaviour can be much more readily explained from their characteristic conscious orientation. Jones is over-estimating the scope of dynamic explanation when he derives from anal-erotic factors characteristics such as: "Marked individuality, determination, and obstinacy, love of order and organizing ability, industry, dependability and thoroughness, refinement of taste and artistic judgement, unusual delicacy and skill in dealing with concrete affairs of the world", and in addition: "irritability, bad temper, hypochondria, avarice, narrow-mindedness and meanness, mental clumsiness, love of power and self-will".

One should speak of obsessional neurotic character-traits only when defence and adjustment have produced a rigid and exaggerated personality. Not all habits of defence and control indicate such rigidity, although their fixity and consistency may look like compulsion to the man less controlled by principles. The distinction

[1] Jones, "Anal-erotic Character-traits", *Papers on Psycho-Analysis*, New York and London, 1928.

[2] Abraham, "Contributions to the theory of Anal Character" and "A Short History of the Development of the Libido", *Selected Papers*, London, 1927; *Psychoanalytische Studien zur Charakterbildung*, 1925 (no English translation).

which is lacking in the psycho-analytical view is that which exists between rigid mechanisms, dynamically explicable, and having a fixed place in the total mental economy, and structural peculiarities which can really only be understood as part of a whole. The obsessional neurotic character, as defined in psycho-analytical psychology, cannot be explained from the mechanisms alone, as indeed the majority of psycho-analysts admit. But their views concerning inherited mental structures are too vague to permit of satisfactory insight into the origin of these characters. This is shown in the variety of types which they include under the conception of the obsessional neurotic character. It seems to me possible to get a better understanding of some of these types, by reference to an inter-action between obsessional neurotic mechanisms and certain types of conscious orientation.

We have already discussed the relationship between obsessional neurosis and introversion. To the introvert, his impulses and their control appear usually as an inner problem to be solved more or less independently of external circumstances. For this reason, reflection, symbolic representation and analogy play a large part in the process of inner orientation. These processes are found in obsessional neurosis in exaggerated forms which fail in their object, but they are not on that account to be regarded as in themselves pathological. Inner insecurity, consequent on certain emotional problems, employs these mechanisms in obsessional neurosis to postpone solution or to make it impossible, and in the case of the introvert a marked effect may easily be achieved in this way upon the whole conscious orientation.

Severe conditions of obsessional neurotic introversion will probably always be found to exist upon the basis of a markedly introverted character, and there are also true obsessional neurotic characters, in whom introversion is the predominant characteristic. The self-absorbed doubter, constantly making ready, but never coming to a decision; the suspicious skinflint, always feeling cheated, his whole life controlled by his compulsive need for financial security; the theorist, whose life is absorbed in his own theories of the universe; the metaphysical speculator, with his belief that he understands the inner relationships of things and his attempts to control them by magical means; the bigoted believer, plagued by religious doubts and fear of condemnation, who has displaced his sense of duty on to internal and external minutiae;—all these manifest a combination of characterological compulsive defences and introversion. The obsessional neurotic evades the problems of his relation to the community and to authority, and his obsessional neurotic mechanisms enable him to dally with them in a way that makes any genuine solution impossible. This unreal approach is found not only in introversion. Obsessional symptoms are also found in markedly extraverted people. But introversion offers a marvellous opportunity for escaping the test of reality, and once this is done, the obsessional defences are elaborated more and more, and it is impossible to estimate how far they really provide security against life. In the introvert, obsessional neurotic manifestations thus show less flexibility than in the extravert, and more easily develop into a kind of fortress into which he withdraws completely. Marked introversion may thus be an important factor in giving obsessional neurotic mechanisms an overweening importance in conscious orientation.

Introversion is not the only factor of conscious orientation which affects characterological development from obsessional neurosis. Just as in hysteria the function of feeling is of special importance for the development of the hysterical character, so it appears to me that two other functions may intensify obsessional neurotic manifestations, namely, intuition and thinking. The intensification conferred on obsessional neurotic mechanisms by these forms of conscious orientation is different in each case, and produces different types of neurotic character. Intuition is related to compulsion, since intuitions have something compulsive about them, owing to the sense of conviction with which they arise. Thinking is related to doubt, since all essential thinking starts from doubt. We will consider these relationships separately.

If we enquire how the patient arrived at the compulsion to use some particular defensive ritual or thought-formula, we shall usually find that it happened in a flash in some particular situation associated with danger. The conscious form of the compulsion is the same as that of an intuition. This is, of course, no explanation of the compulsion, for nothing short of insight into its unconscious foundations will render the content of this peculiar kind of intuition comprehensible. An individual who, on account of his type of conscious orientation, is in the habit of guiding himself by his intuitions, is likely in this situation to have greater difficulty in warding off pathological ideas than one who has never attached much significance to his intuitions. One can understand, therefore, that, once they have gained admission, he will be at pains to find some justification for these ideas, by trying to combine them with the rest of his conceptions. In this type of case, we get the beginning of the development of an obsessional character, as with ever-decreasing criticism place is found, because of the type of conscious orientation, for these peculiar and morbid ideas. How this happens varies according to whether the individual concerned is an introvert or an extravert.

The intuitive extravert perceives all manner of possibilities and tasks in the world which must be realized. The essence of compulsive intuitions is that they do not indicate real tasks, but are a defence against impermissible wishes. The patient himself is, however, unconscious of this distinction. His obsession, on the contrary, obliges him to attach special importance to the urge which he feels to carry out these precautions and operations. Something similar takes place in a more general way in superstition, where an unconscious motive also clouds insight. The way in which the compulsive association arises is, moreover, probably the same in both cases, and indeed it is not always possible to draw the line between superstition and obsessional neurosis. Not every superstitious individual can be reckoned an obsessional character, however, for the mental forms which determine the latter are not always present. In the extravert, the forms that go to produce compulsions are, as a rule, variable, since they are very much under the influence of external circumstances. In everyone they are associated with unconscious problems, but the neurotic differs from others in suffering from severer, and more constant tension on their account, since he has not been able to deal consciously with many of life's problems, and they are accordingly repressed. It is possible, therefore, to maintain the view that obsessional neurotic mechanisms are present in everyone, and that they become of such great significance in obsessional neurosis itself because in this case they serve to conceal important problems of life; and that, in the intuitive extravert, they are less easily recognized as morbid because they accord in all other respects with the conscious mode of orientation. The type of obsessional neurotic character which arises in this way is distinguished by uncertain, inconsistent behaviour, which is governed by peculiar and frequently even bizarre ideas. The conviction with which he maintains these ideas stands in contrast to the uncertainty which is betrayed in the rest of his behaviour. Since intuitive extraverts are always at pains to convince others with their intuitions, this kind of obsessional neurotic abnormality can be occasionally very vexatious.

In introverts, the effect of intuitions takes another form, and obsessional neurotic mechanisms are also dealt with differently in the character. Here, intuitions relate to the nature of man and to the standards of behaviour required, if he is to fulfil this. This insight may be clouded by compulsive intuitions, for the latter are first and foremost intended as a defence and to conceal something. Here again the patient is unconscious of the peculiar use to which he puts his intuitions. There is, in fact, a certain assurance associated with the process, so that he defends himself, should ever the value of his insight be doubted. In individuals of this type of conscious orientation, introversion, coupled with their own strong conviction regarding their intuitions, results in a greater elaboration in conscious orientation of intuitions which are compulsive. Consequently, obsessional neurotic intuitions are in these circumstances more defined and more obstinate than in intuitive extraverts. These people may tie themselves up in infantile, archaic ceremonials and magical modes of thought, to a degree that gives their whole life a peculiar impress. Occasionally they may even be able to convince a group of individuals of the value of their peculiar views. In these characters there is often an extraordinary mixture of the morbid and the worth while, so that it is not at all easy to separate the one from the other. What is typically neurotic in these cases is the playing with mental contents for personal, narcissistic and defensive ends, whereby some of their value is sacrificed.

Thought, moreover, like intuition, is related to obsessional neurosis. Characterological development is manifested here in a somewhat different way. Thought, like intuitive insight, is able to overcome uncertainty, and here again the neurotic, by partly repressing his conflicts, may cling to mistaken forms which provide no real solution, but only produce an appearance of assurance. These obsessional neurotic attempts in the way of thinking are revealed both in exaggerated doubt, in a challenging of intellectual certainty, and in the construction of thought-systems aiming at intellectual order in spheres where this is not possible, or at least not possible at the present time. We may then get, side by side with correct thought-forms, compulsive forms which are not easily identified as pathological. The difference between introverts and extraverts is here less striking than in the case of the intuitives, because thought-forms aim at objectivity and are therefore bound to be in closer agreement. It is possible, however, even here, to distinguish two types of characterological development.

The thought-processes of an extravert of thinking-type tend to assume the forms which are current in the community, and it is not easy for him, therefore, to achieve pathological forms in the face of criticism, except when the defence expressed is a collective one (for example, the attitude of the Church towards Galileo's discovery). Hence it is not easy here for the compulsive element in the thought-process to assume peculiar thought-forms. It is more readily expressed in an exaggerated use of prevailing thought-forms, and in an exaggerated punctiliousness and conscientiousness in the application of certain principles. It is a further mark of extraversion, that peace and assurance can only be attained when some way is found of successfully putting across the particular thought-series that has been arrived at. As in the case of intuitive extraverts, compulsive manifestations may also here become a great nuisance to the environment, and so much the more because these compulsive thought-forms impose on it the whole weight of collective authority which invests the thinking of individuals of this type. In such a case, the characterological development of an obsessional neurosis is not very transparent. In slight cases, it would probably never be possible to reveal to this type of individual, convinced as he is of his normality and objectivity, that his thoughts are themselves influenced by complexes. But even in severe cases, it is no easy task to convince such patients of the neurotic aspect of their character.

The possible development of obsessional neurotic manifestations under the influence of introverted thinking is somewhat more striking than in the case of the extravert. Thought-processes here assume rather more individual forms, which may be partly correct but also partly serve as a defence against repressed tendencies. As a result, one finds side by side with an originality which gives their thinking a certain independence and value, a kind of eccentricity which seeks support in personal thought-systems and principles. Introversion limits the possibility of correction. Difficulties in external relationships are evaded, doubt becomes a habit, and the patient withdraws himself from responsibility for action into a system of deliberations and assurances. These people become extraordinarily skilled in the rationalization of their inadequacy and in the justification to themselves of the inconsistencies in their actions. In severe cases, thought-forms are primarily used as a defensive means to shut out the world. Eccentricities, no longer distinguished from the worth-while origins from which they sprang, come to exert an ever-increasing control over their lives. They seem to be able to overcome their neurotic uncertainty only by insisting more and more on their personal means of self-assurance and their personal constructions of truth, seeking to give these reality, at least in their own personal lives.

There are thus various factors which favour the development of characterological elaborations and compulsive manifestations. The full-blown neurotic character will usually be found where these factors have been in combination, as, for instance, in the intuitive introvert with thought as his subsidiary function, and in the thinking-introvert with intuition as his subsidiary function. In the first case, the intuitive type of elaboration will be more obvious, while in the second, compulsive thinking will colour the picture.

Mild Ideas of Reference and Conscious Orientation

Mild ideas of reference might be described as the neurotic form of paranoia. Although these are often pre-psychotic, they nevertheless sometimes disappear again, or become chronic and represent the main content of the illness. This type of neurotic illness is of less practical significance than hysteria or obsessional neurosis, because it is rarer; but it is theoretically interesting, because it forms a transition between ordinary human reactions, such as mistrust and suspicion, and important pathological manifestations, such as persecution-mania. For our study, mild ideas of reference are also important, because we may perceive here inter-action between mental mechanisms and characterological disposition. Kretschmer,[1] who, in conjunction with Friedmann, gives these manifestations a separate place in psychiatry, expressly emphasizes this inter-action. In the foreground he places the "sensitive" character which he designates as predominantly asthenic, with a contrasting sthenic streak. On the one hand, people of this character manifest an extraordinary gentleness, weakness and ready vulnerability, while, on the other side, there is a certain self-conscious ambition and self-will. "The fully developed representatives of this character-group are complicated, highly intelligent and estimable personalities, altruists of fine and deep feeling, with scrupulous morals and with over-sensitive, reserved feelings, reacting to any harshness in the circumstances of their life, withdrawing deep into themselves in their tense and lasting affects, capable of intricate self-observation and self-criticism, very touchy and self-willed, while at the same time very ready to give love and trust. They have definite self-regard, but are timid and without certainty in personal bearing; they are turned in on themselves, but at the same time accessible and friendly; modest and yet ambitious, aspiring, and extremely proficient socially. The peculiar small-mindedness and pedantry of the obsessional neurotic is lacking in the neurotic with ideas of reference. The emotions of these predominantly serious-minded

[1] Kretschmer, *Der sensitive Beziehungswahn*, 1918. (No English translation.)

people show a tendency to persistent depression which is, however, reactive and not altogether constitutional in character."

Side by side with this characterological disposition, there is a definite mechanism, described by Kretschmer as "suppression with consequent introversion". "In these sensitive people the humiliating experience of their own insufficiency and of their moral defeat has an inevitably pathological effect. This experience drives such an individual, with his lack of robust egotism, his sensitive and deep feelings, and his intense conscientiousness, inexorably and ever deeper into a hopeless, hidden fight with himself. With the compulsive return of the suppressed images, a desperate degree of emotional tension finally transforms the original content of experience into a delusion of reference, which presents a visible, external copy of his own internal self-contempt. In these sensitive people with their mild ideas of reference, the psychological inter-action between character and experience forms the essential cause of their illness. For this reason the illness is precipitated not by any chance set of circumstances but by facts such as would inevitably bring about similar difficulties in a healthy person of sensitive type, although not, in his case, to the point of mental illness. In the first rank it is conflicts in the sphere of sexual morals which have this pathogenic capacity" (masturbators, perverts, old maids falling in love and feeling terribly ashamed about it). Ethical problems relating to professional life may also be a causal factor.

Kretschmer, in thus summarizing the results of his investigation, gives a clear picture of a certain kind of pathological development. All people with delusions of reference do not fall into this group, but only a certain sensitive type. If we compare the sensitive character which is the foundation of the type he describes with our types of conscious orientation, we are immediately struck by its similarity to the introvert of feeling-type. There, also, we saw great sensitiveness in regard to ethical problems, and a tendency to elaborate them. The contrast, also, between great vulnerability and a self-willed assurance in regard to values and opinions resembles the structure of introverted feeling. Friendliness, timidity, modesty, affectionateness, together with aspiration and social awareness, are all traits which mark the introvert of feeling-type. He also makes a great business of ethical problems, and if he cannot solve them, feels the foundations of his life endangered. If we disregard the peculiarities in Kretschmer's description, and overlook the differences in his terminology, there seems to be a complete agreement. But if we look more closely, we shall find some differences in his conception which raise certain questions.

Kretschmer sees the characterological basis of these disorders as a severe hereditary disability, characterized particularly by fatiguability. I, on the contrary, have represented the introvert of feeling-type as a normal variation. This contrast is not insurmountable, since, in my opinion, also, markedly one-sided forms of conscious orientation may give rise to pathological disturbances, as I shall show in greater detail in the chapter on the psychopathic pre-disposition. If a characterological basis were enough to account for the appearance of mild ideas of reference in a sensitive individual, we should have to describe this type of illness, not as a neurosis, but as a psychopathic character-development. Against this, we have, first, the fact that we are dealing here with a definite pathological mechanism, and secondly, that other neurotic manifestations may arise from the soil of this "sensitive" introverted character, while, on the other hand, delusions of reference do not occur exclusively in individuals of this character-type. I should, therefore, be more inclined to regard the mechanism as the centre of gravity, so to speak, in the illness than Kretschmer does, and I should consider the characterological one-sidedness primarily as an intensifying factor. This brings the question of the mechanism into the foreground.

Kretschmer divides the manifestations of pathological sensitiveness into four different groups: paranoid conditions involving delusional systems, delusions of reference, mild ideas of reference, and isolated delusional ideas of an obsessional neurotic character. The first form, in many cases, tends for a time to develop progressively, very much like a true paranoia, and to evolve a system of delusions of reference, having as their content general contempt for the patient, and observation of the way in which he conducts himself, all viewed in the light of the experience which has humiliated him. They may even extend to include a delusion of persecution by the police. In contra-distinction to other paranoid tendencies, for example that of the litigious individual, this type of delusion of reference is characterized by a concentration on, and detailed elaboration of, the ideas of reference, in keeping with the patient's anxious, timid and uncertain spirit. Critical phases of short duration may occur in some cases, when a condition of acute delusional dissociation is present, with extreme emotional tension and pseudo-catatonic ideas of physical control and of thought-transference, and feelings of unreality, yet without immediate certainty in regard to the delusional experience, and without loss of affective accessibility. The less severe forms of delusions of reference are classified by Kretschmer as neuroses of reference and are compared with obsessional neurosis.

Recently a good deal of attention has been given to this "sensitive" type of individual with mild ideas of reference, with its peculiar inter-action between character and experience. It has been compared with Gaupp's "abortive paranoia". But here the emphasis falls more on the paranoid process and less on characterological disposition, so that Bouman,[1] for instance, sees a resemblance to paranoia proper. In the case of mild ideas of reference, the patient's character seems to exert more influence than in real paranoia. It is, indeed, questionable whether the mechanism is the same in the two cases. The structure of paranoia has, however, never been worked out with any great clarity in psychiatric literature. The very gradual transition between mistrust, suspicion and ideas of reference makes it difficult to draw any definite line between the normal and the pathological in this field. Bleuler draws attention to the heightened ego-feeling, which stands in contrast to a sense of inferiority. Lange finds in all paranoiacs a struggle for evaluation of the ego. But in this it is less a question of evaluation by the external world than in the subject's own opinion, and then often in one respect only. "As a rule it is not so much heightened self-regard but rather that the paranoiac sets up this self as the unalterable, rigid pivot round which the external world revolves." [2] Lange points out the similarity between this self-regard and Freud's conception of narcissism. Freud and his followers have, however, given a much more clear-cut description of the mechanism that produces this illness, and the concept of narcissism in itself gives no more than an incomplete picture of it. The essential elements in the Freudian conception may be given in outline as follows: The paranoid disposition is the product of an emotional development which, in spite of having arrived at some measure of equilibrium, nevertheless manifests distinctly abnormal features. There is an excess of narcissistic feeling and with it frequently excessive tension in social feeling (as a result of sublimated homosexuality), while the sexual feelings are relatively under-developed. If at this point a disturbance in equilibrium occurs, sublimation may undergo regression whereby the relationship with the community may be endangered by homosexual (and in my opinion also aggressive) tendencies. The paranoiac defends himself against this by entrenching himself in his narcissism and by projecting and distorting the impulses which he fears. In the light of this, delusions of

[1] L. Bouman, "Paranoia", *Psych. en neur. Bladen*, 1931. (No English translation.)

[2] Lange, "Die Paranoiafrage", *Handbuch der Psychiatrie*, 1927. (No English translation.)

reference are again seen as an attempt to preserve the unifying influence of narcissism, and to re-establish contact with the environment.

These factors in the aetiology of paranoia have been widely confirmed. Westerman-Holstijn, in his very clear review of the subject, mentions 120 cases in the literature in which there is clear evidence of homosexual tendencies in paranoid psychosis.[1] He admits, however, at the same time, that the significance of these factors in paranoia proper is much more difficult to grasp than in dementia paranoides, because the defences are so much more elaborate. Freud attempts to explain from this defence against the threat of homosexual impulses, not only persecution-mania, but also eroto-mania and delusional jealousy, while the megolomania involved represents a successful regressive investment of the ego with libido. This mechanism should be valid for abortive and real paranoia and also for dementia paranoides, even though, in the latter case, the precipitation of the illness is possibly conditioned by some physical process. The question arises, however, even supposing that this hypothesis finds further confirmation, as to whether this same mechanism is the controlling factor in "sensitive" individuals with mild ideas of reference and in litigious persons. As regards the former group, Blok [2] and Westerman-Holstijn answer this question in the negative. The latter points out that in these cases infantile guilt-feelings (Oedipus complex, masturbation, etc.), expectation of punishment and condemnation by those responsible for childhood-training, have produced a complex which the later environment has maintained in a state of latent excitement, and which is then re-activated by certain experiences. Here there is projected only an awareness of guilt, while in paranoia proper there is projection of libido. One might say that in the case of these people with mild ideas of reference there is simply an extension outwards of their inner conflicts, while true projection means that something in the instinctual life is repressed, and is experienced only in the objects of those instinctual drives or in persons connected with them. The patient then imagines that he is accused of homosexuality or is influenced by others, which in schizophrenia may give rise to all kinds of physical experiences. Often it is difficult to say whether the patient hates or loves his persecutor, or does both. Killing or being killed often appear as

[1] Westerman-Holstijn, "Zur Psychoanalyse der Paranoiker", *Psych. en neur. Bladen*, 1931. (No English translation.)

[2] Blok, *Over de waandenkbeelden van vrouwen met een paranoide schizophrene psychose*, 1931. (No English translation.)

expressions of sexual impulse. Eroto-mania and delusional jealousy, on nearer investigation, also disclose themselves as the disguises of repressed homosexuality.[1] The impulse in this case is not simply projected. It is also represented in an altered form, which is what happens, for that matter, in persecution-mania.

This view of the structure of paranoia has met with little recognition outside the group of psycho-analysts, although it has deepened our insight in many cases to a remarkable degree. The problem has certainly not been entirely cleared up by psycho-analytical investigators. It is, for instance, not clear why the repression of homosexuality should in these cases lead to projection, and the limits of this method of explanation have also not been clearly defined. When an explanation of the liability to react in this way is sought, then it seems that, from the psychological point of view, little light can be thrown on the matter. Narcissism is usually mentioned both in paranoia and in dementia paranoides, and also as an explanation of litigiousness, but this factor is less in evidence in mild ideas of reference. Moreover, the characterological sub-structure in these latter cases would seem to be different. For this reason, this form of delusions of reference seems to require a special place, and I have already indicated that here the characterological pre-disposition coincides with that of the introvert of feeling-type.

The question then remains as to how far we must assume a different characterological pre-disposition for litigiousness, paranoia and dementia paranoides. I shall deal with the pre-disposition to schizophrenia, which comes under the last head, in Chapter IV, where I shall study it from the point of view of conscious orientation. As far as litigiousness and paranoia are concerned, it seems to me that there are many common traits in the pre-disposition, while the actual mechanisms differ quite considerably. As far as I know, there has been no psycho-analytical study of litigiousness, and I also have no experience of it, so that I speak here with very great reserve.[2] The characterological attitude which is prominent in both cases might be described in Reich's[3] term as phallic-narcissistic.

[1] Reference on this subject may be made to Freud, " A Case of Paranoia running counter to the Psycho-analytical Theory of the Disease ", *Collected Papers*, vol. ii., 1924.

[2] Carp (*De Psychopathieën*) points to the influence of the hypo-manic temperament in litigiousness. It certainly seems to me that there is here a more extraverted disposition, while in paranoia, and particularly in dementia paranoides, introversion predominates.

[3] Reich, *On Character Analysis*, 1933.

The phallic-narcissistic character denotes a prevailing attitude, comparable with other neurotic characterological attitudes, from the soil of which various pathological forms may arise. Among these forms Reich includes paranoia. "The typical phallic-narcissistic character is in his bearing self-assured, occasionally arrogant, elastic, powerful, frequently impressive. The more neurotic the inner mechanisms, the more conspicuous are these characteristics, and the greater the emphasis on their display. In physical type these characters are predominantly athletic, more rarely asthenic, and only very occasionally do they belong to Kretschmer's pyknic type. Their usual manner is never evasive, as with the passive-feminine type, but generally superior, either coldly reserved or mockingly aggressive, sometimes 'prickly'." "These people are in their daily life in the habit of anticipating any likely attack with an attack on their own part." "When their vanity is wounded, they react with either a frigid withdrawal, deep resentment, or violent aggression. Their narcissism expresses itself, in contrast to that of other character-types, not in an infantile way, but with marked self-consciousness, and an exaggerated emphasis on their superiority and worth, although in essence it is no less infantile." "It is not by chance that one finds this type most frequently represented among sportsmen, aviators, soldiers and engineers. Aggressive courage is one of its most outstanding distinguishing marks. This courage and alacrity in attack in the phallic-narcissist differs from that of the genital character, in having a compensatory element, serving the purpose of defence against opposite tendencies." "Social activity is, in relatively unneurotic representatives of this type, vigorous, impulsive, energetic, appropriate, and for the most part productive, thanks to their free aggression; the more neurotic the character, the more does his activity become wasteful and one-sided; from this point up to the development of paranoid systems there is every grade of transition."

It will have become clear that it is not easy with this type of character to determine where the influence of a possible neurotic disturbance will manifest itself, since the façade is definitely one of vigour and health, although a certain exaggeration and compulsiveness may draw attention to the insecurity which is likely to be concealed behind this self-assured bearing. According to Reich, this insecurity is connected with love-disappointments of early childhood, particularly in regard to heterosexual love-objects, as of the boy with his mother, or the girl with her father; and, moreover, love-disappointments taking place at the very height of the effort to win the object through a demonstration of the phallus.

Analysis reveals a typical identification of the total ego with the phallus, or, in the case of phallic-narcissistic women, a deep-rooted fantasy of possessing one. In men of this type, the penis exists unconsciously less in the service of love than in that of revenge against the woman, as an instrument of aggression. Such men are all the time unconsciously trying to convince women of their potency. At the same time, the sexual act represents for them a piercing and a destroying, more superficially a degrading, of the woman. In other cases, where the compensating mechanism is weakened by narcissistic sensitiveness, potency is fluctuating. The individual concerned cannot accept this, and it leads to an instability of mood. "The phallic-narcissistic character exaggerates his characteristics as a defence against regression to passive and anal reactions." "In the case of moral insanity, active homosexuality and sadism of phallic origin, and also in sublimated forms (e.g. professional sportsmen), this defence is very successful. The passive and anal homosexual forces, against which defence has been set up, are expressed only in various exaggerations. In paranoia, however, these forces break through in the form of delusions."

In litigiousness, as in paranoia, this general characterological constitution can often be observed, and in the first, the activation of this constitution seems to be determined chiefly by external circumstances, while fixation is largely brought about by efforts to compensate for inner insecurity. In paranoia, an internal conflict is probably the actual cause of the illness. Reich's exposition seems to me to have given far greater clarity to the characterological basis of paranoia, and it also brings out much more sharply the contrast between this and mild ideas of reference.

Starting from this basis of understanding, we may once again ask whether the characterological development of this neurotic conflict may be influenced by the predominance of a certain type of conscious orientation. It seems to me that the phallic-narcissistic attitude is encouraged by the predominance of certain functions, and inhibited by others. I have already pointed out the relationship between intuition and narcissism. It also became clear that a predominance of instinct tended to inhibit the development of narcissism, while feeling also in another way worked in opposition to narcissism, because of its pre-occupation with social and moral standards. An aggressive narcissistic attitude may under certain conditions also be encouraged through the primacy of thought, expressing itself here in the form of having to be always right and to secure other people's conviction of this. Under the influence of intuition and thought, this attitude may accordingly be intensified, bringing with it the possibility of development in a paranoid direction. In contrast to the obsessional neurotic character, where we found similar pre-disposing factors, there seems to be a difference in pre-disposition, in the fact that in paranoia there is greater aggressiveness. In obsessional neurosis, moreover, introversion appears, as a rule, to have a greater influence, and polarity to intensify awareness of internal opposites. Paranoia seems to me to have, in general, a simpler psychological basis, which at the same time renders easier a regression to the primitive mechanisms of schizophrenia. This further regression is, in my opinion, reinforced by marked introversion, as I shall establish in Chapter IV.

Masochism and Conscious Orientation

In the literature of psycho-analysis, a certain neurotic characterological development has been described as the masochistic character, and we will now investigate its relationship with conscious orientation. The most remarkable thing in individuals of this character is that they seem to seek suffering and humiliation and to find a certain satisfaction in complaining. In this they are the opposite of the phallic-narcissistic character, where sadistic traits are frequently seen. While, in the latter character-type, it is often doubtful whether these people should be described as neurotic, the neurotic attitude of the masochist is usually fairly obvious.

Reich has probably given the fullest analysis of this type of neurotic character. In his conception he sees the following as typical masochistic character-traits: "Subjectively a chronic feeling of suffering which manifests itself, when it finds objective expression, as a tendency to complain; further characteristics are chronic tendencies to self-injury and self-humiliation, and an intense need to torment others, which causes the subject no less suffering than his object. Common to all masochistic characters is a peculiar kind of awkward ataxic attitude both in their behaviour and their intercourse with others, which in some cases almost amounts to a kind of pseudo-dementia." These people constantly demonstrate how awkward and maladjusted they are, and have an extraordinary gift for provoking others to take up a severe or reprimanding attitude to them. They cannot endure praise or success.

This remarkable behaviour has been variously explained in psycho-analytic literature. Freud's original conception was that masochism is a secondary formation, in which the primary aggressive sadistic tendencies are inhibited in their expression, because of fear of punishment and loss of love, and are turned against the self. The super-ego becomes the punisher and manifests itself in feelings of guilt. This conception, which provides in many respects an explanation of the manifestations in obsessional neurosis and melancholia, proves to be less appropriate for masochism. One scarcely ever finds self-punishment here, and the efforts at self-injury are so immediate that Freud has been compelled to assume here an instinct for self-destruction, a "death instinct". Reich opposes this conception, and in my opinion he is right in this. He shows that the masochist is in the last resort striving for pleasure, just as everyone else is. The difference is, that this striving, under the influence of an intense sensitiveness and certain childhood experiences has taken a peculiar form. The moment some pleasure arouses mental tension, painful, internal excitement and anxiety are produced, and a defence against these feelings is raised by means of typical masochistic behaviour. Any pleasure produces a feeling of insecurity, as if there must be something bad in it, and consequently, fear of punishment and rejection is stimulated. Security is then sought through unhappiness and inferiority, as a way of evading the powers that be. The subject humiliates himself and wallows in suffering as a plea for sympathy and love, and as a way of evading any possible punishment. There is, above all, great fear of being left alone, and the masochist provokes with his torments the very person whose love he desires. His complaining represents a disguised claim for love, and his provocative behaviour is a furious attempt to force love. The whole behaviour of the masochist represents an unsuccessful attempt to rid himself of his inner state of excitement and his susceptibility to anxiety, both of which are constantly at high tension. But since it is the beloved person who is tormented, guilt-feelings and anxiety are intensified. Masochists make their claims of love in this disguised way, because they are constantly in fear of disappointment or rejection. In their compulsion to suffer, there is a veiled aggression of which they are not themselves aware.

In many respects, the masochist is the opposite of the phallic-narcissistic character. In the latter case, the mode of dealing with disappointments is determined by a strongly aggressive trend, while in the former case, there is a great sensitiveness. At the same time, external circumstances will also have an effect on the development of these reactive forms. As far as type is concerned, it seems to me that masochistic attitudes may be developed in individuals of any type, but that only in certain cases do they perpetually dominate the whole character. In marked cases that I have seen, introversion, instinct and feeling were the most important factors in mental orientation. The masochist, by means of a demonstration of his suffering, seeks to escape from his isolating introversion. He alienates people, however, so that his intention does not succeed. The influence of introverted instinct strengthens his passive readiness to wallow in sufferings and unpleasant sensations. The hypochondriacal character, which is related to the masochistic, concentrates on these experiences, while the masochistic character makes use of them to establish a certain emotional attitude and a particular kind of relationship with his environment. In this exaggerated representation of a certain fixated emotional experience, there is a connection between the masochistic character and hysteria. It will probably be possible to distinguish two types of this character, according to whether instinct or feeling predominates. Common to both is the over-weening significance of suffering in any emotional situation, and the fact that the patient concentrates on this in such a way that the result he aims at—the re-establishment of an emotional relationship—fails to be achieved. In the case of the hysterical character, his reactions are in similar situations more under the influence of his relationship with others, and thus his object of influencing them thereby is much more often attained than is the case with the masochist, pre-occupied with his own sufferings. Passive subjection to personal experiences is intensified by introverted sensation and by introverted feeling.

Hypochondria and Conscious Orientation

The hypochondriacal reaction is related to that of conversion-hysteria and to that of neurasthenia. In conversion-hysteria, certain organs and functions express unconscious emotions. This mechanism may be induced or reinforced by incidental bodily ailments (physiological synergism). The organ concerned is, in Freud's phrase, invested (cathected) with libido. Both in physical illness and in hypochondria, the state of the subject's own body is the focal point of interest. On falling ill, the patient withdraws his interest from the external world, and his feelings are concentrated in a narcissistic manner on his own body. To the hysterical patient this, in fact, signifies some emotional relationship which is in fantasy connected with this physical expression. The state of affairs in hypochondria, as in bodily illness, is simpler, because here it is actually the body that is the real centre of interest. Freud sees here a general heaping up of narcissistic libido. In hypochondria, the physical condition is rather the precipitating factor, while the real causes lie in external circumstances and in the mental organization.

In the hypochondriacal reaction, the influence of external circumstances is seen in an emotional withdrawal, under the pressure of difficulties, from the external world. As a rule, there will be found in such a case a basis of inadequate capacity for social contact and excessive (narcissistic) interest in the body. In the organ-neurosis, the libido, which is thus concentrated on the body, expresses itself in the abnormal functioning of certain organs, which in these people are more sensitive than in normal individuals. In asthma and in the intestinal neuroses, this kind of sensitivity is frequently a familiar characteristic. While in conversion-hysteria, symbolism and factors in the development of the personality play an important part, here the relationship between complex and symptom is determined rather by heredity. Mental problems provide merely the energy for the production of illness, but do not determine its form. If the mental situation is altered by external circumstances, or even by being dealt with more adequately from the psychological point of view, the symptoms in these cases will also disappear. The same result may also be achieved in another way, if it is possible to reduce the sensitivity of the organ concerned.

In hypochondria, we get a kind of generalization of all the organ-neuroses. The mental attitude is the same in both cases. This attitude is seen more clearly in chronic hypochondriacal conditions. It may gradually dominate the whole character, until it produces the hypochondriacal character. The latter is marked not only by apprehension and concentration on bodily manifestations, but also by functional disturbances and by a withdrawal of interest from the external world.

When such a characterological change is evolved from an organ-neurosis or from a hypochondriacal state, one may assume the presence of some susceptibility which is particularly liable to reinforce these particular mechanisms. Here again I should like to express an hypothesis concerning the nature of this susceptibility, although I shall have to leave the final solution of the problem to the clinicians and their findings. In some cases, I found an intensification of hypochondriacal characteristics in introverted persons of pronounced instinctive type. It is indeed understandable that an individual of this type, being in any case more intent on his physical experiences, will more readily become fixated on them under the influence of an organ-neurosis or of chronic physical illness. It may be very important for the physician to recognize this danger betimes in individuals of this type, since their attitude may occasionally be modifiable at an early stage, while, once the hypochondriacal attitude is fully developed, the patient is no longer accessible to psychological influence.

In contrast to the masochistic character, feeling seems to me to play no great part in these cases, which makes it considerably more difficult to prevent withdrawal from the external world.

Summary

I think I have now given an outline, from the psychiatric point of view, of the problem of the inter-action between neurotic mechanisms and the structure of conscious orientation. I am far from thinking that I have represented exhaustively the wealth of material that lies to hand here. Neurotic mechanisms are classified clinically according to their outward manifestations, and, since the advent of psycho-analysis, more and more according to their inner development; but this classification is a fairly rough one, even though it is of great practical use in the identification of types. The more exact descriptions of mental mechanisms, which psycho-analysis is rendering ever more possible, will no doubt enable us to recognize still fresh clinical forms. In practice, neurotic forms are generally seen in combination, and their manifestations are named in the light of the most outstanding symptoms. These manifestations are often seen in close proximity to what are actually expressions of the character, and it is necessary to be a little careful in diagnosing the various forms of neurotic character. Only when the character is dominated to a very high degree by hysterical or obsessional neurotic structures is the conception of the hysterical or the obsessional neurotic character appropriate. Moreover, such cases can never furnish a basis for the characterological understanding, or the characterological classification, of normal persons. Although there are cases in which the totality of the personality-structure is dominated by isolated mental mechanisms, so that in describing the personality only the latter have to be taken into account, nevertheless, in the normal individual, isolated mechanisms, naturally found here as well, can never be added together to explain the structure of the whole personality. And although it is impossible to understand the neurotic character without knowledge of its mental mechanisms, yet it is essential, even in these cases, to take into account the typical structures of conscious orientation, in order to attain a right understanding of pathological character-development.

CHAPTER III

CONSCIOUS ORIENTATION AND PSYCHOPATHY

PSYCHOPATHY is a general, somewhat vague field in psychiatry, where very various disturbances, neither neuroses nor psychoses, may be grouped. Certain types of psychopathy have, however, gradually received descriptive form, at first in clinical terms. It was one of the results of the stupendous task which Kraepelin set himself, of classifying all disturbances according to their manifestations, that even the psychopathies came to be described with greater clinical exactitude. The next step in scientific research consists, however, in investigating, here no less than elsewhere, the inner structure of these clinical forms, and, where possible, in establishing the sources and circumstances of their development. The attempt to do this in psychiatry for the psychopathies has been a later development than in the case of the neuroses and psychoses. Only a better differentiation of the varieties of personality-structure will enable us to appreciate the essentials in this problem.

In contrast to the neuroses, where the disorder gives the impression of being something separate from the personality, the various forms of psychopathy reveal difficulties in development and adjustment involving the whole personality. For this reason, static description of structure is of greater significance in this field than dynamic explanation from definite causes, and the investigation of hereditary characteristics, for instance, plays a more important part. In psychopaths, fixated complexes have naturally considerable influence, and blend with other factors deriving from the structure of the personality. In neurotic characters, there is indeed some influence from the personality, but in such cases, the picture is dominated by the neurotic mechanisms. In psychopaths, the main thing is the remarkable personality-structure. In practice, there are thus transitional forms, where it is impossible to determine whether a character shall be classified as neurotic or psychopathic. At the same time, there are many other cases where this differentiation is appropriate and of assistance in clarifying the structure and the causes of the disorder and in determining the indications for treatment. The treatment of neurotically fixated disturbances may under certain conditions be extremely important, even in the cases of psychopaths, but if they are considered only from this point of view, the claims of the personality-structure may be overlooked, and in these cases it is frequently this very structure which calls for very definite measures. In addition to cases in which neurosis is present in the absence of abnormal character-structure, and others where the inter-action between neurosis and character-type has produced a neurotic character, there is a third type of case where the picture is dominated not by neurotic features, but by the psychopathic character-structure.

How can one define what is abnormal in personality? In clinical description there are often two criteria of a practical kind, namely, whether the individual concerned suffers or causes suffering to others, as a result of his make-up, or whether this latter interferes with his satisfactory adjustment to the community. Science, however, looks farther for more objective concepts, and these are found in a clearer description of structure. In this search I associate myself with many others, such as Gruhle, Kurt Schneider, Kahn, Schultz, Carp, Kretschmer, Ewald and Jung. In doing this, I recognize the possibility of understanding such structure from various points of view. In addition to bodily structure and temperamental differences, it seems to me that in this question the type of conscious orientation may be of paramount importance. Looked at from this point of view, many psychopathic types appear like caricatures of the normal types described in the first part of this book. In practice, the description of these types is frequently complicated by the fact of their manifesting in addition certain neurotic characteristics.

In this chapter I shall try to show how certain psychopathic structures are evolved from one-sided structures in conscious orientation, as I have seen it happen with ever-increasing clarity in my practice. In the course of the devèlopment of these views of mine, I realized with satisfaction that my differentiations agreed in important points with the descriptions of other investigators, particularly Kahn,[1] Kurt Schneider,[2] and Carp.[3] Although it will not be possible for me to consider, within the limited space of this chapter, all the other classifications and interpretations, I shall nevertheless try to indicate some important points of agreement with other investigators. It is not my intention to give here more

[1] Kahn, " Die psychopathischen Persönlichkeiten ", *Handbuch der Geisteskrankheiten*, Bd. v., 1928. (No English translation.)

[2] Kurt Schneider, *Die psychopathischen Persönlichkeiten*, 3. Aufl. 1934. (No English translation.)

[3] Carp, *De Psychopathieën*, 1934. (No English translation.)

than an outline of how a consideration of the type of conscious orientation may be of use in the solution of this problem.

Before I pass on to the description of the various types, I shall call to mind a few points that I made in the chapter on complex and type. The one-sided exaggeration of a character-structure is distinguished, not only by a particular kind of mental activity, but also by the characteristic that this kind of mental orientation, and the behaviour consequent on it, are also called into play on occasions when other modes of mental activity would be more appropriate. These other modes are lacking, and this lack of certain modes of adaptation is just as much part of a one-sided development in conscious orientation as is the prevalence of one of the functions. We have seen that whenever one function is dominant, there is another more or less opposed to it, which is in consequence less able to make itself felt, while two further functions are more readily combined and so provide variations in the types. This fact is even more obvious in the case of psychopaths, so that here also certain variations may be explained in this way; for example, the complications which frequently render the character of psychopaths so difficult to understand, such as a paradoxical giftedness in one direction and stupidity in another. The relationship between genius and psychopathy becomes much more comprehensible. With the help of this point of view, it will be possible to get a clearer understanding in regard to the structure of many abnormal characters.

Psychopaths of the Extraverted Instinctive Type

Instinctive orientation is the oldest and most fundamental of the forms of adaptation, and an individual under the one-sided direction of his instinctive function gives an impression rather of something animal and primitive, than abnormal. Very marked extraversion may, however, produce manifestations indicating clearly that there is in certain directions some disturbance in adaptation. Where such extreme extraversion is present, we shall thus expect to find a type of individual who is to a high degree controlled by his instinctual needs, and in consequence reacts primarily to environmental stimuli and circumstances. It is not difficult to find this type among the psychopaths. They are the people who react immediately to any kind of stimulus in the realm of sensuality, manifesting at the same time an alacrity in activity and emotion, which are, however, not lasting, and are easily diverted by other reactions. These psychopaths have been described (first of all by Ziehen) under the name of "Hyperthymics". Kurt

Schneider says of them: "Hyperthymic personalities are cheerful people; not uncommonly they are kindly, industrious, full of outward activity, and possessed of an imperturbable optimism which cannot be shaken by any experience. Closely connected with this characteristic is their frequent lack of depth and thoroughness, and they are usually uncritical, incautious, self-assured, easily deflected and not very reliable." He quotes Kant, who writes concerning the "cheerful temperament of the sanguine man": "He is a good companion, full of jest, and high spirits, unwilling to attach great importance to anything (*vive la bagatelle*) and friends with all men. He is usually not a bad fellow, but a sinner difficult to redeem, very repentant, it is true, but with a repentance that is soon forgotten and never becomes a real grief. Serious business soon wearies him, yet he is constantly busy in play."

As has been said, the abnormality in these characters lies chiefly in their exaggerated extraversion, and there are certain hyperthymics in whom this peculiarity is very obvious. They may be called people without stability. Kurt Schneider speaks of unstable hyperthymics, since instability is also found in other psychopaths and in some neurotic characters. It seems to me, however, that a lack of any stability in life is particularly striking in instinctive people of one-sided development, with very marked extraversion. They are very easily swept along by their environment, and since they are specifically sensitive to simple stimuli, they are easily attracted by people who enjoy life in a simple way. These psychopaths are often good-natured people who are readily led into excess and dishonesty. Temperamental factors no doubt also play a part in their character, but it does not seem to me possible to explain the whole structure by them. Kahn and Carp stress the temperamental factor, but this point of view overlooks the fact that in these people temperament is particularly in evidence, for the very reason that their general mental structure reinforces rather than inhibits its influence.

In accordance with supplementary complications, hyperthymics are classified into various sub-groups. Kurt Schneider speaks of "excited, contentious, unstable, and pseudological hyperthymics". Kahn divides them into: lively, excitable, explosive, irritable, contentious, and gay. These sub-divisions are comprehensible and of considerable practical use. But for a theoretical understanding, explanation from temperament alone is insufficient. The content of the affects, revealed in these cases with great frankness, is often primarily determined by complexes, that is to say, by emphases in the instinctual disposition and by impressions fixated in childhood.

Most of the qualities mentioned by Kahn would probably have to be explained as the product of neurotic features, whose origin may frequently be discovered in the individual clinical history.[1] In somewhat more complicated characters, it is possible to see a further effect of type in the part played to a minor degree by a subsidiary function. In psychopaths, this function will, however, have a less compensatory effect on the limited instinctual orientation of the subject. If the function of thought is developed to some extent, it may be evident in a certain calculation in regard to the gratification of instinctual needs, but also in a lack of response to feeling-relationships. In other cases, feeling may be related in its simpler forms to instinctual needs, and when this is so, there is usually little development in the function of thought. Thus in this group we get stupid, intensely impulsive natures, given to violent outbreaks of emotion. Another variation is provided by the effect of polarity derived from intuition. This may find expression in a certain longing for adventure, in wit, superstition and restlessness, and also in a tendency towards boastfulness and lying. Kurt Schneider probably has this type in mind in his description of the pseudo-logical hyperthymic.

Various combinations of hyperthymic characters with other psychopathic manifestations have been described. Some of them are explicable by reference to the type of conscious orientation. For instance, the connection between this type of character and alcoholism is explained by the desire for stimulation and sociability. In primitive forms of this type, there may easily be a combination with feeble-mindedness, since this instinctive type of conscious orientation is not essentially complicated. The connection between the combative type of individual and litigious persons seems to me to rest only on a superficial resemblance between their modes of expression, for there is great difference in character. In the former, there is not the persistence nor the sourness of the latter. The combative individual can much more readily be distracted, although he may occasionally, under the influence of strong emotion, develop an enormous energy.

Psychopaths of the Introverted Instinctive Type

The same is true for this type of psychopath as for the instinctive extravert: the predominance of instinct produces somewhat primitive forms, what is abnormal being primarily the consequence

[1] Carp also provides a description of much more concrete groups, which do not always bring out the essential factors in causation.

of marked introversion. Where the exclusive predominance of instinctual orientation is very marked, sensory impressions and instinctual needs are felt to be the only reality, and, as a result of intense introversion, we find that less significance is attached to the facts of the world than to the subject's own state. Psychopaths of this type thus react less to external circumstances than to their internal impulses. They are slower and less flexible than the hyperthymics, but resemble these in being strongly earthbound. This characteristic manifests itself in these cases in a great need for special external circumstances and for a special milieu. They are unhappy if their environment does not exactly correspond with their demands, and they show a tendency to dig themselves into it. If they are not successful in this, they find themselves driven hither and thither, and may become tramps and vagabonds. The influence of instinct is manifested also in sudden impulsive cravings for movement, for sexual activities, alcohol, brawls or similar expressions of instinctual drives. In instinctive introverts, these impulses may arise more or less suddenly, in lives that are otherwise simple and retiring. In most cases, however, defence against unexpected changes, likely to threaten their quiet equilibrium, is the most characteristic feature. Differences in temperament are also likely to be important here. Temperament is less in evidence than in the instinctive extraverts, but it would be a mistake on this account to deny the existence of temperament in introverts. The intensity of their impulses may, however, be concealed behind a certain anxiousness and timidity. Differences in temperament give rise here to great differences in behaviour, but we have to be careful not to be deceived by what is a mask. Among these people there are those whose phlegmatic and apathetic attitude is only apparent, as well as genuinely phlegmatic, apathetic and spineless psychopaths. If work can be found for such people, which interests them and gives them pleasure, they may, in an environment which has to some extent been adjusted to their needs, become capable of sustained activity which otherwise, from their behaviour, might have seemed unlikely. Other individuals belonging to this type are anxious, shy, dejected, melancholy and moody. Common to them all is the fact that their mood is dependent on the relationship between their external circumstances and their instinctual wishes. In general, one would say that they react, rather than act, thus giving a somewhat passive impression. They surround themselves with a kind of passive resistance, and are, accordingly, not easy to arouse from their introversion. If one does succeed in establishing a relationship with them, the peculiarity of the instinctive type is evident in that they are less fixed in a pre-conceived attitude. Hence a certain friendliness is often concealed behind their stand-offishness. But where introversion is marked, the reserved, misanthropic elements in their personalities ultimately gain the upper hand.

The various manifestations characteristic of this type may also be influenced by temperament, and thus develop different degrees of tension. Occasionally, also, neurotic traits are found in these psychopaths, which are only explicable through complexes. These give rise to transition-types showing the characteristics of those types of neurotic character in which we found a special connection with the instinctive introverted character, i.e. the hypochondriacal and masochistic characters. Other fixations in emotional development may also give a certain stamp to psychopaths of this kind. Quite frequently one finds defences in the form of a flight to nature and from people, or in a flight to a personal environment with familiar objects (collectors), or a defence by means of possessions (misers), or in certain pleasures (secret gluttony and drinking, cocaine addicts), or in an intense erotic slave-like attachment to a woman. Their physical state usually plays an important rôle in the experience of these people, and when neurotic disturbances take a physical form, there may develop a most obstinate tendency to hypochondriacal brooding. Self-feeling is in persons of this type usually not very highly developed. They quickly become uncertain as to their own worth. They do not compensate for their sense of inferiority by means of a mask, but take refuge in an attitude of indifference and rejection. If masochistic traits are present as a manifestation of neurotic mechanisms, they may easily give the character a special stamp. In impulsive psychopaths of this type, sadistic tendencies may also play a part and lead to impulsive criminal acts, particularly of an aggressive or sexual nature. It seems to me, for example, that the psychology of many sexual murders may be explained by the inter-action of sadistic fixations with this type of psychopathy.

Psychopaths of the Extraverted Intuitive Type

The predominance of intuition is more apt to give rise to a pathological one-sidedness than one-sided instinctive orientation, because it may involve the rejection of certain fundamental adjustments necessary to life. In this case, we get, not simple primitiveness, but a caricature of intuitive adaptation. In the cases we are considering now, there is, in addition, an exaggerated extraversion which intensifies one-sidedness.

The psychopath of extraverted intuitive type is characterized, in comparison with the normal individual of this type, by constantly employing his intuitions for purposes for which they are not appropriate, and by the lack of many other normal forms of orientation and adaptation. Intuition is, and particularly with extraverts, a very flexible function, permitting insight into ever fresh possibilities and associations in the surrounding world. Reaction to stimuli follows as promptly here as in the strongly extraverted instinctive type, but it is worked out in quite a different way, being determined less by sensuous needs than by certain ideas, or pictures derived from the imagination. These people are not usually subject to the dictates of advantage or of personal need, but are carried away, often at the risk of their lives, by plans for adventurous undertakings. Intuitives identify themselves with their ideas, and this enables them to exercise suggestive influence and is combined with strong self-feeling. Extraverted intuitives are always aiming at changing the world in accordance with their ideas, and in psychopaths this becomes both exaggerated and superficial, so that facts are neglected in favour of imaginative notions.

One finds these people in the psychiatric categories of those with a compulsion to assert themselves (Kurt Schneider's *Geltungsbedürftige*) or of those who over-estimate themselves (Kahn's *Ichüberwertende Typen*), but these categories do not clearly indicate their essential characteristics. Vanity is often associated with their projects, but it does not give rise to them. Also, it seems a mistake to me to group these psychopaths with the hysterical characters, as is sometimes done. Although hysteria may be associated with this form of psychopathy, it is essentially distinct from it. The hysterical patient is controlled by fantasies which are laden with feeling, and for the most part unconscious. In the case of intuitive extraverted psychopaths, conscious imagination is uppermost, and feeling comes afterwards, particularly of a narcissistic kind. There are, indeed, transitions to the hysterical character, but at the same time there are many variations in which feeling plays little part. In pathological swindlers who succeed in arousing enthusiasm both in themselves and in others for fantastic inventions and undertakings, feeling is very little developed, but there is usually the most extraordinary intuitive power, giving rise to instantaneous sizing-up of individuals and of situations. In *pseudologia fantastica*, also, one finds a similar capacity, although neurotically fixated feelings are also a factor here. This kind of imagination is most like the play of children. In bragging, also, both in normal people and in psychopaths, imagination plays a part. Kurt Schneider distinguishes, in addition to fantastical liars and braggarts, a type which he calls eccentric *Geltungsbedürftige* (see above). He admits at the same time that there are eccentrics who do not need to make themselves felt. Their eccentricity is related to special intuitions, which in the case of extraverted intuitives are very noticeable, because they control both action and expression. Only knowledge of their complexes can, as a rule, make these comprehensible.

The simple pathological deviation from the extraverted intuitive type is seen in a flexible, nervous personality, leaping from idea to idea, and possessing a capacity for expression sufficiently persuasive to get these ideas across to others as something real. In more complicated individuals of this kind, the effect of a subsidiary function may offer further explanation of the structure of conscious orientation. We may expect to find an association with thought, particularly in men. Their adventurous spirit then finds expression in intellectual and practical fields, in the form of inventions, discoveries, scientific publications, commercial and political undertakings, all of which have in common the propagation of premature intuitions by means of intellectual arguments which do not quite meet the case. Intuitions bearing the mark of genius may with these people occur in the midst of more or less nonsensical speculations. The mixture of acuity and fanciful imagination often makes a bewildering impression on their environment. They are found to be accessible to neither facts nor arguments based on feeling, and it is even difficult to get at them through thought, since, in the main, their thinking is determined by intuitions. If feeling is associated with intuition, we get another variation in this type of psychopath. One often finds this form in women, although it is also represented in men, for example in certain artistic types, particularly in the domain of the theatre, of literature and of music. Here the spirit of adventure appears in the sphere of feeling, which is often expressed and played out with great talent, without the individual concerned feeling himself involved even to a slight degree. The feelings are employed primarily to realize certain ideas and fantasies, but this realization must not be held as binding, since otherwise the sense of freedom would be disturbed. These people live in pictures, and are extraordinarily gifted in compelling other people to adjust themselves to these pictures. When they are not—or cease to be—successful in this, they are extremely skilful in breaking off the relationship, in order, with equal skill, to enter on other relationships, in which they will be able to exert influence with their ideas. It is in the nature of these psychopaths that they must always be striving to exert influence, taking part in intrigues, without assuming any responsibility for their activities. Hence they are usually excellent actors and actresses, both in ordinary life and on the stage. The effect of their marked extraversion is that they may be content with superficial success, but their intrigues often bring about great confusion. Women of this type make use of their physical and intellectual charms more to play a part than in the search for a feeling-relationship. One-sided intuitives are after the image only; they flee as soon as it becomes too real.

A third, rarer variation, explicable from this type of conscious orientation, occurs when instinct exerts a strong influence of polarity. This gives rise to great oppositions in consciousness, which may on the one side compel a suspension of the conscious one-sidedness, but on the other hand, in the event of this not succeeding, it may lead to somewhat chaotic states. Intuition remains the main guide in life, but in this case the instinctive sphere is always interesting to some extent, and whereas with most intuitives it is neglected, to the individual of this type it causes disquiet. There is something peculiar in the way in which these people interest themselves in nature or in machines, in sexuality or in nutrition. They do not have the natural attitude towards the facts involved that the instinctive man has, but must always do something special with them. Where gifted with something of genius, they may thus become discoverers or inventors, but the ordinary individuals of this type give the impression of something not very real: they play with the objects that interest them and have no proper relationship with them. This is most clearly seen in psychopaths. In the world of instinctual interests they find ever fresh possibilities, but they are carried away by other concrete images, before they have created anything real. They bring a fantastic element into ordinary things, and thus know how to give a certain charm to life, but they do not adjust well to reality, employing it as an adventurous game, and remaining outside all real relationships.

Many further peculiarities in this kind of psychopath are to be explained by reference to neurotic mechanisms. We have already seen that the predominance of intuition may intensify narcissistic tendencies, and it is understandable from this point of view that psychopaths of this type have been described as having a need to assert themselves (*Geltungsbedürftige*). One frequently finds among them intensely ego-centric personalities who have no use for anything that does not serve their own ends. They are apt to proceed recklessly with their plans, and are occasionally unable to understand why others do not immediately accept their ideas. They then accuse these others of being hostile. Here we find transitional types extending to the litigious type and to paranoid characters. When obsessional neurotic mechanisms are present, there develop on the one hand uncertainty in regard to the subject's own intuitions, but on the other hand an exaggerated and primitive use of them, which may lead to a superstitious attitude in regard to them and to chance circumstances. As a rule, these characteristics in extraverted intuitive psychopaths are inconstant and variable, but in somewhat more complicated cases, obsessional neurotic mechanisms may give rise to transitional types extending as far as the definitely obsessional neurotic character. In individuals of this extraverted intuitive type, in whom feeling plays a greater part, hysterical traits may also complicate the picture. This leads both to a certain insecurity, and also to increased emotional tension in intrigue, and the living-out of fantasy. Hysterical complexes act in a more disguised way here than with the hysterical character, because the greater adaptability of this type makes it possible for them to disregard the emotional tensions involved. In a normal person of extraverted intuitive type, the opportunities and plans which he envisages permit him to avoid repressed tensions. In psychopaths of this type, intuitions tend to be superficial and inconstant, and the repressed emotional tensions of the hysterical mechanisms increase this tendency. The liking for intrigue and for co-operative arrangements is then expressed primarily under the influence of emotional complexes. There is much play-acting in order to conceal personal difficulties. Although there are transitions between this type and the hysterical character, this type of psychopath has its own typical structure. In my opinion, *pseudologia fantastica* comes under this head.

Other neurotic mechanisms may, of course, equally well occur in these psychopaths, but they are less firmly welded into the whole character. Their manifestations are likely to take on the stamp of the character, however. For instance, hypochondriacal fears will suddenly spring up with great intensity, and be elaborated in a plastic manner by the imagination, only to disappear with equal suddenness after a short period. The characteristics of these psychopaths are altogether exceedingly variable and various. It would be hardly possible to classify them according to their behaviour alone, without taking into account the type that is the basis of the superstructure.

Psychopaths of the Introverted Intuitive Type

Psychopathy arising from a one-sided exaggeration of introverted intuitive orientation, is, as a rule, less striking in its expression than is the case with extraverted intuition. If we penetrate into the inner life of these people, however—never an easy matter with intense introversion—we shall often find very remarkable and curious contents and motives. There is often an inter-action between intense introversion and an exaggerated evaluation of strange intuitions, since the latter are subjected to no correction, and the imagination encourages a further retreat from the external world.

Introverted intuition gives rise to an inner insight in the individual concerned, by means of which he comprehends certain connections in life. This insight finds approximate expression in pictures and images, and although it is held with very great conviction, it is not always easy to communicate it. If, as a result of taking the images too literally, these intuitions are extended to spheres where they do not apply, much confusion and superstition may arise. Thus alchemy was in the beginning a mixture of scientific postulates and rules for the conduct of life.[1] In the earliest scientific forms, and in many religious cults, this confusing of truths, extracted from inner and outer experience, may be encountered. This function of intuition renders possible the deepest insight into the meaning of life, and at the same time gives rise to the strangest imaginings and conceptions. In psychopaths of this type, we find many symbolic forms which have played a similar rôle in the history of mankind. They have a peculiar feeling for symbolism and are fond of employing it, usually in a somewhat obscure manner. For these people, their own intuitions have the significance of a standard. The form which they take is not, owing to the extreme degree of introversion, tested against the opinions of others, with the result that what is the product of chance is given full play. A relatively subsidiary aspect of a person or of an event, interpreted in a somewhat capricious manner, may thus result in the attachment in a very definite manner of significance to that person or to that event. This significance assumes some importance in so far as there do exist these aspects in human life, but the judgment made in these circumstances is frequently inappropriate to the objective state of affairs, because only one aspect, and that not the most important, objectively speaking, is brought forward. The extremely intro-

[1] On this point see H. Silberer, *Problems of Mysticism and Symbolism*, New York, 1917.

verted intuitive is only able with difficulty to correct these mistakes, and remains obstinately of his own opinion, even if others do not share it. In this way, crazy ideas may be developed. Side by side with occasionally startling insight, we find many conceptions of a whimsical and bizarre kind. Personal destiny is, as a rule, envisaged in much too close association with insight into the general meaning of life. Small self-seeking interests are then given absolute significance. There is a constant insistence on the relationship between individual life and cosmic happenings. Collective forms of this kind, as seen in superstitions and in cosmic systems (such as that of Theosophy), are very closely related to the mental orientation of these people.

Among the psychopaths of this group are found fantastic figures of very different kinds. In clinical descriptions they have not been included in a single group. Kahn's "queer" psychopaths, as also Kurt Schneider's "fanatical" psychopaths, probably belong mostly to this type. How far Kretschmer's "Schizoids" come under the same head, I will discuss in the next chapter. Kraepelin finds the distinguishing characteristic of the group of "queer" people in a lack of inner unity and consistency in their mental life, and Kurt Schneider has pointed out that this characterization holds good for their perversity of expression, behaviour, clothes and manner of speech, and also for the peculiarities of their thought and aims. The introverted intuitive finds expression in these ways for his inclination to value small peculiarities as symbols. The negative aspect of the description also agrees with the special character of our type. These psychopaths have a particularly poor relationship with the instinctual side of experience, with their bodies and instincts and with all practical and technical matters. Where these things are concerned, they give an impression of helplessness and ignorance. "These queer people", says Kahn, "are unbalanced in regard to their instinctual life, they never fail to manifest some signs, greater or less, of feebleness or uncertainty of instinctual impulse." "All these queer people find themselves, in regard to temperamental and instinctual make-up, in more or less direct opposition with their environment, which throws them back on themselves." He also describes their poverty in things of the heart and lack of capacity to make contacts, and a kind of "autistic thinking", peculiar to the type "which may show a varying mixture of pure logic and incomprehensible inconsequence". Kraepelin writes: "The activities and mode of life of these patients appear to be without plan, contradictory, and in part quite incomprehensible. They lack a feeling for reality and the capacity for consistent evaluation of factual relationships." "They do not guide themselves by the experience of others, but try to go their own way, occupying themselves with schemes that will get them nowhere and are quite beside the mark. Since their attack is always inappropriate and peculiar, they never have any luck and never get on."

The variety of forms in which this type is seen is partly the result of differences in temperament, but also of neurotic mechanisms and of complications in conscious orientation. The activity and tension which characterize its manifestations seem to me to be dependent on temperament. Kurt Schneider distinguishes between fighting fanatics and faint-hearted fanatics, Kahn describes active and passive types of "queer" folk. The content of the eccentricities is usually determined by complexes. Narcissism, which is particularly related to intuition, and is, moreover, encouraged by introversion, plays an enormous part in many of these people. It is often associated with mental contents, as in the case of pseudo-prophets, would-be world reformers, and sectarians. These people usually manage to impress a group of supporters of similar type. They are convinced that they possess special magical powers and are in touch with spiritual forces. In artistic or social fields, also, these psychopaths over-estimate their abilities, but they frequently create an impression, by attributing colossal significance to all the small peculiarities of their lives. Their love-relationships are not infrequently affected by their narcissism. In addition, other kinds of fixations, such as father- or mother-fixations, or perversions (here often manifested in fantastic, symbolic, more or less disguised forms), may, as in other types, come to expression. Consistency is never a strong point with intuitives, and the most glaring oppositions are frequently found side by side: the man who regards himself as a saint may commit dishonest and immoral acts without feeling the slightest disturbance in himself about it.

There are transitional types in the direction of the paranoid character, which may, where introversion is marked, resemble cases of dementia paranoides. Here the type of conscious orientation is complicated by typical mechanisms. How far there may be an unbroken transition to schizophrenia, I will discuss in the following chapter. When obsessional neurotic mechanisms are present, they may have an effect on the character of this kind of psychopath. Compulsive acts and ceremonies will then, under the influence of introversion, take on very remarkable forms. Here, also, there are transitional types where it is impossible to decide which factor is the stronger in producing the manifestations, the character-structure or the mental mechanism. Hysterical traits seem to me rarely to play an important part in these psychopaths. One is more likely to find evidence of hypochondriacal mechanisms in the character. In contrast to the hypochondriacal character proper, these mechanisms are often bound up in a fantastic manner with intellectual ideas.

More complicated forms of this type of psychopath may be rendered more comprehensible by recognizing the effect of a subsidiary function in conscious orientation. Where this function is thought, we get more or less systematically constructed theories and systems, deriving from certain spiritual conceptions. Thought stands in the service of certain intuitions. These people are less influenced by criticism than are thinking-introverts, because errors in logic are less important in their eyes. The main thing for them is to explain everything, human and inanimate, by means of some visionary conception of the essence of being, and with psychopaths great significance may be attached to incidental factors in the way things are explained, and in the images used. One or two ideas of some significance are then swamped in waves of fantastic systematization. In psychopaths of genius belonging to this type, it may be a matter of great difficulty to distinguish the essential from the inessential in their thought. If in introverted intuitives of very one-sided orientation feeling does gain any influence, it is dominated by the customary attitude. Feeling will not be directed towards the concrete personality of the other person, but towards the idea for which he stands. Relationships with other people are indeed of considerable importance in the life of these intuitives, but they are not quite real: a kind of symbolic play is made of them.[1] Concrete things appear as images, which may reveal a secret meaning. These people may live in a world of poetic dreams. Intuition renders their feelings inconstant and inconsistent. The same people will appear on different occasions in very different form. Sudden convictions may take complete possession of them, both as concerns their relationships with others and their experience of their own mental life.

The polar function may also exert some influence on the structure of these psychopaths. Imagination is then directed on the instinctive sphere, which is then not simply taken in its material aspect, but has special intents and associations superimposed upon it. These "back-to-nature" people [2] do not simply live with nature, but are compelled to express their relationship with her by means of ideas

[1] Oscar Wilde's *Picture of Dorian Gray* may serve as an instance.
[2] For example, Jean-Jacques Rousseau.

and symbols. "The 'back-to-nature' representative explains himself by going barefoot and with long hair", says Kurt Schneider. When these people turn their attention to sexuality, they are apt to make out of it a mixture of lasciviousness, asceticism and intellectual ideas and principles, whereby the whole thing is often, by their narcissism, exalted into a sphere of solemn ceremonial.

Psychopaths of the Extraverted Thinking-Type

At first glance, it is not easy to see how this type, with its entirely objective attitude, can take on a pathological form. People of this type generally regard themselves, even more than others do, as normal, and in their orientation they always attempt to take the normal as their pattern. But in their case, one-sidedness may consist not only in their measuring everything by the norms of thought, but in their one-sided extraversion, which makes them take the standards of their environment as absolute. In the psychopaths of this type, we get, in addition to an extreme one-sidedness, an absence of compensating factors. This latter is seen particularly in the absence of any influence of feeling. The general one-sidedness of extraverted thinking consists in the equal evaluation and acceptance of all forms of classification and all conceptions based on rationalization, so that life appears to consist of a vast multiplicity of facts and opinions. The starting-point has to be that which can be simply demonstrated and reckoned on. Side by side with this there is frequently found a rationalistic view of the world, sometimes simple, sometimes complicated, which in these days often appears linked up with some scientific theory. But even in this case, the forces which determine life are not altogether rational, and orientation by means of thought determines only its form and not the use which is made of it. One of the results of orientation according to thought, however, is that other modes of orientation are not considered to be worth anything, and hence are less able to make themselves felt.

If we look around for clinical descriptions of psychopaths showing these peculiarities, we find that Kurt Schneider mentions psychopaths lacking in feeling, and F. Scholz speaks of "moral anaesthesia": "The man with moral anaesthesia is perfectly aware of the laws of morality; he perceives them, but he does not feel them, and hence does not act in accordance with them." The expression "moral insanity" has come to have a special significance. The concept does not, indeed, entirely correspond with that of the psychopaths whom I am trying to describe, but anyone who, like me, regards a moral orientation as an expression of the function of feeling, will be likely to attribute a lack of this kind of orientation to extreme thinking-types. Failure to distinguish between emotional tension as an expression of temperament, and behaviour which is swayed by feeling, may frequently produce confusion here. Kahn, for instance, describes people who are deficient in feeling from the point of view of temperament. There may, however, be intense emotionalism in cases where orientation by feeling is very poorly developed. In thinking-types, this will, however, usually be concealed under the domination of reason. Kahn has also described another type deficient in feeling as active, cold-hearted egotists, driven by powerful instincts. He says of them: "Their activity and mobility on the one side, with their coldness or heartlessness on the other, bring them into an attitude towards their environment characteristic of the type—active hostility to society." It seems to me that most clinical descriptions tend to confuse neurotic traits here with the description of a character-structure. Moreover, the pure type is here less striking, since there is usually quite a good adaptation to the social sphere, whether high or low, and their heartlessness and coldly calculating egotism do not permit these people to come themselves to much suffering. Other people may, however, doubtless have to suffer as a result of the one-sided development of a character of this kind. But there are also harmless examples of the type, people with a craving for collecting and reading scientific books, who pass one examination after another without getting anywhere, and who are only happy if they are left alone with their schedules, statistics, red tape, card indexes and calculations. Such people should only be called psychopaths if this mode of orientation stands in the way of practical life, or causes disturbances in work or in family life. As a rule, this only happens as a result of neurotic factors. But the effect which these have may also be partly determined by the one-sidedness of the type.

Complexes in the form of fixed mechanisms originating under the influence of some emotional constellation may then also play a part, if conscious orientation is only slightly influenced by feeling. If this happens with people who are very one-sided in their extraverted thinking, they are often very little aware of it, but the use which they make of thought reveals this background in an indirect manner. Among emotional attitudes which (consciously or unconsciously) may employ a certain mode of thinking are the following: narcissism, a tendency to dominate and compel others, and hostility to society. Narcissistic influences are to be found in pedantic defences, which may occasionally prove to be obsessional neurotic defences against unconscious tendencies. In such cases, thought, in itself correct and taking ordinary forms, is exaggeratedly emphasized at the expense of other experiences and points of view. This produces a type of psychopath who pesters himself and his colleagues with every kind of rule and regulation. There is a continuous transition to the obsessional neurotic character, but there is no doubt that there are certain types whose structure is more one-sided than neurotic. Another type employing thought for the purpose of dominating over other people corresponds with the type of character described by Freud as anal-erotic, but does not exactly coincide with it. The concept anal-erotic covers a group of mental attitudes of which the desire to dominate is only one, and this tendency may be expressed in other forms than those characteristic of extraverted thinking. In psychopathic individuals of this kind, there is a tendency to force themselves and their whole environment into a certain mould, and to exclude from life everything that is not rational. In doing this, they exert strong pressure on their environment. Sometimes different systems are tried out one after another, or simultaneously. The real psychopaths of this kind are most conspicuous when their emotional adjustment has brought them into conflict with prevailing moral standards, in which case they regard the latter as a kind of humbug. Thought-forms are then employed in the service of the most reckless egotism. In these cases, the term "moral insanity" is frequently appropriate. A belief in personal objectivity is, moreover, expressed in the assertion that everyone is by nature the same as they are, and is prevented only by fear and convention from true self-expression. Many intelligent, cool and cunning criminals in various grades of society probably belong to this type. The influence of temperament is seen in these people in so far as it determines the inner drive of instinct and the amount of tension.

Besides temperament and mental mechanisms, complications in conscious orientation may offer explanation of more complicated forms of this kind of psychopath. If instinct plays a part as subsidiary function, thought will be noticeably directed towards the practical and the factual. If intuition plays a part, thought will be more flexible in its orientation, but at the same time more speculative. The psychopathic character of an exaggerated extraversion is revealed in the uncertainty produced in these people by the mass of opinions and points of view, so that in their nervousness they feel obliged to cling with persistence to some theory or principle. The classifications of thought seem sometimes to be more of a burden to these people than a help. Neurotic traits will also complicate the picture. If feeling, acting as the polar function, exercises a strong influence on conscious orientation, the exaggeratedly extraverted attitude will be constantly disturbed by extremely subjective feelings, and rendered uncertain thereby. These people will then talk a lot about emotional problems, but it will all be very theoretical. What is psychopathic in these thinking-types, is in fact, that they never, with all this theorizing, come into real contact with life. The individual who is affected by polarity is more aware of the fact that his feelings are starved, and he is disquieted by this. As a result, there is less one-sidedness in such a case, but more unrest and conflict.

On the whole, it may be said of markedly extraverted thinking-types that they are less likely to assume psychopathic characteristics, since the characteristics of modern culture are extremely helpful to them in enabling them to make suitable adjustment; but in their exaggerations and limitations they show up the weaker aspects of our culture.

Psychopaths of the Introverted Thinking-Type

Introverted thinking can appear more obviously pathological in its one-sidedness than extraverted thinking, because the forms it takes do not automatically correspond with the current forms. In the psychopathic deviations, we frequently find, in addition to extreme introversion, a further outstanding manifestation in the form of peculiar personal modes of thought, which are clung to with great conviction. Personal original thought-systems and conceptions are often evolved in opposition to generally current forms. As a result of their obstinate insistence on their own objectivity, these people may come to doubt the generally current forms of objectivity, judging these from the same point of view. Pedantry and hobby-horse riding may be regarded as the consequence of such an attitude. In these cases, a personal element enters into intellectual concepts, as a result of which there is a tendency to impose their own views on others. Abstract questions, of little value, are often investigated with pedantic exactitude, so that their whole way of thinking will often appear ridiculous to others. In the pathological forms of this type, we may find, in addition to one-sided positive manifestations, the lack of other normal human traits. Feeling in particular may be wanting, so that their lives appear peculiarly cold and dull. Contact with facts, and understanding of others, may likewise be very inadequate, which gives rise to a type of remote, fanatical theorist.

In the clinical description of the various psychopaths, this type is not often represented, because adjustment is usually sufficiently adequate, and there is no feeling of illness. The term "crank" would appear to be most applicable to them. Certain variations of the type may also be described as heartless or fanatical. Kahn says of the "crank" type that they tie themselves up in a train of thought, and cannot get away from an idea they once get hold of, so that for them the whole of life consists in fanatical fighting and suffering for this idea. Such a description may occasionally equally well apply to one-sided introverted intuitives. When in an introvert thought and intuition are combined, it is not always easy to decide which function predominates. There is, however, a considerable difference between the introverted intuitive, full of his one idea which came to him as a revelation, and the introverted thinker, dominated by systems and principles and endeavouring to find a foundation for the truth he has perceived. Both types may under certain circumstances be found among the "enemies of society". But, as a rule, they are too little interested in society to express any affective reaction against it. It is not possible to regard these people forthwith as egotists or ego-centrics, since their interest is focussed more or less outside themselves in systems and principles. In any clinical description of this type of psychopath, the emphasis will usually fall on their neurotic attitude, which in some way intensifies their pathological characteristics. But even here the neurotic element may in many cases be entirely subsidiary to the one-sidedness of the mental structure.

Complexes which are particularly likely to find expression through thought are the same as we found in thinking extraverts: lust for power, narcissism and hostility to society. Narcissistic influences lead to the over-valuation of personal methods and principles. Neurotic defences are here directed inwards more than outwards. Endless work is carried out on the details of thought-forms, theories and methods, with pedantic emphasis on personal forms. In this way, eccentrics are produced, pursuing their lonely ways, undisturbed by differing opinions. Their thinking tends to remain unfruitful, and lack of recognition frequently leads to an irritated, somewhat paranoid attitude to their fellow-men. This irritated attitude may in a misanthrope, under the influence of complexes, dominate the whole picture. Thought is then employed either to tie himself up in theories, or for the purpose of a reckless imposition on others, according to temperament. Temperament does, in fact, play an important rôle in this connection. The psychopath of this type is characterized by an extreme heartlessness and by a lack of contact between his own thinking and generally current principles and systems. When the hostility to society is expressed in crime, then we get the type of criminal who is secretive and makes long and careful preparation, to whom his crime has become, so to speak, a principle. If thought is employed primarily as an expression of domination, it produces in its simple, one-sided forms a type of dogmatic pedant, always ready with an exact argument, insisting that everything must be seen as he sees it. As a result, there are constant conflicts with colleagues and superiors, and the family also lives under an intolerable tension. Since affective contacts are not acknowledged, all relationships are determined from the point of view of thought. An unbroken transition is found between this type and the obsessional neurotic character. In other cases, there may be a transition to the paranoid character, in which case mistrust is the prevailing attitude.

Complications in conscious orientation give rise here also to more or less typical forms, in which the one-sidedness is to some extent modified, but at the same time takes on more precise forms. An association with the sphere of instinct leads to thought on concrete objects, criticism being directed particularly towards exactitude, and the careful application of methods. These people are often crippled in their adaptation, because they stick too much to small details. They are uncertain and pernickety in their relationship to the external world, and try to compensate for this uncertainty by systematic preparation. As a result, they have no energy or interest left for more important problems. Where intuition has been developed as the subsidiary function, thought is, in introverts, directed more on to spiritual problems. This kind of brooder shows some correspondence with the one-sided forms of the introverted intuitive type. Abstractions, defended with fanaticism, suppress all other interests. Such people become ever less fit for the ordinary relationships of human life. Where feeling, as the polar function, exerts some influence, thought will be directed on to mental and moral problems. Attempts to bring order by means of thought into the feelings do not always succeed, and here also we may get a caricature of what is intended. Intense primitive feelings constantly lead such people into involved relationships with others, followed up by much theorizing and speculation. The contrast between passion and the need for order according to principles may then offer a tragi-comic picture.

In these more complicated cases, pathological and valuable characteristics may exist side by side. Markedly psychopathic forms will usually also reveal obvious neurotic features.

Psychopaths of the Extraverted Feeling-Type

In these days, feeling finds less support in the forms that are in common use than does thought. Forms in which feeling finds expression are not valued much, and frequently fall into disuse. As a result of this, primitive and pathological forms come more easily to light, and when this happens in an individual of feeling-type, these forms readily gain a certain significance in the character. The feeling-extravert finds confirmation for these forms by means of a milieu in which they are generally accepted. Exaggerated attachment to such a group or to certain individuals may hinder development and adaptation, and give an impression of something pathological, in the same way as would a fixation or abnormal expressions of feeling. Extreme extraversion in itself may also have, as a consequence, that every fresh relationship is greeted in a rapturous manner, as offering an ideal outlet for feeling, whereupon deep disappointment soon follows. Such an individual revels in his emotions and is constantly at pains to rouse feelings in others. Relationships usually remain superficial and are soon broken off, so that they offer no secure foothold. Fixations or maladjusted and primitive modes of feeling, which may in addition be the source of pathological manifestations, bring us to the problem of how far these fixations are identical with neurotic fixations.

The problem of the dividing-line between neurosis and neurotic reaction may be raised in regard to every individual. Theoretically no sharp line can be drawn, since in everyone unconscious fixated attitudes are a factor in emotional life. The degree to which feeling-relationships are determined by the past varies greatly, however. In people of extraverted feeling-type, all feelings find plastic expression, those that are well adjusted, as well as those that are fixated. Fixated forms may be expressed directly or indirectly. For example, there is direct expression, when a suppressed feeling of hate breaks through in some affective reaction; or an indirect expression, when it is unintentionally revealed in the whole attitude and in small manifestations. Such direct and indirect manifestations, even when they are unconscious, are still well within the bounds of normal emotional life. When outbreaks become very frequent and violent, or when indirect expression takes incomprehensible forms in the way of inhibitions or peculiar reactions, then the bounds of the normal are overstepped. These abnormal manifestations may be regarded as neurotic, or as the expression of a psychopathic character. Wherein lies the difference? In the case of neurosis, they are felt to be in conflict with the rest of the personality, and form an independent mental structure. The patient does not, as a rule, himself understand why he has reacted in this particular way. In the hysterical character, also, the morbid manifestations remain incomprehensible, as far as their real meaning is concerned, even though an explanation for them is sought. On the other hand, exaggerated or abnormal expressions of feeling (for example, scenes) are felt by psychopaths of feeling-type as belonging to their personality. Opposition between emotional expression and the demand of ideals is less great, and demands of various kinds are not so much part of a hierarchical system. Regarded from outside, there may in certain cases be much similarity between the emotional outbursts of hysterical patients and of psychopaths of feeling-type, but the place that these manifestations take in the total personality is different in the two cases. Apart from this differentiation, the transition between the normal feeling-type and hysteria would be eliminated, which is very apt to give rise to a devaluation of the function of feeling (and of female psychology by men).

Kahn describes as one of his more complicated psychopathic types the "hysterical personality". He does not regard the hysterical manifestations as symptoms of illness, but as mental reactions, potentially active in everyone, and realized in a great number of people, provided only that the pressure from without upon the equilibrium of the total psycho-somatic organism is sufficiently strong. He states "that there exists in various psychopathic types a certain predilection for the realization of hysterical mechanisms, and indeed in those who manifest a defect in their conscience as regards health there may be a tendency to flight into illness". In my opinion, the "evasion of the demands of life" is not characteristic of true hysteria. Freud has clearly shown that this is not to be regarded as a cause, but as a secondary gain from illness. Kahn adds, it is true, that under the wide heading of hysteria there are also found personalities who "either never, or only occasionally, make use of hysterical symptoms, but who seem to be only distinguishable by the psychopathic peculiarity of their attitude in general. Since, however, they reveal in this general attitude much that is common to psychopathic personalities in whom hysterical manifestations have been grouped and observed over many years, they have kept the designation of hysterical personality." This common factor he then proceeds to find in their lack of genuineness. He quotes Jaspers: "The hysterical personality needs to appear before himself and before others as more than he is, to experience more than he is capable of experiencing", and Bumke, who calls the artless bearing of the hysterical personality, his pose. In my opinion, these attitudes belong to the hysterical character in the narrower sense, although they do not cover the most essential characteristic of hysteria, as I have already stated. In the case of the primitive, and often to some extent abnormal, emotional manifestations of the psychopathic feeling-types here referred to, this designation of lack of genuineness and of pose does not apply. It would be nearer the mark to accuse these people of a lack of unity and durability in their feelings.

I have already stated that Kurt Schneider's psychopaths who need to assert themselves (*Geltungsbedürftige*) are related to the extraverted intuitives more than to the feeling-types. Attempts to connect hysteria with peculiarities of bodily structure of an intersexual kind seem to me to be of doubtful value in the case of these psychopaths, although I should not like to deny the possibility of a connection with bodily structure. A disordered instinctual disposition is also, from Freud's point of view, not impossible, but it is somewhat too convenient as an explanation of all hysterica manifestations.

In discussing the hysterical character, we saw this as the product of an hysterical mechanism and a characterological constellation, particularly in the case of extreme extraversion of feeling. In this type of character, we thus find well-marked traits belonging to this kind of feeling-type, and we may also expect to find them in the psychopaths I am now describing. The difference is, however, that in the psychopaths, neurotic mechanisms play a subordinate rôle, while simple and exaggerated expressions of feeling dominate the abnormal mental structure. Kahn mentions fantasy, untruthfulness and lying as the protective and defensive measures of the childish purposive system, and regards them as originally normal and natural manifestations, which under the influence of the community, and as a result of education, have been gradually given up. Not only these infantilisms but others also belong here, such as exuberance, affectation, coyness, exaggerated piety, playing with ideas of suicide and illness, etc. I have already repeatedly referred to the exaggerated significance of fantasy in the orientation of feeling-types. The tendency to establish relationships full of feeling is more important here than an actual need to make themselves felt. The latter occurs more frequently in true hysteria (but also in other neuroses) as a compensation for insecurity, arising there from condemned and repressed wishes. The insecurity which impels the psychopaths to superficial and fantastic expressions of emotion arises rather from repeated disappointment, and usually soon reappears in fresh guise.

Psychopaths of extraverted feeling-type are thus characterized by vigorous, lively and flexible expression of feeling, reacting exaggeratedly to every situation. Both the way in which they are carried away by emotional storms, and their exaggerated attachment to loved objects, may give an impression of something pathological. Variations of the type are determined by differences in temperament, by various complexes, and by complications in the type of conscious orientation.

When temperament gives rise to acute tensions, the result is a primitive type, dramatically expressive, found chiefly among women. Where tension is less, feelings are expressed in a more passive form, and people of this kind seek to ingratiate themselves or to create an impression in a childish manner.

Complexes and neurotic traits give rise to very various emotional attitudes, which in the case of psychopaths find very one-sided and exaggerated expression. The kind of complex is not the prime factor here, and sometimes various fixated attitudes dominate the picture in turn. But often certain manifestations predominate. For example, as a very early fixation, we find a tendency to cling to some mother- or father-figure, so as to be taken care of, in which case helplessness and a using of despair and complaints to keep a hold on this person are important factors. A contrast to this form is offered by an attitude of paternal or maternal domination in people who want to tyrannize over others with their love. Yet another type is the misunderstood woman, always the loser, always ill-treated, for ever demanding compensations. Relationships with others usually assume a passionate character with this type of psychopath, so that both attachment and jealousy and misunderstandings are expressed with dramatic violence. Such people may powerfully attract others by their sincerity and the strength of their feelings, but they may also cause confusion and anxiety. Occasionally, perversions are found side by side with normal sexuality, but these arise less from strongly fixated or accentuated sensuality than from a striving after attachment, or as an expression of disappointment and the search for oblivion. In some cases, this attitude of seeking oblivion and ruin may dominate the whole life and lead to degeneration and crime. In this way, we get, for example, the development of the "interesting" type of ne'er-do-well or prostitute, as described in novels. In comparison with the hysterical character, the fixation of attitudes of this kind is determined less from the unconscious than from a habit of letting go and a lack of other forms of adaptation. In these cases, moreover, these uncontrolled attitudes, and the tendency to give themselves up to their feelings, are usually found to have been present from an early age.

If markedly hysterical structures are present, the transition to the hysterical character may be unbroken. Hence it is possible for a psychopathic character, under the influence of certain experiences, to become more and more hysterical. There is yet another connection with the masochistic character. With the predominating tendency in these psychopaths to give expression to their feelings and to work on others, one may expect to find in them a peculiar talent for getting themselves humiliated and injured by others, in order to raise continual complaint as a consequence. Sadistic traits are a less constant constituent in these characters, although strong aggression may break through in their affective outbursts. It is possible, of course, to find every other kind of neurotic structure in these cases, which may in certain situations come to very striking expression as a result of their capacity for plastic expression; such as, for example, paranoid or hypochondriacal attitudes. These are, however, not so easily maintained as permanent expressions of the character.

When a subsidiary function exerts influence on the conscious orientation, somewhat more complicated forms arise. Combination with instinct gives rise to a more hardy, strongly emotional, sensual form, in which the instinctual orientation gives to the feelings a practical and solid foundation, but may also be the cause of powerful attachment and violence. Intuition as subsidiary function gives to the feelings, on the other hand, something adventurous, a charming unreliability, an enchanting and irritating frivolity. People of this type rush into every kind of relationship and take nothing seriously. The difference between them and extraverted intuitives with feeling as subsidiary function consists in the greater reality of their relationships with others, which are less dramatized. Although feelings in these cases rarely come to maturity, they are at least genuine, and may indeed carry the subject hither and thither, both in joy and in suffering. Fantasy provides here an element likely to lead astray. When thought, as the polar function, helps to determine conscious orientation, the effect produced by emotion is less convincing, because reflections and calculations step in the way. Opinions and principles are, it is true, supported to a very great extent by emotional attitudes, but these are less adequately expressed. Hence it is not uncommonly the fate of these people not to be taken seriously, and occasionally to irritate others. Because, as feeling-types, they seek relationship with others, they are constantly striving to attain agreement with others in matters of theory and principle, and the disappointments which they suffer are apt to make them quarrelsome.

Psychopaths of Introverted Feeling-Type

Introverted feeling-types develop structurally pathological forms by their exaggerated introversion and by the one-sided predominance of infantile or primitive unadapted reactions. It is not easy with people of this type to decide how far pathological elements play a part, because, more than other introverts, they conceal themselves behind a mask. In simpler individuals of the type, with less capacity to develop compensations through other functions, and where tension is considerable, the one-sidedness of their orientation is more clearly revealed. Their inability to give expression to their inner ideals frequently produces a feeling of inadequacy and loneliness. Relationships with others are tried out with painful exactitude, but with his inadequate power of expression, such an individual often arouses quite different reactions from those he desired. This results in an anxious, uncertain attitude of reserve. Psychopaths of this type reveal their sensitivity in much the same way as do psychopathic feeling-extraverts, in primitive and infantile behaviour. But in these cases, corresponding to their introverted attitude, there is more emphasis on defence and indirect influence. Sulking is a typical example of such an indirectly expressed intention. Defence is seen, for example, in aggressive behaviour when feelings are touched. While in healthy people of this type there is often great inner security, psychopaths of this kind find less support in their ideals, because these are often mainly expressed in the negative form of criticism and condemnation. They suffer not only with their own moral problems, but because of the moral insufficiency of the world and the lovelessness and cruelty of other people.

If we search in clinical descriptions for types corresponding to this general sketch, we find points of agreement with Kurt Schneider's "psychopaths lacking in self-confidence", with the "sensitive psychopaths" and also with the "anxious" and "sad" people described by Kahn. Included by Kurt Schneider under the psychopaths lacking in self-confidence are the "sensitives lacking in self-confidence" and the self-styled outcasts (*Anankasten*). The latter types, dominated by compulsion, belong, in my opinion, to the obsessional neurotic characters, whereas the former seem to me to be in the main conditioned by character-structure. In his description, Kurt Schneider agrees with Kretschmer, who finds the distinguishing mark of these people in their "conscious retention of strongly affective groups of ideas, with lively intrapsychic activity, and deficient capacity for performance"; which means that their capacity for receiving impressions from every kind of experience is intensified, but they are unable to discharge these, and their mode of coping with them is entirely directed against themselves. These sensitives always look first for the fault in themselves. They are ambitious in the ethical sphere, and conflicts in regard to the ethics of sexuality are frequent with them. The opposition between strict standards and unbridled desire is usually played out in fantasy. I have in an earlier chapter written about one mode of dealing with this problem, described by Kretschmer in patients with mild ideas of reference. Kurt Schneider points out the important part played by compensation in these people: "A correct social formality is frequently the means of concealing inner insecurity and constraint." Kahn writes about his sensitives: "Not uncommonly in these sensitive people there is over against their self-depreciation an over-compensating dramatization to themselves and to others of their susceptibility and vulnerability. 'I am so finely made that all others in comparison with me are clumsy louts; life is brutal, I am the exception'." The anxious and depressed psychopaths, described by Kahn, seem to me to be more explicable by neurotic accretions. Kahn regards them as caused by temperament, but in my opinion this is to give too wide a connotation to temperament. When he states that many of these sad people possess "an extraordinarily deep emotional responsiveness", that they are sympathetic and kind and particularly receptive to the suffering of others, and, in addition, that in self-protection they conceal this responsiveness, then it seems to me that all this exactly corresponds with the introverted feeling-type of person.

By means of this concept of the one-sided development of the introverted feeling-type, it is possible to get a more accurate grasp of the nature of this type of psychopathic character and to define it more clearly. The essence of it is the exaggerated inner preoccupation with emotional problems, i.e. with the conflict between wishes and ideals, and this introversion has as its consequence an uncertain and helpless attitude towards the world. The expression of this attitude may vary very considerably as a result of temperamental differences, of neurotic mechanisms and of complications in the type of conscious orientation.

Temperament gives rise in these cases to differences in tension, which by many investigators is expressed as the contrast between sthenic and asthenic types. A sthenic quality is seen in the fighting for ideals, whether this takes unpractical forms or whether it is carried out by means of more or less extraverted efforts. Even passive resistance takes on a more aggressive form in these cases. Asthenic types are apt to be more defenceless, and give an impression of being too delicately made for this world.

Here again the outstandingly psychopathic forms may occasionally be complicated by fixated neurotic reactions, in which case certain mechanisms are found, which on this soil have a particular influence on the character. Hysterical, masochistic and to some extent paranoid mechanisms may in this way come to have special significance. The difference between this type and the hysterical character lies in the fact that the hysterical manifestations are here merely indicated, or are variable in their appearance, and on the whole dominate the picture less. But they may complicate the manifestations, for example, by adding to the general sensitiveness and scrupulosity a peculiar resistance in sexual matters, or a strong attachment to the father or the mother. Fear of the external world is then expressed in an exaggerated prudishness, and in a propensity to self-sacrifice for the sake of an older person, as a consequence of which a certain irritability or hysterical conversion-symptoms and flight into illness cloud the picture of a delicate, over-sensitive personality. Religious scrupulosity also occurs in marked forms in these feeling-types. These manifestations are more related to obsessional neurosis, and signify rather a compulsive emphasis on ideal feelings as opposed to the demands of the instinctual life. When a masochistic attitude lays stress on suffering and to some extent causes it to be sought, we get another caricature of introverted feeling. Personal susceptibility then becomes a god to which the happiness of the self and of others is sacrificed. Anxiety concerning spiritual and bodily welfare, and insistence on the slightest disturbance in this, cause irritation in their environment. Suffering is less consistently the pivot of everything, as it is in the case of the masochistic character, and introverted feeling usually brings a moral factor into the picture. Exaggerated self-criticism tends to modify aggressiveness, so that this is expressed only indirectly in complaints and grumbling against the environment. Even in paranoid mechanisms this trait is seen, the alleged persecutions and talk being examined again and again to see if any personal fault could have given occasion for them. Many cases, described by Kretschmer as mild ideas of reference, seem to me to belong here, although this psychological development cannot in itself be explained from the type. Less severe cases, however, often show most clearly the influence of one-sided orientation by feeling. Suspicion, arising from a morbidly bad conscience, drives these people ever more deeply into their introverted brooding.

In addition to the neurotic mechanisms which render different variations of the type comprehensible, there is also the possibility here of explaining more complicated cases by their orientation through a subsidiary function. Instinct, here as elsewhere, provides feeling with a more realistic foundation, which may, however, in the case of psychopathic one-sidedness, express itself in violence and passion. Emotional problems land these people in great confusion, so that they sometimes become physically ill. They escape from emotional situations by assuming an abrupt and stand-offish manner, since these simpler psychopathic types are not able to evolve a more complicated mask. Their need for a relationship permits them to fall an easy prey to deception, since in their estrangement from the world they do not easily see through other people. One-sided introverted feeling-types, who make use of intuition as a subsidiary possibility in orientation, show greater flexibility, but also greater adherence to fantasy. The contrast between the inner world of feeling and its expression is sometimes very great here. Intuition favours the finding of indirect means of expression. This gives rise to a fictitious, diplomatic, not altogether honest attitude, which may be more or less typical of sensitive, introverted women. They seek to fulfil their ideals and intentions in regard to others without any direct exposition. In the psychopathic forms of this type, the controlling fantasies are often chaotic and confused, and influence conduct on the one hand in the direction of dissembling and shyness, and on the other by intrigues and secret adventures. As a third, rarer possibility in the way of a subsidiary function, thought may even here play a part. Scientific points of view and "absolutely objective" principles will then be brought forward to compensate for insecurity in feeling. The polar function will not easily provide a true compensation, however, and more especially not where development is psychopathically one-sided. A thought-system will be taken over wholesale, and feeling defends itself against any possible alterations, so that it serves more or less as a creed. The conscientious accuracy of introverted feeling-types makes them anxious about details, which in this case gives rise to ponderous and pedantic theorizing. These people thus give the impression of not being quite up to life. They protect their sensitiveness in wrappings of science and theory, but their emotional needs, which are for them the most important of all, are not thereby satisfied. There is something exaggeratedly careful and suspicious about them, they do not readily enter upon any relationship, and they frequently remain stuck in their deliberations.

Here, also, we find very great differences among the psychopathic forms of this type of conscious orientation. Very complicated and gifted people, and also simple, somewhat undefined natures, may, by means of the concept of this mode of orientation, be better understood. Common to them all is the underlying self-criticism, the intensive elaboration of emotional problems, and insecurity in the face of stark reality.

Some General Remarks on Psychopaths and their Treatment

A more thorough understanding of many psychopaths seems to me to be rendered possible by means of the point of view here outlined. Nevertheless, a few forms have been described in the literature on which the structure of conscious orientation can throw little light; for instance, those described by Kurt Schneider as the asthenic psychopaths. He himself adds that asthenic traits occur in widely differing types of psychopath, particularly in those who are depressed, without self-confidence and without will-power, and that it is doubtful if one is justified in distinguishing another special psychopathic type, characterized perhaps by nothing else but asthenia. He is of the opinion, however, that everyday clinical experience requires such a category, in order to include in a scientific classification nervous people showing the signs of neurasthenia and psychasthenia.

The question of physical and mental tone is certainly, in my view, connected with constitutional structure, but with the temperamental aspect of this, not with the type of conscious orientation. There is a connection, in so far as the mode of orientation may simulate, or even mask, tone. Where there is diminished tone and a more passive mode of orientation, as is found in feeling and in instinctive types, asthenia will be more obvious. Also, an important point in the estimation of tone is that, although it is to some extent dependent on constitution, it is strongly influenced by physical and mental factors. It is true that often, for the sake of convenience, this factor has been made use of to explain both characters and disorders.

The viewpoint taken by Kahn, who considers psychopathic personalities both from the temperamental and the characterological aspects (not to mention the instinctive aspect), seems to me to offer great advantages. Only, I regard it as incorrect to derive the feelings from the temperament. A somewhat deficient conception of character is the result. What he describes as instinctual influences, I have, in the case of psychopaths, described as the effects of complexes and neurotic fixations. My way of describing these influences is more complicated, because I adopt here the findings of psycho-analysis. The influence of instinct is, according to this point of view, complicated by early childhood experiences. In its main outlines, the principle of classification which I employ agrees, however, with that made use of by Kahn. Only, I prefer to classify characters in which the picture is dominated by the effects of complexes and neurotic fixations, not among the psychopaths, but as neurotic characters.

The distinction between neurotic and psychopathic characters lies, in the first place, in their different foundations. Like the neuroses, neurotic characters are originally the product of faulty mental mechanisms, one might say of bad mental habits, which have for the most part taken their particular impress in early youth. As a result, their manifestations are localized to a certain sphere. Psychopathic characters, on the other hand, are the product of a special structure, which is more or less evident in all their reactions, is occasionally found in other members of the family, and suggests a stronger hereditary influence than do the neuroses. Although the distinction is not always sharp, although inherited factors play a part in many neuroses, and although, on the other hand, most psychopaths are in their mode of life greatly influenced by circumstances, this distinction nevertheless remains of great significance, whether the subject is to be studied mainly from the dynamic, or mainly from the static, point of view.

Moreover, this distinction is extremely important for the treatment of the different disorders. Although simple, faulty mental mechanisms can occasionally be influenced by suggestion, for more complicated fixated complexes psycho-analysis is the most suitable method of treatment. In the case of neurotic characters, psycho-analysis can do quite a lot, but it seems to me important here to take the characterological structure into account, since otherwise too much will be laid to the account of the neurotic mechanisms. In psychopathic personalities, the abnormal character-structure is the main thing, and in treatment, education of the abnormal personality comes into the foregound. As a result of the development of psycho-analysis in recent times, this aspect of psychotherapy has aroused less interest. If one has in mind mainly the severe forms of psychopathy as seen in institutions, then this aspect of psychotherapy appears as a very unfruitful undertaking. But when one recognizes that there is every kind of transition between out-and-out psychopaths and normal character-types, and that an understanding of the structure of conscious orientation can help in the understanding of both kinds of manifestation, there arises a connection between the education of the normal and the treatment of the psychopath, more especially the young psychopath. Modern education is characterized by a much greater regard for the individuality of the pupil than was formerly the case. An attempt is made to develop spontaneous efforts along correct lines and to build up the guiding ideals in association with these efforts. This change of attitude has opened up new perspectives for the education of abnormal personalities. That hostility towards society which is so often found in psychopaths is probably partly founded on the poor understanding of their personalities which they have received from other people. Such a fixed emotional attitude might thus in many cases be avoided. I cannot here work out in detail how education might become more successful by taking into consideration peculiarities of mental structure, and how psychotherapy would be furthered thereby, since these practical applications lie outside the bounds of this book. There are many problems here which await more thorough treatment.

CHAPTER IV

CONSCIOUS ORIENTATION AND PSYCHOSIS

THE problem of the relationship between certain psychoses and certain character-forms has attracted the attention of many students. Lately, as a result of Kretschmer's researches on bodily structure and character, it has again become the centre of interest. Kretschmer, as is well known, took as his starting-point schizophrenia and the manic-depressive psychosis, and he discovered in large groups of normal people, as significant factors in their make-up, the same bodily and mental peculiarities that he found in these psychoses. This point of view differs from that previously adopted, since attention had hitherto been concentrated on the relationship between psychosis and smaller groups of abnormal characters, as, for instance, between paranoia and the paranoid character, and melancholia and the melancholy character. In Holland, Jelgersma [1] has stated this relationship with great clarity. Kretschmer, however, described normal people in the light of the distinctive characteristics of these psychotics. A study of his psycho-physical types suggests that we are here dealing with differences which are deep-rooted in human nature, belonging to a realm which lies far deeper than the conscious personality. This agrees with the general conception, that in the case of the psychoses, mental forms and contents break through from the depths, to break up or destroy the structure of personality. These forms and contents will therefore scarcely be explicable from peculiarities of the conscious personality. One may assume, rather, that they point to peculiarities in the deeper structure, and that this structure will also determine certain characteristics of the conscious personality. Kretschmer agrees with this, and has mentioned, in addition to physical qualities, certain mental peculiarities which point to such a structure.

It seems to me that Kretschmer with this conception points to some essential distinctions. Hence he raises for us the question as to whether any correlation can be found between the psycho-physical types as described by Kretschmer, and certain types of conscious orientation. Both modes of classification seek to

[1] G. Jelgersma, *Leerboek der Psychiatrie.* (No English translation.)

understand peculiarities of ordinary human structure, although they start from different points of view, and it would seem quite probable that they are complementary.

If Kretschmer's description of schizothymes and cyclothymes is compared with Jung's description of introverts and extraverts, points of agreement are obvious. This should not tempt us to regard the manifestations immediately as identical, for the source of the two conceptions is very different. In the case of Kretschmer, it arises from a clinical description of behaviour, while for Jung, the source is provided by differentiation of inner states based on phenomenological psychology. Kretschmer starts with the most abnormal and incomprehensible mental manifestations, while Jung turns his attention to normal people and creative personalities. Kretschmer speaks of cycloid and schizoid "temperaments". It appears doubtful to me, however, whether the forms he describes can be explained by temperament. Moreover, in that case, agreement with the Jungian types would scarcely be possible, since the latter, in my estimation, depend on a difference in conscious orientation, and conscious orientation cannot be derived from temperamental differences. If the prevalence of introversion or of extraversion is to be ascribed to temperament, this concept would have to be carried farther than I take it. I prefer to explain only the type of reaction (strong or weak, transient or persistent) by temperament, but to regard the direction and form of conscious attention as a separate factor.

The psychological foundations of Kretschmer's differentiation are not very clearly worked out. A separate consideration of the type of conscious orientation, in addition to consideration of temperamental differences, may encourage him to find a better psychological foundation for his types. The first question to arise will then be, whether for a more exact observation there exists a connection between schizothyme and the introverted type, and between cyclothyme and the extraverted type. I am only able to refer briefly to the description of Kretschmer's types, and must refer my readers to his writings [1] for a closer study of his differentiations. If, following the description given here of extraverted types, one reads Kretschmer's descriptions, one is struck by the resemblances. Cycloid people are "predominantly sociable, good-natured people, easy to get on with, fond of fun, taking life as it is. They give themselves naturally and freely, and one is soon friends with

[1] E. Kretschmer, *Physique and Character*, New York, 1915. F. Kehrer und E. Kretschmer, *Die Veranlagung zu seelischen Störungen.* (No English translation.)

them; they frequently have something gentle and warm in their temperament". Either manic or depressive characteristics are in the ascendant. The hypomanic type is gay, humorous, lively and ardent, the depressive still, quiet, serious and gentle. Both aspects are always to some extent combined: "in many hypomanics there is a little depressive component, and in most cycloid melancholics a dash of humour". "Most cycloids have a particularly good, responsive emotional attitude, manifesting all shades of transition, from the sanguine quick-silver temperament of the hypomanic to the deep and warm-hearted sensitiveness of the more melancholic natures." "The word 'heart', perhaps even more, 'good nature', expresses most nearly the factor which is common to the majority of these natures, right through their different habitual moods: a gentle, warm, kind-hearted, friendly temperament, capable of spontaneous oscillations both in joy and sorrow."

This emphasis on "the heart" in cyclothymes must to some extent surprise us, since we certainly do not immediately connect feeling and heart with extraverts. At the same time, there is in the description of cyclothymes much that will remind us of the extravert. We may therefore suppose that Kretschmer in the first place recognizes only extraverted feeling, and that in the second place he includes in the concept of "the heart", to which he attaches a somewhat vague significance, much more than I do. What he calls "the heart", I should prefer to call the responsiveness of the emotional nature. In fact, much that in extraverts goes by the name of kind-heartedness is at bottom merely a certain capacity for getting on well with people.

In Kretschmer's description we doubtless find an evaluation expressed which may be connected with his own type. He assumes without question that extraverted expression is genuine. The average cycloid individual appears to him, "especially in the quieter intermediate phases, as manifesting an equable sociability, as friendly, realistic and adaptable. Since his temperament follows the dictates of his circle, there is for him no rude contrast between himself and his environment, no rejections on grounds of principle, no rigid need to criticize according to hard-and-fast rules, no tragic working up of conflicts, but a living in, and a pre-occupation with, things; he takes his part in life, with feeling and with sympathy. There is something of a childlike naïvety in what, in hypomanics, is called their egotism, which finds its true counterpart in a frequently exaggerated pleasure in giving presents, and in the pleasure of others. This hypomanic self-feeling is no rude opposition of their own personality to a hated or indifferent world, but a case of 'live and let live', a placid enjoyment of the world and of the self, an almost comic conviction of the value and the rights of their own individuality." "An inclination towards a certain materialistic attitude, to enjoy things, to love, eat and drink, towards a simple acceptance of all the good gifts of life, is unmistakable, not only in hypomanics, but can be traced as a character-trait all through the intermediate cycloid phases, right down to that of the deepest depression." "Cycloids are not rigidly consistent, and follow no thought-out systems and schedules." "Mood is everything, reflection of no account." "Hence we find everywhere among cycloids much ardent pleasure in work, a ready and practical energy; but we do not find among their strong points that hard, purposeful energy, carrying on inflexibly right through to the end, which is characteristic of certain schizoid temperaments. High ambition is rarely found in cycloids." Asocial characteristics are extremely rare. "Their positive characteristics are in particular an inexhaustible energy and pleasure in work, temperament, a ready wit, ardour, daring, amiability, adaptability, a free unhampered mind, skill in the handling of people, a wealth of ideas, eloquence, and an astonishingly quick eye for the golden opportunity." The negative qualities are, according to Kretschmer: "a tendency to superficiality, inactivity, inconstancy, over-valuation of the self, and rashness".

If we compare the above qualities with those of the types which I have described, a few important comments may be made, which may help us in elaborating our point of view. We find with Kretschmer a somewhat idealized description of extraverted people, in which "the heart" is particularly emphasized. The mode of feeling characteristic of introverts seems to be entirely unknown to Kretschmer. The more detailed description of his extraverts shows that his "heart" is different from what I have described as "feeling". It is also noticeable that while in his description we can recognize obvious elements of extraverted instinct (for example, a materialistic attitude) and of extraverted intuition (for example, an eye for the golden opportunity, wealth of ideas), extraverted thought and feeling play scarcely any part. Anything systematic is ruled out, as far as cycloids are concerned. In extraverted thinkers, however, it is the most important factor. The attitude to morality is not dealt with in detail. These comments give rise to the supposition, which we will examine further, that Kretschmer's description of cycloids applies mainly to extraverted instinctives and intuitives. We must, however, first consider somewhat more closely his description of the schizoids.

While cyclothymes appear with Kretschmer to be idealized, the picture of schizothymes is that of a not very pleasant type of being, and one that can scarcely be regarded as healthy: "Cycloid people are simple, uncomplicated beings, whose feelings appear directly, spontaneously and undisguisedly on the surface, so that in general they are soon correctly understood by everyone. Schizoid people have both surface and depth. Ruthlessly harsh or sulkily gloomy, stingingly ironical or shy as a mollusc, touchy, withdrawn—that is the surface. Or the surface presents nothing at all; we see a person who stands before us like a question mark, we are aware of something dull, boring, and yet somehow perplexing. What are the depths behind all these masks?" According to Kretschmer, we find there, not only affective deficiency—an empty heart, a lack of soul—but also wild fantasies, leading to incomprehensible deeds. Kretschmer's description passes from here straight on to serious cases. "The products of the inner life of the schizophrenic cannot be studied in country yokels; kings and poets are just good enough for the purpose. There are schizoid people with whom one may live ten years and still not be able to say with certainty that one knows them. A shy girl, of lamb-like piety, is in service for months in the town; she is gentle and obedient to everyone. One morning the three children of the house are found murdered. The house is on fire. She is not demented; she knows all about it. She smiles uncertainly as she confesses the deed. . . . A young man fritters away his golden youth. He is so awkward and clumsy that you want to shake him. Put him on a horse and he falls off, smiling disconcertedly, somewhat ironically, but saying nothing. One day a volume of poems by him appears: the most delicate feeling for nature, and every push given him in passing by some clumsy fellow worked up into a tragedy of the inner life, in polished numbers, full of style. . . . That is what schizoid people are like. Bleuler calls it 'autism': a living within the self. It is impossible to know what they feel, sometimes they do not know themselves; or only uncertainly, three things mixed up together, and yet packed with feeling, in some supposedly mystic association; or the most intimate and the most blatant things forced together with numbers and figures in some purely personal scheme. But what they feel, whether it is a banality, a crotchet, something mean and vulgar, or a collection of fairy tales, that is nobody's business, but theirs alone."

Kretschmer adds that among schizoid types it is even more difficult than with the cycloids to separate the healthy from the diseased, character cases from psychotics. My reason for quoting him in some fullness is also to show how his psychiatric differentiation, in spite of the literary excellence of his descriptions, falls short of the mark. We find strongly introverted personalities thrown together with people showing obvious schizophrenic manifestations, the incomprehensibility of both having to serve as their common factor. One's inability to get inside the feelings of a certain person provides the characterological diagnosis. While with cyclothymes what is positive and understandable provides the link between manic-depressive psychosis and the normal type, the common characteristic, according to Kretschmer, in the external manifestations of schizophrenia and of the schizothymic individual is their incomprehensibleness. "The schizoid individual presents to us, so long as we do not possess the key, only the surface of his psyche, just as do schizophrenic psychotics." "Bleuler was the first to find the key to the inner life of the schizophrenic, and in so doing to open up the approach to an astonishing wealth of psychological knowledge, of which probably only a tiny part has so far been divulged. For the key to the inner life of the schizophrenic is at the same time the key to large tracts of normal feeling and activity." Kretschmer sees very clearly the way that must be followed here. "We can only get connected information concerning the inner life of schizoid temperaments from the self-revelations of gifted and educated schizoids, and above all from the objective psychological documents that have been bequeathed to us by schizoid and schizothymic geniuses, more especially the poets. The deeper characterology of schizoids can thus only be fully revealed to us through the detailed, careful and sympathetic analysis of individuals."

Kretschmer gives one the impression that he finds it much more difficult to get into the mind of the schizothymic individual than into that of the cyclothyme, so that he constantly compares this difficulty with that which one feels in the face of schizophrenics. I, with others, seem to find less difficulty here, which would seem to point to a difference in type. It is probable that those who themselves belong more to the schizothymic type will pick up more from indications offered by ordinary people of the type, so that ultimately they would come to understand this aspect of psychology even without the help of poets. Nietzsche is apt here, when he says: "Many souls you will never understand, unless you first invent them." For those who can more easily get into the mind of this kind of person, the gap between him and the schizophrenic must, however, seem much greater. Although one must admit that there are many resemblances between schizophrenia and the schizothymic character, yet a sympathetic understanding will reveal differences which will make us enquire whether there is not, after all, in schizophrenia a further non-characterological factor at work. This factor may be discovered in some physical disorder, as well as in a mental one. In the present state of research in this field, it must be recognized as an important possibility that a greater or smaller number of schizophrenics have fallen ill as the result of some physical process, and that this process either takes place more easily on a certain psycho-somatic soil, or may even produce mental peculiarities, otherwise found in a certain characterological pre-disposition. If this were so, the manifestations of schizophrenia would draw attention to a certain group of characterological manifestations, without being identical with them. It seems to me wiser to let this possibility of explanation take its place alongside that of the gradual development of schizophrenia from a certain psycho-somatic pre-disposition.

When we ask ourselves what mental peculiarities, usually found in schizophrenia, draw our attention in schizothymic characters, we may again follow Kretschmer. He states that the most common characteristics of the schizothymes are that they are unsociable, reserved, serious (without humour) and strange. In addition, the following are found in various combinations: over-sensitiveness, expressed in timidity, shyness, fine feeling, touchiness and nervous excitement; and a lack of sensitiveness, which shows itself in slowness, good temper, docility, indifference, dullness and stupidity. Most schizoids are over-sensitive and cold at the same time. Occasionally in the course of their lives they change over from the one group of characteristics into the other, usually from the hyper-aesthetic towards the anaesthetic. Their autism is, according to Kretschmer, frequently a symptom of over-sensitiveness, but it may be a simple heartlessness, a lack of affective resonance. "Schizoid people are either completely unsociable, or eclectically sociable within a small enclosed circle, or superficially sociable, without any deep mental *rapport* with their environment. This disinclination for social intercourse varies from the mildest anxiousness, shyness and timidity, through ironic coolness and a gloomy crotchety indifference, to a cuttingly brutal, active misanthropy." "Schizoid good temper is something fundamentally different from the corresponding characteristic in cycloids. Cycloid good temper is a good-heartedness, it has something really friendly about it, a sharing of joy and sorrow, an active goodwill or a friendly tolerance of others, whose ways are understood. The good temper of the schizoid child, however, is made up of two components: shyness and impoverished affect. It means a yielding to the wishes of the external world from indolence, mixed with a timid fear of opposing it." "An aristocratic quality in these schizoid natures is expressed even in simple people in a need for distance, an emphasis on being different from, and better than, their fellows." "The essence of this characterological tendency is their exclusiveness, a striving for inclusion in the closed circle. When they are among people like themselves, their autism extends to the group as a whole. Friendship with such schizoids is a keenly selective friendship with an individual." "It is the same thing with the love-life. There is no warm spontaneous attraction, but either ecstasy or utter frigidity. There is no looking for a pretty girl, but for 'Woman', the 'Absolute', Woman, Religion and Art in one single figure." There is a superficial sharing in the life of society without any deeper mental *rapport*; the schizoid is not absorbed in his milieu. "In the hyper-aesthetic types there is often an abrupt antithesis: me against the world; a constant overstrained self-analysis and comparison: what effect am I making? who is being unjust to me? have I compromised myself in any way? how shall I manage?" "A harsh and frigid egotism, pharisaical self-satisfaction and an over-weening, over-strained self-feeling are frequently found in all forms and degrees in schizophrenic families. But these are not the only forms in which autism is found. Another form consists in the striving after theoretical benefaction, for principles based on schemes and dogmas, for world reform, for some specially designed education for their children, frequently accompanied by a stoical disregard of personal needs. An altruistic self-sacrifice on a grand scale, especially for universal, impersonal ideals, is almost specific for certain schizoids."

I do not propose to go into greater detail concerning the variations of the schizothymic types as described by Kretschmer. It would probably be possible to find correspondences here with the various types of conscious orientation, but we are primarily concerned with the question as to how far schizothymia may be identified with introversion. As I have already remarked, it is possible to perceive in Kretschmer a certain sympathy with cyclothymes, and a tendency to criticize schizothymes rather severely. Although he cannot help but recognize the accomplishments of the schizothymes with genius, nevertheless they all appear in his description as primarily strange and abnormal people. This may in part correspond to general opinion, since people whose nature it is to adjust themselves to other people appear in general more attractive than those who are guided by inner standards of their own. There are, however, great differences in general opinion, according to the attitude of society. In North Germany or Scotland, the introverted individual is regarded as normal, while in the South of France or Austria, extraverts set the standard. In the first-named countries, a strongly extraverted person is readily considered hysterical or manic, whereas in the extraverted countries, an introvert is apt to be classed as an obsessional neurotic or a schizophrene. Even the psychiatrists are not always aware of the subjective basis of their point of view. This suggests various corrections to Kretschmer's views.

The biggest mistake seems to me to be that Kretschmer regards autism as without question a symptom of the schizoid temperament. Even if the concept of autism is to be confined to introverts,[1] the necessity for a differentiation between autistic and non-autistic introverts would still arise in the consideration of these cases. Bleuler originally described the concept of autism as dependent on two factors, detachment from reality, and a relative and absolute preponderance of the inner life.[2] Kretschmer, in his differentiation, relies primarily on the second factor. To me, however, it appears that not only external reality is meant by Bleuler in his use of the term "reality". An introvert who takes as his chief guide inner reality (for example, logic and a moral code) is not, in my opinion, to be regarded as an autist, even though in doing so he confines himself to his own experience. Also the introvert, who approaches the world from inner points of view, is not on that account to be taken as an autist. Even when the inner aspect of things preponderates, reality may still be taken seriously. I should only describe as autism that state of mind (usually introverted) in which neither internal nor external reality is taken seriously, and the imagination is entirely under the domination of fixated feelings. In this case, it is clear that autism signifies a disorder, while orientation that is exaggeratedly from the inner aspect may only be described as one-sided.

In Kretschmer's description, the effects of introversion and those of complexes are constantly confused. When, for example, he writes that the good temper of schizoids is made up of shyness and impoverished affect, of indolence in regard to the wishes of the external world, and fear of opposing them, there is expressed in this description only the defence of the feelings, only the external

[1] Which seems doubtful to me, since there are also extraverted autists, ego-centric fantasists, who will not allow the validity of reality, if it conflicts with their ideas.

[2] E. Bleuler, *Dementia Praecox*, 1911, p. 52. (No English translation.)

aspect, and from this external aspect impoverishment of affect is deduced. But behind this defence there may be concealed strong affects and subtle feelings, having a far-reaching effect on the life of the individual concerned. What Kretschmer calls "extending their autism to the group" has nothing to do with autism. There certainly are autistic communities where an idea, maintained by fixated feelings, e.g. a religious notion, temporarily holds a group of people together by means of mutual identification. If the introvert prefers a close personal relationship with a few persons to the general good cheer of a larger community, his conduct should not be invested with pathological modifications. Kretschmer seems to intend a reproach when he concludes: "The schizoid is not absorbed in his milieu." But many would consider this an advantage. Also, it does not seem right to me to represent the schizothyme simply as unsociable, quiet, reserved, serious (without humour) and strange. Many introverts are extremely sociable within a small circle, and sometimes manifest good humour. Strangeness often means that a person is not understood. To the introvert the extravert may often seem a strange fellow. The basis of strange behaviour is usually found in fixated complexes, expressing themselves indirectly and indistinctly. In autistic people, these are the cause of their queerness. Since in everyone fixated attitudes play some part, probably everyone has some incomprehensible ways, which are, however, in the case of men of the world, more easily concealed. They are not, indeed, obvious in strongly introverted people, but the latter are more likely to give the impression of concealing something.

Kretschmer's mistake in his description of schizothymic types seems to me to consist in his mixing up the morbid and the normal, as a result of not taking varieties of inner orientation sufficiently into account, and not clearly distinguishing between the effects of feeling in its normal and in its pathologically fixated forms. We found a similar vagueness in regard to the feelings in his description of cyclothymes. He lacks here the more precise insight which psycho-analysis has given us. It may be that psycho-analytical psychology has too much neglected the problem of pre-disposition in favour of fixated developmental forms, but its more exact description of fixated feelings has enabled us to raise also more precise questions concerning pre-disposition. The problems which Kretschmer has overlooked in his enquiry concerning the psychological peculiarities in the manic-depressive psychoses and in schizophrenia become, in view of this, more obvious.

Let us turn, therefore, first of all to the difficult question as to how far we can point to a definite mental mechanism as specific for mania, melancholia and for schizophrenia. The problem has been most clearly stated in psycho-analytical psychology. It is probably not yet ready for actual solution. It is, moreover, only my intention to consider the problem from the point of view of investigating the relationship between the type of conscious orientation and psychosis. In doing so, our intention is first of all to formulate the scientific problems more distinctly.

The distinguishing mark of psycho-analysis is that it sees pathological manifestations in the light of personal development, and associates them with errors which have usually been made very early in this development. The problem in the study of mental disorder is therefore particularly sought in the developmental phase, in which false mechanisms first arise. In the case of the neuroses, psycho-analysis has often succeeded in describing these early forms, and in showing how the peculiar forms of the later disorder may be explained from these early situations. This mode of study was then applied by Freud and his pupils to the psychoses as well, and an attempt was made to isolate certain mechanisms and to explain them from mistakes in the processes of development. Hence we must here go into the question as to how far a similar mode of study to that which has been laid down for the neuroses is suitable for the psychoses. We found in the case of the neuroses that with a certain pre-disposition, certain mechanisms may give rise to characterological disorders, and that they are furthered by this pre-disposition. In the case of the psychoses, both the mechanisms and the inherited pre-disposition are little known, so that here, more than with the neuroses, we are on hypothetical ground. We will confine ourselves here also to the problems of the manic-depressive psychosis and of schizophrenia.

Concerning manic-depressive states, Freud, Abraham, Radó and Helene Deutsch have more especially shed light from the analytical standpoint. Abraham first pointed out [1] that melancholia represents a mourning comparable with the reaction to the loss of the loved object. Freud subsequently went more deeply into the problem,[2] by showing how, in this mourning, the lost object is clung to, and by assuming the same thing to happen in melancholia, with the difference, that the kind of loss is here not always clearly recognizable, and that an aggressive attitude towards the lost object

[1] Abraham, "Notes on the Psycho-analytical Investigation and Treatment of Manic-depressive Insanity and Allied States", *Selected Papers*, London, 1927.

[2] Freud, "Mourning and Melancholia", 1917: *Collected Papers*, vol. iv.

is expressed in melancholia in self-reproaches. "If one listens patiently", writes Freud, "to the many and various self-accusations of the melancholiac, one cannot in the end avoid the impression that often the most violent of them are hardly at all applicable to the patient himself, but that with insignificant modifications they do fit someone else, some person whom the patient loves, has loved or ought to love." "So we get the key to the clinical picture —by perceiving that the self-reproaches are reproaches against a loved object, which have been shifted on to the patient's own ego." "The behaviour of the patients becomes now much more comprehensible. Their complaints are really 'plaints' in the legal sense of the word; it is because everything derogatory that they say of themselves at bottom relates to someone else that they are not ashamed and do not hide their heads. Moreover, they are far from evincing towards those around them the attitude of humility and submission that alone would befit such worthless persons; on the contrary, they give a great deal of trouble, perpetually taking offence and behaving as if they had been treated with great injustice." Narcissistic identification with the object is stimulated by the fact that the original choice of object has in these cases frequently been made on a narcissistic basis. (Freud refers also to the first development of the mechanism of identification, which belongs to the oral or cannibalistic phase of libido development.)

"The occasions giving rise to melancholia for the most part extend beyond the clear case of a loss by death, and include all those situations of being wounded, hurt, neglected, out of favour, or disappointed, which can import opposite feelings of love and hate into the relationship or reinforce an already existing ambivalence. This conflict of ambivalence, the origin of which lies now more in actual experience, now more in constitution, must not be neglected among the conditioning factors in melancholia." "The self-torments of melancholiacs, which are without doubt pleasurable, signify, just like the corresponding phenomenon in the obsessional neurosis, a gratification of sadistic tendencies and of hate, both of which relate to an object and in this way have both been turned round upon the self. In both disorders the sufferers usually succeed in the end in taking revenge, by the circuitous path of self-punishment, on the original objects and in tormenting them by means of the illness, having developed the latter so as to avoid the necessity of openly expressing their hostility against the loved ones." The love cathexis of the melancholic has taken the regressive form of identification, returning at the same time to ambivalence and sadism. Some years later, Freud[1] expanded his view on this problem, after he had postulated his tri-partite division of mental life into Id, Ego and Super-ego. This more complicated conception shows that in melancholia it is not so much the ego that rages against itself, as an exaggeratedly powerful super-ego that is in control of the conscious self and attacks the ego. The super-ego has in these cases a sadistic attitude, to such an extent that it may sometimes drive the ego to death. How is it, we may ask, that in melancholia the super-ego comes to have such a sadistic attitude? At first Freud explained it by the occurrence, in identification, of processes of desexualization and fusion of instinct. Later he returned to the problem,[2] to go into it more closely, and he investigated more thoroughly the aggressiveness of the super-ego and of the conscience.

At a certain stage in early childhood, the authority of the person who is responsible for the training of the child is internalized by the establishment of a super-ego, conscience representing this inner authority. The super-ego is able to torture the sinful ego with the same feelings of anxiety as this educator was, and it "lies in wait for opportunities to get it punished by the external world". The severity of the super-ego may arise from various causes. In the first place, it may simply perpetuate the severity of external authority, which it to some extent suspends and replaces. In the second place, both the sense of guilt and the condemnation of the super-ego may be intensified by an awareness of conflicts. External authority compels a material obedience, while the authority within demands submission on grounds of principle, and since the latter is scarcely ever attainable, there must always be a residual sense of guilt. "Here the denial of the impulse is not enough, for the wish remains and cannot be concealed from the super-ego." The wicked deed and the wicked intention are felt to be the same, hence a sense of guilt and a need for punishment. Conscience, it is true, is originally the cause of the denial of impulse, but later the relationship is reversed. "Every denial of impulse now becomes a dynamic source of conscience, every fresh denial intensifies its severity and intolerance", because the tension of the suppressed impulses is intensified thereby and a still stricter defence becomes necessary. Freud is here demonstrating a remarkable inner process. When wishes have to be suppressed, there may readily arise an aggressive attitude, which has then itself to be suppressed. This may happen by the child's (or the adult's) identifying himself with

[1] Freud, *The Ego and the Id*, 1923.
[2] Freud, *Civilisation and its Discontents*, 1930.

the unassailable authority, so that it becomes the super-ego. The aggressive attitude is now transferred to this authority. There it finds a safety-valve, but at the same time a sadistically inclined super-ego may become a source of inner torment. This mechanism is of universal significance in human life, but it is particularly important in melancholia.

Abraham has dealt with the question as to why this mechanism comes to have so much influence in melancholia, and in doing so has brought out more clearly the influence of a disturbance in early development as the source of illness later on.[1] He confirms the view that the object-loss in melancholia is bound up with an introjection of the beloved person. He then proceeds to investigate the characterological state of manic-depressive patients in the intermediate phases of the illness, and his ideas on this subject are of particular importance for our investigation. Abraham states that in his experience "a definite differentiation of the melancholic character from the so-called obsessional character is impracticable". "We find in our cycloid patients in the intermediate phase the same peculiarities in regard to tidiness and cleanliness, the same tendency to obstinacy and defiance alternating with abnormal submissiveness and excessive amiability, the same anomalies in the attitude to money and possessions, that are familiar to us in the psycho-analysis of the obsessional neurosis." Since there are side by side with this similarity great differences, Abraham concludes that the anal-sadistic phase, in which he seeks the point of fixation for both illnesses, must include two different phases.

In order to render what happens at the outbreak of an obsessional neurosis or of an attack of melancholia more comprehensible, Abraham takes as a starting-point the periods in the patient's life when he was symptom-free. "A remission in the case of the obsessional neurotic, or the intermediate phase in a manic-depressive, appear to be periods during which anal and sadistic impulses are successfully sublimated. If at this point the danger of the loss of the object arises, there follow violent reactions in the case of patients of both groups. The whole strength of the libidinal fixations rises up against the threat of domination by impulses which are antagonistic to the object. If the conservative tendencies —composure and control—are victorious, the conflict with the love-object will call forth compulsive mental manifestations. If, on the other hand, victory lies with those anal-sadistic tendencies which aim at the destruction and expulsion of the object, then the

[1] Abraham, "A Short History of the Development of the Libido", *Selected Papers*, London, 1927.

individual concerned falls into a state of melancholic depression." From this difference in fixation one may draw the conclusion that the relationship with the object in the earlier anal-sadistic phase is slighter than in the later phase, with which obsessional neurosis is connected. In melancholia, therefore, the break-up of the relationship with the object may easily lead to still further regressions. There may be, for instance, a further fixation at the oral-sadistic level, this being the level at which ambivalence is expressed in its earliest and particularly acute conflicts. A heavy degree of ambivalence is, according to Abraham, characteristic of the pre-disposition to melancholia. The devotion of these people is of an overwhelming and compulsive kind, and carries within itself the danger of a sudden rupture. "The effects of ambivalence in the clinical course of melancholia are still more far-reaching. After the libidinal cathexis of the object has been withdrawn, it is applied to the ego, while at the same time the object is introjected into the ego. The ego is now ruthlessly exposed to the ambivalence of the libidinal drives. Only a very superficial kind of consideration would permit us to think that the melancholic is filled with nothing but a tormenting self-contempt and an exclusive craving for self-disparagement. Attentive study teaches us that we may with equal justice say the opposite about them." "In general we may say that the melancholic carries within himself a feeling of superiority, which in the period of remission may be demonstrated for what it is." In the picture of melancholia, manifestations of positive and negative narcissism stand in abrupt and immediate juxtaposition.

Abraham sees the influence of various factors at work in the development of melancholic depression. As a constitutional factor he postulates a constitutional intensification of oral erotism, which, happening to coincide with special circumstances, may determine the fixation of libido at the oral level. Added to this there is severe damage to childish narcissism through coincident disappointments in love, usually by both mother and father, giving rise to the impression of being completely abandoned. This first great disappointment takes place before the Oedipus complex has had time to build up solid relationships in the emotional life. As a result, there is developed a susceptibility to disappointments in later life, to which the individual concerned reacts with introjection and regression.

The point of view thus evolved enables us to understand many factors in the development of melancholia, but the part played by characterological pre-disposition, and the compulsiveness of the mechanisms, do not seem to me to find quite adequate explanation.

At this point Radó [1] has tried to see farther into the problem. He finds in characters pre-disposed to depression an intensified narcissistic hunger and considerable narcissistic intolerance. It is observable that these people react to even slight injuries and disappointments with an immediate diminution of self-feeling. The ego may be entirely absorbed in them and crippled in its activities. "Moreover, these pre-disposed depressives depend for the maintenance of their self-feeling entirely on other people; they have not attained that stage of independence at which self-feeling is firmly based on personal accomplishment and criticism." Hence passive-narcissistic instinctual goals predominate in their object-relationships. In this their behaviour is peculiar. They are indefatigable in their courting of the favour of their beloved objects, and in seeking tokens of their love. "But as soon as they have become certain of the affection and devotion of someone, they accept the love-offering of the beloved person with a positively sublime matter-of-factness, becoming more and more domineering and autocratic, and letting loose an increasingly unbounded egoism, until their behaviour becomes completely tyrannical." To any counter-aggression, or to the threat of withdrawal of love, they react with embittered violence, and take the loss of the object as the greatest injustice the world has ever known. Radó points out that a melancholic reaction is usually preceded by an indignant revolt, and in the subsequent broken-heartedness he sees a reaction to the break-down of the rebellion. "The ego repents, pleads for forgiveness, and seeks in this way to regain the lost object." It is true that this is not always evident, for the struggle for forgiveness is internalized and directed towards the super-ego. A reaction from the period of the development of the super-ego is reproduced in this, in which the child, by punishing itself, seeks to regain the parents' love. Why, and for what, does the ego actually feel guilty? The melancholic usually gives open expression to this: he feels guilty, because by his aggressiveness he has himself incurred the loss of the object. Aggression against the object has now been wholly directed against the ego. The ego "can in its helplessness never get free from the hope of a saving forgiveness, it takes on the rôle of the object, takes on itself also the whole guilt of the object, and submits without struggle to all the cruelties of the super-ego. The ego has succumbed to the indestructible infantile illusion of the possibility of escape from its narcissistic distress, but by no other means than submission and expiation."

[1] Radó, "The Problem of Melancholia", *Int. Journal of Psycho-Analysis*, vol. ix., 1928.

In the inner conflict of the melancholic we find simultaneously two different identifications: on the one hand, the repentant ego assumes in part the guilt of the lost object; on the other hand, the super-ego and the object are identified as the punishing agents whose forgiveness is besought. As in the case of many other neurotic and psychotic mechanisms, we reach an understanding of this process by comparing it with a primitive infantile mechanism. In the beginning, the child has no comprehension of his own ego nor of another person as entities, which is expressed in the fact that he is able to see both himself and others as the bad and as the good child, as the bad and as the good mother, as the bad and as the good nurse, etc. At the beginning, the situation probably is that under the domination of a more powerful love-urge, his whole actual knowledge of the bad aspect of the mother is simply wiped out, and the opposite occurs if an impulse of hate breaks through. It is impossible to speak of any real ambivalence at this stage. This only arises later, after he becomes able to see more as entities the various expressions of his own personality as well as those of others. Then the idea arises that the bad mother may be turned into the loving mother, by punishing and so to speak destroying the bad ego. The image of authority, the super-ego, will now see to it that the love of the parents is not imperilled by the bad ego. This situation helps us to understand how lack of love, as felt by the child, may reinforce the severity and sternness of the super-ego; and also how an early love-disappointment in mother or father or others, such as Abraham assumes as the basis of a depressive pre-disposition, may give rise to a sadistically inclined super-ego. The extraordinary exaggerations of melancholia, in which the patient expiates not only his own sins, but those also of the lost object, and the forms taken by the efforts at self-punishment, may also be partly explained from the characteristics of the period when the conflict of ambivalence first arose. For a complete understanding we still require many more detailed investigations.

The problem of the psychological significance of mania has received less study from the psycho-analytical point of view. In contrast to the situation in melancholia, Freud [1] has depicted mania as a fusion of the ego with the ego-ideal, in which inhibitions, discretion and self-reproaches all disappear. The maniac shakes off the domination of the ego-ideal. The latter is no longer opposed to the ego in the rôle of critic, but has been absorbed in it. Abraham [2] points out that the libido, no longer consumed in the inner conflict,

[1] Freud, *Group Psychology and the Analysis of the Ego*, 1921.

[2] Abraham, "A Short History of the Development of the Libido", *Selected Papers*, 1927.

turns now, in the manic phase, with great eagerness to the world of objects. The maniac has a peculiar craving to take everything to himself, but he readily rejects what does not suit him. Erotic craving in the maniac, too, soon gets over earlier inhibitions. He returns to the state when the super-ego did not yet exist. The origin of this state is, however, not easy to understand from the psychological point of view. Helene Deutsch [1] has tried to penetrate more deeply here. She treated a case in which periods of revolt, such as occasionally precede, according to Radó, the depressive phase, alternated with manic phases. These aggressions proved to be reactions to disappointments in love. After a brief interval, a hypomanic state was then developed, in which "abundant object-relationships were revealed, but only in the form of a narcissistic ecstasy: 'How they do all love and admire me!'" In this state, aggression is avoided, the injuries and disappointments which have been endured being put right, as it were, in the person of the environment. "A massive mechanism of denial, making it unnecessary to hate the world and then to suffer punishment for that hate. The result is another economic gain in the way of freedom from a sense of guilt." Helene Deutsch thinks that this mechanism of denial lies at the base of all manic states. She finds it also in hypomania and thinks its origin lies in the defence against the castration complex. Both unpleasant aspects of the external world and certain impulses of the id are, in mania, successfully denied. "In some cases, this process can only begin after the severity of the super-ego has been overcome by melancholic suffering (manic triumph); in others, it temporarily suppresses, by means of periodic remissions, the depressive-aggressive impulses (periodic mania). Occasionally, the defence-mechanism of the ego succeeds in so stifling the germ of melancholy that it never comes to light; the constant activity of the defence-mechanisms is betrayed in chronic hypomania. That it is a question of a defensive process is manifested in that little something more, in too much expenditure, in a restlessness and exaggeration. If the actual value of the products of manic activity is subjected to closer observation, it is seen how peculiarly pale these appear in comparison with the output of energy, how, in spite of apparent passion, the love-relationships of these people lack warmth, how sterile their actual performance is, in spite of constant productivity. This is the consequence of the claims made on the psychical energies by the necessity for suppress-

[1] Helene Deutsch, "Zur Psychologie der manisch-depressiven Zustände, insbesondere der chronischen Hypomanie", *Int. Zeitschr. für Psychoanalyse*, 1933. (No English translation.)

ing narcissistic wounds, aggression, and reactions to a sense of guilt. As far as this latter is concerned, mania attains its end."

Helene Deutsch states clearly that the question of the origin of mania cannot be answered by reference alone to the libidinal disposition. As a factor in pre-disposition she mentions, like Abraham, a peculiarly oral disposition. But even with the insight which the psycho-analysts have given us in regard to this point, it is not quite clear how this disposition can give rise to such powerful and persistent consequences as manic and melancholic states present. Moreover, "oral character-traits" have not been very clearly described in psycho-analytical psychology, and in the melancholic pre-disposition there are also anal-erotic fixations to be taken into account. Here, also, the weak point in psycho-analytical psychology seems to me to be its inadequate conception of pre-disposition. It is probable that the inherited pre-disposition to manic-depressive psychosis depends not only on emphases in the instinctual pre-disposition, but also on factors in the structure of conscious orientation. If we compare Kretschmer's description of cyclothymics with those quoted from Abraham and Radó concerning the character of depressive patients in the intermediate phase, we find very little agreement. The good-hearted, good-natured pyknics, who understand a joke and take life as it is, are then revealed as people with strong ambivalence, endlessly courting, it is true, the love of others, but then proceeding to domineer over them, becoming irritable if they resist. Agreement is more easily found from another point of view. The person whose character has been mainly formed under oral influences is described by Abraham [1] as an incurable optimist, expecting, like a child, to find everywhere some kind person to take care of him, and therefore not exerting himself much. If their wishes are not fulfilled, these people display a kind of incessant exaction. They exert pressure, are insistent, and seem positively to suck at other people. "They are particularly afraid of being left alone, even for a very short period." Besides this constant exaction, there is a persistent urge to communicate themselves to others by the oral path. "The result is an obstinate urge to talk. Added to this, there is in most cases a sense of being ready to overflow; such people feel they have an inexhaustible supply of thoughts, and ascribe special value to their spoken utterances." This means, also, that hostile tendencies find oral expression; the mouth is the organ of aggression, aiming at the destruction of the opponent. Talking may be substituted for any other function. Abraham distinguishes

[1] Abraham, *Psychoanalytische Studien zur Charakterbildung*, 1925. (No English translation.)

two stages in the oral phase of development, according to whether sucking or biting has most influenced emotional attitudes. Fixation at the former stage tends to give rise to a carefree optimism, generosity, a gay attitude; from the second phase we get greed, envy, a grudging spirit, hostility and spitefulness. People with oral fixations show in general, according to Abraham, impatience, haste and restlessness. They talk a lot, hate to be alone, and enjoy the pleasures of the senses, particularly those of eating and drinking.

This description comes much nearer to that of cyclothymes, although it gives a less idyllic picture than Kretschmer presents. It also shows that the pre-disposition to manic-depressive disorders is primarily connected with fixations at the second oral phase, in which ambivalence first develops, so that the pre-disposition of the pyknic type and that of the manic-depressive patient according to the psycho-analytical conception are certainly related, although not immediately identical. In psycho-analytical psychology it is not quite clear how this question of pre-disposition is regarded; whether, for example, fixations at the oral phases are dependent on the emotional significance of the mouth quite apart from anything else, or whether certain activities are accentuated as a result of the pre-disposition. In the first case, it would be possible to group together pyknics and manic-depressives, as far as disposition is concerned. In the second case, the disposition would vary (the pyknic being associated more with sucking, the manic-depressive more with biting). Also, it might be asked whether an inborn high degree of sadism did not lend to the ambivalence conflict of the manic-depressive its peculiar significance. The problem of definite emphases in the instinctual structure seems to me to be in any case important, and the psycho-analytical investigations into the mechanisms of depression and of manic states offer an approach to the understanding of psychosis. But it is certainly not possible to say that our psychological insight on this point is complete, and it seems to me, therefore, important to take into account as a factor the constellation of conscious orientation.

My experience of the manic-depressive character is not sufficient to allow me to do more than make a few passing remarks, whose intention is to stimulate further research. If we compare Kretschmer's clinical observations and the analytical views of the psycho-analysts with our ideas concerning the types of conscious orientation, the striking point in both descriptions is that extraversion forms a predominant factor in pre-disposition. We have already seen this clearly in Kretschmer's types. Abraham's comparison of the manic-depressive pre-disposition with the obsessional neurotic character is somewhat confusing, because we have discovered particular connections between this character and introversion, although a similar characterological elaboration of obsessional neurotic mechanisms may also occur in extraverts. Radó's and Helene Deutsch's descriptions indicate particularly the extraverted attitude of these people. Radó shows how the pre-disposed depressive relies for the satisfaction of his narcissism, so important to him, entirely on other people, and that he takes enormous pains to develop his relationships in accordance with his desires. Helene Deutsch unmasks the lack of genuineness in the manic attitude, but at the same time makes it clear how much store these patients set by their relationships with other people. The question then arises as to whether the great significance of the mechanism of introjection, which plays such a great part in melancholia, can be explained as a product of a predominantly extraverted state.

In order to answer this question, we must first formulate more distinctly what we understand by the concept of introjection. This concept has gradually assumed a narrower meaning in psychoanalysis than was first given it by Ferenczi.[1] At first it coincided with the concept, at that time equally vague in its formulation, of transference. Abraham gave it a more precise meaning. In contrast to identification, a process showing similarity to that of introjection, there is in the latter case not only an incorporation of another person or attitude, but the subject's relationship thereto is also internalized, so that both attitudes, related as they are to each other, persist within, in opposition to each other. In fantasy, also, an external relationship may take on an inner form, but in that case identification with the various attitudes is less compulsive. Fantasy forms a semi-neutral zone between the external world and the actual self, and may therefore throw light on the feeling which is determining a state of mind. Introjection is more primitive and more tragic. A similar conflict, which in the hysteric gives rise to a luxuriance of fantasy, and in the obsessional neurotic causes brooding and compulsive assurances, will in the person pre-disposed to manic-depressive insanity stir up a primitive conflict with the internalized authority. These people seem not to have settled their ideals in the sphere of feeling, which thus have little independent significance, and the result is that in any difficult situation they fall back on the more primitive mechanisms belonging to the history of the development of the super-ego. Introjection in Abraham's sense is such a primitive mode of internalizing an external authority.

[1] Ferenczi, "Introjection and Transference", *Contributions to Psychoanalysis*, Boston, 1916.

According to the view offered by the psycho-analytical investigators, we should most likely expect to find this mechanism in people in whom the later modes of dealing with internal and external problems, i.e. thinking and feeling, are less well developed. Also, it would be reasonable to expect that this mechanism would be more likely to acquire considerable influence in extraverted people than in introverts. In extraverts, modes of adaptation are primarily expressed in an outgoing direction, while the inner elaboration of problems seems to have much less differentiation. Introjection as a mental mechanism belongs to a stage of development at which an independent inner life is only beginning to arise. An introverted person would have to have a fairly primitive internal structure, if this kind of mechanism played an important rôle in his psychology. That does not, of course, exclude the possibility of its being found in association with other mental mechanisms, even in introverts. But one would more likely expect to find hysterical or obsessional neurotic forms of depression. An extravert may attain a fairly high degree of mental development, while his inner adjustments remain primitive. This is particularly true of instinctive and intuitive extraverts, who tend more to the simpler mental mechanisms. According to this view, we should most likely expect to find severe manic-depressive states developing in extraverted instinctives and in extraverted intuitives. In practice, I have found this idea confirmed in some cases, but it requires the control of larger numbers. Hence it is important that we should compare it with Kretschmer's idea, and I think we shall find that it confirms mine.

I have already drawn attention to the fact that in the description of cycloids we find very few characteristics pointing to a predominance of thought or feeling. Certainly, according to Kretschmer, "the heart" plays a large part, but in his description this characteristic appears to be more an emotional responsiveness than feeling in my sense. Also, they are "not people of rigid consistency or thought-out systems and schemes". On the other hand, Kretschmer emphasizes their materialistic disposition, their inclinations in the direction of enjoyment, love, eating and drinking, and of the natural acceptance of all the good things of life, which corresponds to the attitude of instinctive people. Other characteristics, such as a wealth of ideas, an eye for an opportunity, ready wit, daring and over-estimation of the self, remind us of the extraverted intuitive. We have already pointed out how extraversion stands out in the description of cycloid types. It seems to me, therefore, that in Kretschmer's description of cycloids we find a confirmation of my assumptions.

Let us now turn to the question of the pre-disposition to schizophrenia. I have already stated that, in my opinion, Kretschmer is too apt to equate a general pre-disposition (which he calls schizothymic) with the disease of schizophrenia, thereby confusing the contours both of the congenital character and of the mechanisms of the disorder. A possible inter-action between these two factors can only be studied through an attempt to understand both aspects more clearly. It is, however, not easy to fulfil this requirement in the present state of our knowledge. I propose to try to suggest in outline the direction in which insight is likely to develop. In doing so, I shall confine myself to the mental aspects.[1]

Since Bleuler directed his genius to the investigation of schizophrenia,[2] its psychological manifestations have become an important object of research in psychiatry. Kraepelin had given us the general concept of dementia praecox. This laid down the main clinical features of the disease, but its real meaning remained quite incomprehensible. Bleuler next undertook the great task of bringing us nearer to an understanding of these enigmatical manifestations. In his view, schizophrenia was distinguished by certain fundamental symptoms. First of these was a definite splitting of the mental functions; where the disease is marked, the personality loses its unity; first one, then another mental complex represents the person, the reciprocal effects of the various complexes and impulses being insufficient, or completely lacking. Even ideas are only in part thought out, and fragments of ideas are incorrectly combined into some fresh idea. Associations lose their connections, and the idea they were to lead up to sometimes gets lost altogether in the process. All the connected threads in the thought-processes may, in fact, get broken, giving rise to a state of stupor or block. This associative confusion brings about such manifestations as lack of concentration, condensation, stereotypies, monoideism. Bleuler considers the second fundamental symptom to be that of a deadening of feeling. In the severest cases, expressions of feeling are practically imperceptible. This defect is usually most pronounced in relation to the higher interests. Even in cases coloured by a prevailing mood, there is usually a lack of unity in the affects. Their expression is, moreover, stiffer, and lacks modulation. Affects are superficial and labile, show capricious variations, and are often inadequate in relation to their causes. Simple affects, such as wrath and rage, are

[1] In saying this, I do not in the least intend to suggest that I do not appreciate the importance of the physical aspect of the disease. Study of the brain and of endocrinology both offer clues in this respect, but they have not yet brought any definite results.

[2] Bleuler, *Dementia Praecox*, 1911.

usually preserved. Feelings regulating ordinary human intercourse are frequently lost at a very early stage. Ethical characteristics are, it is true, usually blunted, but do not altogether disappear. Schizophrenes vary very considerably in character, although their indifference, when the disease is advanced, gives them all similar external features. The lower instincts and the feeling-tone of the bodily processes usually suffer less than the higher affects. There is generally strong ambivalence in the feelings. In comparison with these disturbances, it is striking to note that perception, orientation and memory have suffered no damage.

Bleuler sees the cause of these fundamental symptoms in a tendency to place personal fantasy above reality, and to withdraw from the latter. He calls this morbid preponderance of the inner life, autism. Through it the schizophrene gets away from reality, and is pre-occupied solely with the images of his own fantasy. This makes his outward indifference understandable. Other things are more important to him. Misunderstandings arising from his autistic thought-processes are difficult to correct, owing to his deficient associative capacities. He lives in a different kind of reality, which has for him more significance than the outer world of normal people. Such schizophrenes frequently no longer believe in the testimony of their own senses. The content of autistic thinking consists of wishes and fears. In this way, a typical form of dementia may arise, in which the patients become enclosed in their own thoughts, without any interest in the external world.

All other manifestations, lending to this disease its peculiar variety, colour and strangeness, are lumped together by Bleuler as accessory. Here we get the hallucinations, delusions, changes in personality, language and writing, physical symptoms and catatonic manifestations. The contents of the extraordinary mental life of these patients finds to some extent expression through these phenomena. Bleuler explains these contents as primarily the consequence of the associative disturbance in their thinking, as a result of which affects assume a relative preponderance, and there is a rupture in the psyche, determined by complexes which are invested with feeling. The split in the associations leads, according to Bleuler, "also to a pathological ambivalence, as a result of conflicting feelings or thoughts flowing side by side, without influencing each other". Thus, in Bleuler's view, these powerful effects of complexes are caused by a primary breaking-up of the stream of associations. Affects, which in any case have a tendency to split off, are then more readily detached from the personality.

Side by side with this conception another has developed, which gives full recognition to Bleuler's psychological differentiations, but ascribes, in explanation of the disease, the first place to disorders in the emotional life, and seeks to trace its remarkable associative structures back to emotional influences. These attempts began with Jung,[1] Abraham [2] and Freud,[3] and have opened up interesting vistas in the psychology of schizophrenes. Psycho-analytical investigation then proceeded to concentrate mainly on the problem of the delusional formations, and it has shown how here certain complexes and fixations have considerable influence on the clinical manifestations.[4] In schizophrenes we find the extraordinary phenomenon, that on the one hand the typical disturbances, whose origin Freud has found in fixations, are much easier to demonstrate than in other mental diseases; while, on the other hand, it is peculiarly difficult to explain their connection with mental development. Incestuous attachment to the object, auto-erotic manifestations of every kind, sadistic and masochistic impulses, often appear undisguised on the surface. Before the development of the psychoanalytical point of view, this aspect of the manifestations received little attention from the psychiatrists. The discovery of infantile sexuality first made it possible for us to perceive in these manifestations indications of regressive forms from early developmental phases, and to seek a connection between them and the life-history. This study is, moreover, helped by a recognition of the significance of symbolism. Freud has clarified for us the language of the dream and of the symptoms of neurosis, revealing at the same time the tremendous importance of symbolic forms for modern civilized man. In his laws and in his customs he retains unconsciously many characteristics which correspond with those of primitive mental life, and with the manifestations of schizophrenia. Freud's influence on our conception of schizophrenia is also revealed in the much more thorough consideration which is now given to the connection between mental contents and the individual life-history.

Bleuler's distinction between primary and secondary mani-

[1] Jung, *The Psychology of Dementia Praecox*, New York, 1909.

[2] Abraham, "Über die Bedeutung sexueller Jugendträume für die Symptomatologie der Dementia Praecox", *Zentralbl. für Nervenheilkunde*, 1907 (no English translation); "The Psycho-sexual Differences between Hysteria and Dementia Praecox", *Selected Papers*, London, 1927.

[3] Freud, "Psycho-analytical Notes upon an Autobiographical Account of a Case of Paranoia (Dementia Paranoides)", 1911: *Collected Papers*, vol. ii.

[4] These investigations have been further prosecuted in different countries, e.g. in Switzerland by Jung, Maeder, Spielrein, Grebelskaja, Nelken, Itten; in Austria by Schilder, Nunberg, Bibring, Brunswick; in France by Claude, Laforgue, Minowski; in Holland by G. Jelgersma, Muller, Stärcke, Rombouts, Carp, Endtz, H. C. Jelgersma, Westerman-Holstijn, myself and others.

festations is also found with Freud. For the latter, the primary factor is regression to a specific fixation in mental development, while the secondary manifestations represent an attempt at restoration, based on a lower mental plane. Here, also, the question arises as to whether typical fixated forms can be laid down as causes. For the paranoid forms of schizophrenia, Freud has postulated a fixation in libidinal development as the cause, and his views in this respect have been confirmed by various investigators. This fixation is sought in the narcissistic phase, in which the child "begins by taking himself, his own body, as his love-object, and only subsequently proceeds from this to the choice of some person other than himself as his object".[1] Fixation in this phase may have as a result that the choice of object is influenced by the subject's own genitalia, and thus a homosexual object-choice may occur before heterosexuality is established. "After the stage of heterosexual object-choice has been reached, the homosexual tendencies are not, as might be supposed, done away with or brought to a stop; they are merely deflected from their sexual aim and applied to fresh uses. They now combine with portions of the ego-instincts and, as 'anaclitic' components, help to constitute the social instincts, thus contributing an erotic factor to friendship and comradeship, to *esprit de corps* and to the love of mankind in general." "Persons who have not freed themselves completely from the stage of narcissism, who, that is to say, have at that point a fixation which may operate as a disposing factor for a later illness, are exposed to the danger that some unusually intense wave of libido, finding no other outlet, may lead to a sexualization of their social instincts and so undo the work of sublimation which they had achieved in the course of their development. This result may be produced by anything that causes the libido to flow backwards (i.e. that causes a 'regression'); whether, on the one hand, for instance, the libido becomes collaterally reinforced owing to some disappointment over a woman, or is directly dammed up owing to a mishap in social relations with other men—both of these would be instances of 'frustration'; or whether, on the other hand, there is a general intensification of the libido, so that it becomes too powerful to find an outlet along the channels which are already open to it, and consequently bursts through its banks at the weakest spot. Since our analyses show that paranoiacs *endeavour to protect themselves against any such sexualization of their social instinctual cathexes*, we are driven to suppose

[1] Freud, "Psycho-analytical Notes upon an Autobiographical Account of a Case of Paranoia (Dementia Paranoides)", 1911: *Collected Papers*, vol. ii.

that the weak spot in their development is to be looked for somewhere between the stages of auto-erotism, narcissism and homosexuality, and that their disposition to illness (which may perhaps be susceptible of more precise definition) must be located in that region. A similar disposition would have to be assigned to patients suffering from Kraepelin's dementia praecox, or (as Bleuler has named it) schizophrenia." Freud then proceeds to devote the acuity of his genius to the study of the forms adopted as defence in paranoia, and points out how projection impresses one as being the most important of these.

The mechanism of projection has a special importance in the psychological foundation of paranoia. Freud describes it as follows: "An internal perception is suppressed, and, instead, its content, after undergoing a certain degree of distortion, enters consciousness in the form of an external perception. In delusions of persecution the distortion consists in a transformation of affect; what should have been felt internally as love is perceived externally as hate." Freud adds that it would be tempting to regard this process as pathognomonic for paranoia, but that it does not play the same part in every form, and that it always has a share in our attitude to the external world. "When we refer the causes of certain sensations to the external world, instead of looking for them (as we do in the case of others) inside ourselves, this normal proceeding also deserves to be called projection." Freud then decides to postpone the study of projection for the present, and unfortunately he has never returned to it. It is true that, in the case of Schreber, Freud proceeds to demonstrate very clearly that another process precedes the development of projection, which he calls a detachment of libido from the object.[1] This detachment of the libido is a phenomenon which also regularly takes place in normal mental life, without leading to any psychosis. Normally, the freed libido may, it is true, remain in the psyche as a fluctuating tension, but, as a rule, it finds a fresh object, although there is a possibility that it may give rise to neurotic manifestations. In paranoia, the libido, when withdrawn from the object, is employed in a special kind of way. It is withdrawn into the ego, leading to enlargement of this and to megalomania. It is from this fact that Freud deduces a regression from sublimated homosexuality to narcissism. It is true that the notion of the end of the world shows that the whole relationship to

[1] It is true that in the case of Schreber the delusion of persecution (an attempt at a return to the objects) came before the fantasy of the end of the world (which represents this detachment symbolically), but Freud explains this by saying that the detachment takes place by stages, with a constantly recurring attempt at restoring the connection.

the external world is threatened, so that we have here more than a mere disturbance in the libido, but Freud offers the hypothesis in explanation that there may be reactions from the libidinal disturbances upon the ego-cathexes. The hallucinations also are seen as the result of a struggle between repression and an attempt at cure, which has as its aim the return of the libido to its objects. Even in the motor stereotypies Jung has recognized the compulsive retention of one-time object-cathexes. In these hallucinations and catatonic phenomena, the attempt at cure does not, as in paranoia, employ projection, but the mechanisms of hallucination, and of magic gestures. These mechanisms indicate a further regression than that of projection, and to fixations which must lie at the very beginning of the child's development, when it first turns from auto-erotism to recognize an object. Common to the various forms of schizophrenia we might assume, therefore, a more predominantly narcissistic relationship to the external world (partly in the form of conscious and unconscious homosexuality), and secondly, the fact that object-cathexes never attain the same importance as compared with narcissism that they do in normal people. Stärcke has further pointed out yet another circumstance,[1] namely, that the predisposition to psychosis consists sometimes not so much in an intensification of narcissism as in its infantile character. We found a similar observation confirmed in the case of manic-depressive psychosis, when we perceived in the introjection of the person with authority a primitive, narcissistic mechanism. This brings us to the question as to whether in mechanisms such as projection, hallucination and the magical catatonic gesture, we are not dealing with similar primitive mental mechanisms.

If Freud came to a standstill in his study of projection, the reason seems to me to be partly because he has associated a pathological mechanism with the problem of the normal experience of an external world. Freud regards it as projection, "when we refer the causes of certain sensations to the external world". He and others who take a similar viewpoint do not realize that something of a general metaphysical conception of the world is implied here, and a conception which is open to criticism. There is, as a matter of fact, a presumption that an inner life exists first, and that it renders possible deductions in regard to experience of the external world. It has, however, become increasingly clear from the study of the child and of the savage that a phase, when there is no distinction between the self and the external world, precedes the clear

[1] Stärcke, "Psycho-analysis and Psychiatry", *Int. Journal of Psycho-analysis*, 1921.

differentiation made by civilized man. Moreover, phenomenological researches, such as Husserl and Heidegger have made, have shown us the importance of the unity of conscious experience as the basis of all conceptual distinctions. Association Psychology, which dominated the objectification of mental life for a long period, has created many erroneous ideas, as a result of its atomistic point of view. Moreover, the problem as to why certain perceptions (the corner-stones of mental life according to this point of view) have been associated to form an external world, while others make up the self, has never been solved by Association Psychology. Luckily we do not need to torment ourselves with the solution of this insoluble problem, because neither the external world nor the self have been constructed in consciousness along these lines. It is true that we find in thought the association of isolated ideas, but it would be absolutely wrong to regard this mechanism as dominating the whole of mental life. Experience of the world and of the self exists in the child, as in the human race, long before thought seeks to construct objectifications of either. Before we can approach the problem of projection, we must try to get an idea as to how the differentiation of the world from the self does come about, since we reject the intellectualistic account of the process as erroneous.

Even if we agree that the unity of experience precedes isolated ideas, the question remains as to how from this lack of differentiation more precise concepts of the world and of the self are evolved, ontogenetically and phylogenetically. Ferenczi has on this point given us views which are of extreme importance for this problem.[1] The child's general experience of the connection between himself and the external world passes through various stages which determine his sense of reality. Ferenczi describes the condition of the unborn child as a period of unconditional omnipotence, because during it every need is satisfied without the child having to make any effort. It is questionable if we can speak of experience at this stage. But in any case, this wish-fulfilling influence of the external world is maintained after birth in the care of the infant, when the child finds that he can obtain restoration of a comfortable state of affairs by yelling and kicking. Ferenczi speaks here of a period of magical and hallucinatory omnipotence. (Whether his assumption that the child hallucinates satisfaction is justifiable, I prefer to leave over for the moment.) As the life of the infant becomes more complicated, he finds it more difficult to satisfy his wishes. He learns to express these wishes by means of certain gestures, and thus

[1] Ferenczi, "Stages in the Development of the Sense of Reality", *Contributions to Psycho-analysis*, Boston, 1916.

gains a new mode of influencing the environment: the period of omnipotence by means of magic gestures. The conditions for the fulfilment of his wishes continue to become more difficult. "The outstretched hand has often to be withdrawn empty; the longed-for object does not obey the magic gesture. An uncontrollable hostile power may even oppose this gesture by force and compel the hand to take up its former position. The child is obliged to isolate from his ego certain malicious things, which refuse to obey his will, which become the external world." Only at this stage can we speak of introjection and projection. In this phase, the self, as the thing which one can control, assumes great significance, and a similar self, with its organs and activities, is found again in the things of the external world: the period of the animistic conception of reality. Symbolic representation now comes into being, particularly through language. The symbolism of gesture is resolved into the symbolism of language, making it possible to exert a more precise influence on the environment, which at first is assumed to be magical. Ferenczi calls this period the period of magic thoughts and magic words. The limits of this influence are, however, soon learned. Side by side with an exaggerated feeling of omnipotence, feelings of inferiority arise, and disappointments compel a recognition of the conditional nature of personal wishes and thoughts, and the objectification of reality. With this the stage of the predominance of the reality-principle is reached.

Ferenczi proceeds to point out that the development of sexuality may take place to some extent independently of the development of the sense of reality, particularly if its manifestations are suppressed and find a way, through auto-erotism and fantasy, to perpetuate the omnipotence phases of erotic development. Hence regressions are more easily made here, although they may be much more obvious in the adaptation to reality. There is always, however, in neurosis some lack of adjustment to reality, but it will be confined to certain libidinal situations. Ferenczi expresses here the hypothesis already made, that the wish-content in neurosis is dependent on the point at which fixation in libidinal development took place, while its mechanism is probably determined by the stage of ego-development which the subject had attained when the pre-disposing frustration took place. He adds that it is quite reasonable to suppose that when the libido regresses to earlier stages of development, that phase in the development of the reality-sense which prevailed at the respective fixation level is also resuscitated in the mechanisms of symptom-formation.

These regressive forms of reality-sense have still greater significance in the psychoses, because regression is visible here not in single manifestations, but dominates the whole picture of the psychosis. A general regression of the ego is found only in the psychoses, and the stages of development described by Ferenczi may help us to give greater exactitude to our description of the forms taken by this regression. The weak point in Ferenczi's formulation seems to me that he relates regression only to infantile development, and neglects the phylogenetic aspect. But it is permissible to assume that not all these regressive forms are determined by the relationship with the environment, but that a good deal must be attributed to pre-disposition. Under this head, I would include the various modes in the conscious elaboration of experience, as I have described them in this book. It seems to me, also, that by taking these factors into account, one is in a better position to give a clear account of the mode of regression as regards reality-sense. We will try to do this more exactly in the case of the mechanism of projection.

Westerman-Holstijn [1] has pointed out that Freud uses the term projection in two different senses, which he does not sharply distinguish. On the one hand, he regards projection as a perception of something within, which is not recognized as such but is attributed to the external world; on the other hand, he seems to mean by it a return of the libido to its objects. Of course, the regressive and progressive forms assumed by the libido and the sense of reality may affect one another, but they also occur separately. Both libidinal reinvestment of objects and the reference of inner perceptions to the external world are regularly found in normal people. This fact, and the above-mentioned differentiation, impel me to suggest a limitation of the concept so as to avoid what might become a terminological confusion. I should like to use the term projection only for a certain situation in the sense of reality, and only for those cases in which it is clear that there is an error in the objectification of the external world. Jung describes projection as "a process of dissimilation, in which a subjective content is separated from the subject and to some extent incorporated in the object".[2] He writes: "Projection depends on the archaic identity between subject and object, but is only to be called projection after the need to resolve this identification with the object has arisen: the expression projection indicates, therefore, a state of identity which is noticeable and as such has become an object of criticism, whether by the subject himself or by another." In my opinion, it would be better to

[1] Westerman-Holstijn, *Streven en waarneming bij paranoide psychosen*, 1929. (No English translation.)

[2] C. G. Jung, *Psychological Types*, 1921.

substitute for the expression "identity" that of "fusion" (*Ungeschiedenheit*), but otherwise I would agree with this sharper definition of the concept. Projection would thus mean that a false separation between the external world and the self is noticeable, namely, one by means of which contents of the self are ascribed to the external world. The concept then means something primitive and pathological, although it must be recognized that the boundary between it and what is normal is undefined, owing to the limitations of our minds.[1]

Psycho-analytical observation has given us the view that projection indicates a somewhat undeveloped state of reality-sense, which may be determined by regression or by primitive development. This does not explain, however, why this mechanism attains such significance in certain cases, or why in the psychoses it assumes such extraordinary forms. Can it be that this particular regression is encouraged by the prevalence of a certain mode of conscious orientation, and is it possible from our recognition of the conscious functions to throw a clearer light on the structure of regressive forms? We will begin with the second question.

Westerman-Holstijn has made an important observation concerning the nature of this regression, namely, that this has nothing to do with external perception (which many analysts equate in a one-sided way with adaptation to reality), but with inner perception. According to him, inner perception avails itself of external perception, and of feelings, impulses, etc. Unfortunately he does not enlarge on this observation. It would, for instance, have been very important to define the developmental stages in inner reality, in comparison with Ferenczi's stages in the development of reality-sense. I have tried in this book to show how there is between instinctive experience and a conceptual understanding of the world and the self, derived from conscious perception, an important phase, in which intuition is operative. Hence I cannot possibly accept external and internal perception as the simplest expression of consciousness, as Westerman-Holstijn and others do. Moreover, it does not seem easy to me to explain from such a point of view the development of a differentiated external and internal perception, from a state in which neither is differentiated from the other. Recognition of the significance of intuition enables us to give a more exact account of the stages in adaptation to reality. With

[1] In accordance with this point of view, it would be possible to confine the concept of introjection in a similar way to contents and mechanisms which are erroneously ascribed to the self, while it is obvious that they are derived from external influences.

the help of this recognition, we shall try to get a better understanding of the regressive manifestations in schizophrenia.

At first sight, Westerman-Holstijn's idea that we are dealing here with a regression in inner perception does not seem very acceptable. What strikes us first of all in schizophrenia is a certain inner change, which we may describe as dissociation or inner confusion, but along with this, perception of the external world soon becomes distorted. Suspicion, delusions of reference, persecution-mania, and above all hallucinations, disturb objective perception. At the same time, external perception is found to be intact, so that it is not possible to assume without further evidence a disorder of the sense-organs or of the brain. Moreover, we find in ordinary life, and particularly among savages, manifestations showing similarity to those of schizophrenia. Among savages, real perception is not very objective, although this fact is concealed under a good instinctive adaptation, giving an impression of good sense. The first evidence of insight, standing out from undifferentiated instinctual experience, can be described as neither objective nor subjective. The earliest concrete intuitions grasp connections in the world, in which the self is also involved. Whether the lightning flash of intuition is turned more on circumstances in the world or on attitudes in the self, the other aspect will also frequently form part of the picture. Only very gradually do there develop from these pictures, as they lay the foundations of conscious experience, real perceptions and ideas. The starting-point of their development is, however, always intuitive insight. Intuitive insight into an inner happening is not yet perception, any more than is insight into an external connection. Only when an insight has been tested can it be regarded as perception. Thus the important point is the problem of classification and testing, and it seems to me extremely important that there are in the beginning no separate modes of testing for the data of the external world and for those of the self. Side by side with undifferentiated instinctual experience, there exist intuitions concerning data in the external world, concerning relationships between the self and the external world, and concerning the self; and with the development of thought there is added to this a testing of these data by comparison of them with ideas which have already been consciously elaborated. A differentiated inner world and outer world are at first perceived and conceived only, as it were, by chance.[1] A separate testing of external and internal data takes place only fairly late in the development of mankind, and the first sciences

[1] It must be regarded as a consequence of this state of affairs that savages ascribe concrete significance to their dreams.

(astrology, alchemy) still show clearly how slightly the various forms of testing are differentiated one from another. Simple perception is, it is true, subjected to the test of thought, but the forms assumed by the testing processes are still very undeveloped. What we are accustomed to call internal and external perception are complicated processes, capable of revealing every kind of transition down to simple observation. External perception first evolved more precise forms in the natural sciences. It would be a mistake to think that internal perception played no part in these more developed forms, since the objectivity of one's own attitude must be just as thoroughly examined as external facts. It is true that this inner control is mainly employed to exclude subjective influences.[1] Scientific perception is thus anything but a simple process. The same is true of internal perception. This is only now beginning to develop as a science, although the development of phenomenology may be said to have laid firm foundations for further structures on these lines. Critical observation of the self can no more deny the existence of the external world than can objective perception of the world take place without some reference to the self. The majority of internal processes are directed towards the external world, and are themselves illuminated by this reference. Many people regard as really true about themselves only that which is mirrored in the opinions of others. Many kinds of art express what is within only by means of what is without, although there are forms, such as music or lyrical poetry, which seek a direct communication of inner contents.

Inner perception has been much less systematically developed by modern man than external perception. Hence in many people it retains very simple forms, unless there is some special talent in this direction. In schizoids and schizophrenes we occasionally see such special gifts. Even quite simple people of this type may astonish us with deep, introspective observations, and we know that many schizophrenes, even while ill, will show great gifts in abstract thinking or in artistic expression. As a rule, however, they express themselves in some intricate symbolism, having only a vague correspondence with mature forms of expression. Should we regard these confused forms as an expression of regression in internal perception? I believe it is possible to choose a better expression, in the first place, because it is clear that these forms are no longer a matter of actual *perceptions*, but of something which preceded them: the intuitive understanding of inner happening; and secondly, because only a qualified reference to regression is

[1] I have gone into this in more detail in Chapter I of the philosophical section.

possible, since only a few cases will show evidence of a previously superior form of internal perception, while these regressive forms usually occur in some realm which has previously held little interest for the patient. If these intuitions referring to the self occur in a form which is ascribed to the external world, we may then speak of projection. The fantastic forms of these intuitions are certainly to some extent caused by the circumstance that comparison with other forms has ceased, so that thought no longer has any authority. And not only thought, but feeling also, exerts a certain control over spontaneously arising mental forms. Retrogression in emotional life in schizophrenia is probably recognized by everyone. Thus we find here something similar to what we found in the manic-depressive psychosis, where we also found the operation of more primitive mechanisms in the place of a higher conscious control. There we described these forms as an introjection of an external authority and of the relationship to it. The content of projection is not so easily summed up, but what we should expect in the case of the healthy person is always the same, namely, a better way of dealing inwardly with problems, so as to give greater inner unity, thereby rendering possible an improved understanding of the external world. We get the impression, both with schizoids and schizophrenes, that experience of the self is very obtrusive and not easy to escape, as it is, for example, for the hysteric. In the melancholic, the mental mechanism depends on a regression to the earliest mode of adjustment to the problem of good and evil, at a period when these principles are still closely bound up with reward and punishment. The mechanisms of schizophrenia are more connected with adjustment between anxiety and a feeling of security, between being lost and being saved. Side by side with the feeling of omnipotence, emphasized by Ferenczi, there is the experience of absolute dependence. If the hallucinations and delusions were in the service of the former principle only, it would not be possible to understand why their content is in most cases highly unpleasant. This contrast between omnipotence and being lost is felt less acutely in normal people, because established relations with the environment, dependent on feeling and reason, bring some correction to bear on the extremes of both attitudes. When feeling and thought are for any reason excluded, and the representation of collectivity in the inner life thereby suspended, the adult, like the child or the savage, stands before chaos within himself and all around him, equipped with only two mental tools: instinct and intuition. But while, in the case of the savage, intuition is guided by collective images, and is therefore much more of a collective function; and while, in the case of the child, intuitions are often understood and explained by the environment—translated, as it were, into feeling- and thought-forms, and modelled on these—the adult, having nothing but intuition to fall back on in a difficult conflict, which has cut him off from his environment, finds himself helpless and alone in the world. He tries to get some sort of grasp of his internal and external situation. Surmises and notions begin to organize themselves into definite delusional pictures. The question arises here as to whether we should not regard the hallucinatory voices as a simple form of concrete intuition. It does not seem possible to me, in the present state of knowledge, to answer this question, but experience of "*eidetische*" people (Jaensch), who, in my opinion, belong to the intuitive type, may offer some important indications in this direction.

A further problem, belonging here, is raised by the extraordinary *forms* taken by schizophrenic intuitions. Jung has laid particular emphasis on the fact that the mode in which intuitive contents are expressed occasionally reveals archaic influences, which led him to the hypothesis of the collective unconscious. The images in which our intuitions come to light would, according to this suggestion, be partly determined by some influence from the inherited structure of the brain, which would be all the more obvious in the absence of normal control by conventional thought and feeling. Jung finds this influence in many normal people as well, although it is most obvious in illnesses such as schizophrenia.

I cannot here go farther into the interesting problem of the archaic determination of intuitive forms. For our investigation, it is sufficient to regard the forms assumed by schizoid projection as primitive intuitive forms. Since these forms are most likely to occur where there is little control by thought or feeling, we should expect to find them more readily in intuitive and instinctive people. In the case of the intuitive, it should be observed that in him intuition is a well-developed function, so that primitive forms must be regarded as an expression of regression in this function. I am conscious that I have given only a very general indication of the relationship between the prevalence of function and the development of schizophrenic manifestations, but it does not seem possible to me, in the present state of our knowledge, to say much more about it. There is yet still another problem to be discussed.

I have stated that it seems better to me to describe the phenomena of projection, not as a regression of internal perception, but as primitive intuitions. In doing so, we have found that the indefinite distinction between inner and outer is implicit in this primitive mode of comprehension. Must we therefore reject not only the concept of perception, but also the predominance of the *internal* aspect of things in projection? On the contrary, it seems to me that Westerman-Holstijn has got hold of something right when he emphasizes the inner aspect here, i.e. the significance of introversion in the development of the phenomena of projection.[1] I have myself [2] already drawn attention to this relationship. In my opinion, the mental attitude, whether it be one of introversion or of extraversion, does not in itself imply regression or progression. It may indeed be said that either attitude may encourage certain forms of regression (or progression). This is true for both regression of libido and regression in the adjustment to reality. Where there is a turning inwards, regression to narcissistic and auto-erotic gratifications will be more probable, and personal, spontaneous points of view are more likely to be over-valued. Where the state is one of extraversion, former objects, or their "*imagos*" will attach the feelings to themselves, or old, infantile wishes will be directed either towards the latter, or towards the objects themselves. In the latter case, the subject's own inner reality is even liable to be denied in the face of the influence of external reality. Everyone has at his disposal good and bad forms, both of extraversion and of introversion. It is not, therefore, possible to label forthwith every less well-adapted, more infantile form as regressive. The introvert, in an introverted state, will have at his disposal better-adjusted forms than the extravert; in an extraverted state, on the other hand, the less well-adjusted aspect of the introvert is more likely to come to light. With the extravert it will be the other way round. A regression in mental forms will strike an individual most where he finds his greatest security, while infantile forms elsewhere will, in any case, not be taken very seriously. A markedly introverted person will attach little value to external forms, in so far as he has not himself elaborated them from within and pronounced an opinion on them. If by chance he should get into a state of extraversion (e.g. drunk, or in love) and somewhat infantile forms should come to light as a result, he may possibly look upon it as abnormal or

[1] Westerman-Holstijn is partly committed to this point of view, because he holds the same view of introversion that Freud does, in which a turning away from the external world must always be regarded as associated with a certain regression, which, in my opinion, is not always the case. For this reason, Jung's concept of introversion is preferable to the psycho-analytical one, as being more precise.

[2] Van der Hoop, *Een geval van Schizophrenie*, 1924; "Über die Projektion und ihre Inhalte", *Int. Zeitschr. für Psychoanalyse*, 1924. (No English translations.)

pathological, but will not feel it to be really part of himself. If, however, he is at variance with himself about something, he will not find it easy to get away from the problem. He will try to get a clearer grasp of the difficulty, and in so doing, he will, according to his pre-disposition, make use of his powers of thought, of feeling or of intuition. Most problems have, however, not only an inner, but also an outer aspect, and for their correct solution it may be necessary to take the latter into account as well. When, as a result of exaggerated introversion, this latter is not adequately done, the individual concerned may become involved in endless brooding, in the way that Kretschmer has so clearly described in relation to his cases with mild ideas of reference. From this there may arise a tendency to assume the existence of one's own doubts and accusations in others, and thus an inner conflict is imposed on one's relationships with others. Surmises, assumptions and suspicions come into being, and there is an intuitive attempt to grasp the situation. The more introverted an individual is, the more difficult will he find it to control his mistaken judgments in this respect. We may ask ourselves why the introvert is not content with his own inner adjustment of the matter (as is indeed the fact with many cases). There are, in my opinion, two reasons for this. In the first place, there is something in the facts of the case which he will not look at and has repressed, but without complete success; and in the second place, there is in him, in spite of everything, a dim inclination somehow to take external facts into account for the solution of his problem. There is justification for both ideas, not only in the manifestations in delusions of reference and in schizophrenia, but also in the behaviour of introverted people. Freud has shown how in the projections of the schizophrenic there is a return of the repressed in a disguised form, for instance, homosexual wishes in the fear of homosexual aggression or in hostility towards the beloved person. It is, moreover, a well-known manifestation that people lay emphasis on characteristics in others which they are unwilling to see in themselves, and condemn them with particular severity. One finds, in addition, in schizophrenics a particular attention to external matters and an exact noting of facts, not explicable on emotional grounds. Similar simple forms of extraversion are found occasionally in strongly introverted persons in the form of curiosity, an inclination to collect things, and a painful exactitude in matters of etiquette. These expressions of simple extraversion may occasionally be understood as a compensation for an attitude which is felt to be one-sided, which in schizophrenia agrees with the Freudian idea, that an effort towards cure and a re-establishment of contact with the external world is expressed in the pathological manifestations.[1]

If we ask why a regressive reality-sense in one case takes the form of projection (for example, a schizophrenic delusion), and in another case that of introjection (for example, an hysterical dream-state), the answer seems to me to be that the regression in the first case is in a strongly introverted person, and in the second case in an exaggeratedly extraverted one. In both cases, the reality-sense regresses to a stage in which the contents of the self and of the world are not clearly differentiated. The situations are different, however. In the schizophrenic state, the life within penetrates into an external world, which otherwise remains the same. Occasionally one gets the impression that the external aspect of the conflict (for example, the persecution) is not really taken very seriously. The essential thing is the adjustment of the various aspects of the inner life, which is seen in fantastic forms. Extraversion—an interest in the external world—is only apparent. It is the strongly introverted state which is the source of the pathological manifestations, and regression is here controlled by the introverted state.

In an hysterical psychotic state, external life penetrates in fantastic forms into the inner life. This inner life does not itself appear to undergo much alteration, but it feels itself to be overwhelmed, and reacts with anxiety or bewilderment. In an hysterical dream-state, contact with the external world is dominated by fantasy, which is, however, no longer recognized as such. The origin of these fantasies lies in this case in unresolved conflicts with the environment, and there is usually to be seen in the hysterical manifestations an effort to influence the environment (as in the schizophrene one frequently finds an effort to come to terms with the self). Hence there is usually manifest in hysteria a theatrical factor, even in the regressions of the reality-sense, while the products of schizophrenia are more comparable with artistic creation, in their attempt to give form to inner happenings. The schizophrene will, so to speak, make use even of the external world in order to represent, and to change, what is within, while the hysteric sets the forces

[1] In one-sided predominance of extraversion the opposite occurs. Internal problems are scarcely considered, and are concealed in external difficulties. When these become insoluble, owing to a failure to recognize a personal attitude, the tendency may arise to incorporate external forms in the form of very vivid fantasies. What is internal is then expressed entirely in terms of the external. At the same time, many incidental and unsuitable forms are also incorporated, and these erroneous forms I should describe as introjection (in contrast to Ferenczi, who applies this term to the whole process). Here, also, we find two reasons for the process: the return of the repressed in disguised form, and the tendency to compensate for a one-sided attitude.

of the inner world in motion, in order to make the external world look different and to influence it. The source of the pathological state in hysteria lies in the failure to establish harmonious contact with the environment, at the same time satisfying personal wishes. In schizophrenia, the starting-point is a failure to establish inner harmony and to create a personal mode of existence from within outwards. In all this, it is without a doubt true that the failure in both cases is connected with a one-sidedness in orientation, and that for a solution of the problem the other aspect would have in both cases to be developed. Instead of developing this other aspect from its primitive forms to others more appropriate, the schizophrene tries to impose his own personal forms on the external world, and when unsuccessful, feels that he is similarly being imposed upon by external forces. The hysteric, on the other hand, should develop better modes of internal adjustment, instead of which he takes the external world to himself in fantasies, in which it corresponds with his various desires.

In both cases, the manifestations are determined by two factors: first, by the inadequate, infantile modes of adaptation in a certain domain (to wit, the relationships with external or with internal facts), and second, by a regression of developed mental forms. The alteration in the contact with reality is mainly the consequence of regression, and in schizophrenia this is related to the introverted functions. This regression means that introverted thinking and feeling, as the more recently developed functions, recede in favour of introverted intuition. This makes confirmation of the correctness of intuitions more difficult, and the mistakes which arise in this way give rise first of all to the manifestation of projection, since inner experience is for these people the most important, and since criticism (in the form of inner perception) still is more readily applied to intuitions relating to the inner life. Criticism of intuitions relating to the external world is, in any case, not specially developed in strongly introverted people.

Let us return, after this long discussion, to the question as to how far, in the present state of our knowledge, certain types of conscious orientation may encourage the development of schizophrenic mental mechanisms. Although these mechanisms are still not quite clear, it is nevertheless possible for us to suggest that they are connected with mistakes in differentiating between what are the effects of the internal, and what the effects of the external, world, As a result, images in internal experience, intuitively grasped, serve to cloud experience of the external world. It is immediately clear from the descriptions of Bleuler, Kretschmer and other investigators, that in schizophrenia we are dealing with intensely introverted states. Also, the descriptions of the illness make it clear that feeling and thought come, during the course of the illness, to have less and less importance for the control of action and of mental orientation. Where these functions have been developed to greater independence, stronger resistance to schizophrenia might be expected. In the same way, it might be assumed that strongly extraverted people are less likely to fall into a state of schizophrenic introversion than introverts. Both these assumptions will have to be tested by further observations; as far as our knowledge extends today, it seems to agree with them. From a clinical point of view, the strongly introverted intuitive seems to offer the closest comparison with the manifestations of schizophrenia, and when there are strong influences derived from complexes in persons of this type, they sometimes resemble very closely Kretschmer's schizoids. It seems probable to me, judging from my experience, that this type will be most likely to offer transitions between normal and schizophrenic manifestations, so that persons of this type will more easily, under difficulties, fall into states resembling schizophrenia, but perhaps also be more able to get out of them again. The regressive forms of reality-adjustment in schizophrenia, and the forms in habitual use with these people, are nearer to each other than is the case with other people. Moreover, schizoid mental mechanisms are, in my opinion, more easily explicable from the point of view of the psychology of the introverted intuitive than they are from that of any of the other types.

By this I do not mean to say that schizophrenia can only develop in introverted intuitive persons, but I would certainly deduce from the facts that people with strong introversion are more pre-disposed to this kind of regression than are others. In introverted thinking- and feeling-types there would have to be a far-reaching exclusion or destruction of the prevailing function before the schizophrenic mechanisms could gain the ascendancy. In introverted intuitives, as has already been said, this would not be the case, or at any rate it would be less so than with thinking- and feeling-types. The more highly developed forms of intuition are distinguished from the simpler forms by being in continuous contact with the culture of the times (i.e. with the current forms in the realms of thought and feeling). Here also, in the case of a schizophrenic regression, the relationship is gradually severed, as a result of which, intuitions assume more primitive, more archaic forms. In introverted instinctive people, where intuition, as a differentiated function, has least independent significance, one would expect to find that even primitive forms of intuition would be unlikely to gain much significance in the conduct of life. But one must recognize here, that even in these cases instinct provides only a partial adjustment, social contacts employing to quite a large extent forms which belong to thought and feeling. When a regression in these forms of adaptation sets in, intuitive forms may in their place attain a greater significance. The lack of understanding, which is in general shown in regard to intuitions, intensifies the alarming force with which the schizophrene's experiences are brought to expression. If, in the case of introverted instinctives, thought and feeling are only slightly developed, they are defenceless in the face of their intuitions, both as far as they themselves and others are concerned, since the possibility of control is very deficient.

If we compare this conception of the relationship between the disease-process and pre-disposition in schizophrenia with that offered by Kretschmer, we find, as in the case of the manic-depressive psychosis, points of agreement. In the manic-depressive psychosis, we drew the conclusion that the primitive forms of introjection, and a defence against external authority, are most readily developed in extraverted people with instinct or intuition as the predominating function. We found both these types combined without differentiation in Kretschmer's cyclothymic people, and the domination of instinctual tendencies over the function of feeling coincided to some extent with the descriptions of the psycho-analysts, in which the prevalence of oral and anal forms over the genital is emphasized. The influence of narcissism as a factor in pre-disposition would correspond rather with the predominance of intuition. Manic and depressive reactions may, according to this conception, occur under certain circumstances in everyone, but they will only be fixated in a manic or depressive state, where these mechanisms are, as a result of developmental conditions, particularly liable to come into play, and where the personality-structure has at its disposal no other modes of coping with the situation.

We may bring a similar point of view to bear on the relationship between mental mechanisms and characterological structure in schizophrenia, even if we take into account that here, as a last cause, a physical process may take place which may account both for the regression of the mechanisms and for the change of personality. Even if we confine the concept of projection to faulty or pathological mental happenings, there do nevertheless exist transitional stages to normal psychology, and the same is true, if in a less degree, of the magical influences and of the hallucinations. We may also assume here that, on the one hand, disturbances in development have led to fixations, increasing liability to the development of regressive forms under certain conditions. We do, in fact, find in certain people such manifestations, without any real schizophrenia developing as a result. On the other hand, we can understand that these mechanisms will most likely assume great significance in cases where there is no better way of dealing with the problems, or where such a better way no longer exists. Modern man is helped to make a better differentiation between internal and external influences by means of constant adjustments to the criteria of thought and feeling. We cannot imagine how our world would look apart from these collective influences. The ideas of the schizophrene give us some indication, but no clear picture, since he has not entirely abandoned his old conception of the world, and certain emotional problems are primarily expressed in it. Certain dreams give the clearest indication of the kinship between manifestations of the psychology of normal people and schizophrenia. In them also, introverted intuition plays the chief rôle in the formulation of certain emotional problems.

Primitive forms of projection arise most easily in a strongly introverted state, and where there is little differentiation of criticism and comparison, and we shall more readily expect this state of affairs in introverted people with instinct or intuition as their primary function. It seems to me that here also we can associate ourselves with Kretschmer in his description of the schizoid, although the correspondence is less clear than in the case of the cyclothymic character. The most obvious clinical point is that we cannot expect to find a well-developed emotional life in schizoids, and that spontaneously arising "crazy" notions often have powerful influence. In many cases, the function of thought seems to be retained longer, but on closer observation their thinking is usually found to take remarkable autistic forms, having as origin certain imaginations, and paying little attention to any current explanations. From the psycho-analytical point of view, these forms are related to the thought-forms of the obsessional neurotic, in which a similar play with thought is carried on. We may speak here of a regression of thought in the direction of more intuitive pre-forms. As far as instinct is concerned, we find in many manifestations, particularly in the stolid type of schizoid, clear indications that instinctual interests have profound influence (for example, in the hypochondriacal symptoms).

Here also the ideas of the psycho-analysts find a place, in their demonstration of the narcissistic and auto-erotic factors in the pre-disposition. Projection, as a means of escape from an intensely introverted state, is then seen as a regression to a situation in early childhood, when the sense of reality was still undeveloped, and feelings of omnipotence and of being abandoned led to a concept of the world in particular forms. In strongly introverted people, these forms remain always more or less in evidence, while the extravert has developed the representation of the world in his psychology into such a wealth of varied forms that he is not likely to linger for long over primitive concepts. From various directions we have been informed that we can sometimes get a better understanding of the schizophrenic mode of experiencing if we take primitive psychology as our starting-point, since there are here clearer manifestations for purposes of comparison than in childhood.[1] Here we can see, for example, how the personality does not begin as a unity, but is rather composed of parts (the different "souls"), which agrees with my conception, that aspects of our being are at first grasped by more or less concrete intuitions. There is still room for much investigation concerning this relationship between primitive psychology and the manifestations of schizophrenia, since we realize again and again how difficult it is for the modern man to imagine himself into primitive man. In this connection, it would be a sign of some advance if we gave up talking, without further evidence, of primitive "thinking".

It becomes more and more obvious in modern, less rationalistic psychology that many of our physical forms are related to primitive forms of experience. In introverted people, these forms come more readily to light, because their consciousness is less entirely subordinated to collective, conventional forms. In schizophrenes, these forms are given very much greater validity than in the healthy, or even in healthy introverts. This would make it appear that the boundary between the introverted individual and the schizophrene is a very ill-defined one, in which case the designation "schizoid" would be justified for the former. It seems to me probable, however, on closer observation, that the manifestations of schizophrenia demand a somewhat more complicated interpretation, since regression does not simply mean the re-establishment of a previous state. And in the second place, it should not be overlooked that the introverted mental mechanisms have undergone just as much development as have the extraverted, so that it would be wrong to represent the introverted individual as dominated by primitive (schizoid) mental mechanisms.

I should like, in conclusion, to sum up the results of this examina-

[1] Storch, "The Archaic Forms of Inner Experiences and Thoughts in Schizophrenia", *Nervous and Mental Diseases*, Monograph Series, New York, 1924.

tion of the significance of the types of conscious orientation for the psychoses. Kretschmer's differentiation of the cyclothymic and the schizoid character has great importance, but from the psychological point of view it proves to be too vague, and it confuses the boundaries between healthy and pathological manifestations. In contrast, the efforts of the psycho-analysts towards an exact description of the morbid mechanisms form a useful counter-balance. Both in the manic-depressive psychosis and in schizophrenia these mechanisms appear to be of a primitive kind. In the former case, they concern the introjection of external authority and its rejection, thus representing the earliest form of internalization. In schizophrenia, the mechanisms aim at a clearer, figurative distinction between internal and external, and they attempt in a rough way to draw the line between omnipotence and being abandoned. In all this, it becomes clear that the manic-depressive mechanisms assume great significance most readily where there is a predominance of extraversion, with little development of thought and feeling. Schizophrenic mechanisms also develop more easily when thought and feeling are little developed, but they are usually promoted by an intensely introverted state.

These conceptions link on to Kretschmer's descriptions, if we see in the schizoid type a combination of the introverted intuitive and instinctive types, and in the cyclothymic type a combination of the extraverted intuitive and instinctive types. If we realize that in the psychoses the psyche is overwhelmed by more primitive forms, we shall not be surprised to find in them the more primitive forms of intuition and instinct. These forms are readier to hand in the psychology of those types in which they, together with similar forms, have, in any case, the greatest influence.

PART III

A PHILOSOPHICAL COMMENTARY

CHAPTER I

THE OBJECTIVE BASIS OF PSYCHOLOGY

VARIOUS views are extant concerning the problem of whether psychology has an objective basis, and if so, where this lies. This being so, it would not seem superfluous for me to treat my views concerning the subject independently.

In considering this question, many investigators start from the fact that perception may be external or internal, and they proceed to postulate that the latter is specifically employed in grasping the material of psychology. This fact does not, however, seem to me to be an altogether suitable starting-point, for it assumes a good deal that would appear to require some investigation first. It seems to me that it is necessary first of all to enquire what perception is, and in what relation it stands to experience. We will accordingly first enquire what is the actual significance of experience.

Here I agree with Husserl's view, according to which the physical and the mental originate as extracts, extruded, as it were, from a single unified experience which is the basis of every possible kind of differentiation. This fundamental "phenomenological" experience is not identical with what I have named "instinctive experience", but includes this experience, together with every later development in the way of intuitive insight and its images, and of structures of thought and feeling. Phenomenological experience thus comprises both subjective and objective elements in a combination which is, at this stage, undifferentiated, although capable of differentiation.

It is, however, clear, that out of the totality of this experience we may select and observe certain contents and connections in isolation,[1] for example, the scientific aspect of some particular object. I regard perception as such a selection of a part of experience, originally made intuitively, and then tested in its relation

[1] As I have already stated, the possibility of differentiation and classification appears to me to have originated through spontaneous intuitions, and only later in the development of mankind has this possibility evolved into an organized body of knowledge concerning established mental forms.

to other perceived contents, and so becoming an object of thought. The question then arises, how far is this process of perception different for psychology from what it is for the natural sciences. There is a wide difference in the answers to this question. For some investigators, both the mode of perception and the mode of constructing perceptions into a scientific system are the same for psychology and for the natural sciences. Others see fundamental differences here. Let us first consider these two opposing conceptions independently. They appear in the form of two schools of psychology: the psychology of consciousness, and biological psychology, or psychology as a natural science.

For the psychology of consciousness there is an essential distinction between psychology and the natural sciences. This distinction is seen in an entirely different mode of selection in regard to phenomenological experience. While all the natural sciences leave out of account the whole of the subjective side of experience, in their attempt to exclude anything "merely subjective", the psychology of consciousness is pre-occupied with this very aspect, and neglects the external world, whose objects are recognized only as "my perceptions and ideas", not as having any actual existence. Since the work of Brentano, the essence of subjectivity is seen in a special kind of attention. The psychology of consciousness, or phenomenological psychology, thus studies that part of conscious experience which remains when the whole external world is excluded. This kind of independent "mental" experience is known to us all in the form of that immediate experience of the self by means of which alone we are able to express anything concerning ourselves. It seems to me of considerable importance to emphasize here, that this experience of the self is not identical with inner perception, nor with introspection. This experience of the self is an intuitive experience which selects from phenomenological experience certain associations related to the ego. And here also intuitive experience precedes any perception. When, in our experience of the self, we know that we are sad, or that we desire or intend something, this cannot be called a perception in the self. Real perception arises here, just as in experience of the external world, by means of something questionable, through oppositions in the realization of experience, whereby testing and comparison are stimulated. The evidence provided by intuition now gives place to doubt, and thought begins. Introspection belongs to the sphere of thought, and, for the psychology of consciousness, study begins with introspection. It will thus be clear that, in my view, introspection does not mean inner perception, but the perception of inner intuitive experiences.[1] The psychology of consciousness studies by means of introspection those associations or relationships in the immediate experience of the self which have been grasped intuitively. As in every evolution of knowledge, this means, not only the comparison of every fact of experience, once isolated, with a fixed body of knowledge, but also, as a result of questioning this, the possibility of stimulating a fresh point of view. But the latter is usually successful only with those having a special bent in this direction.

It is possible thus to investigate one's self, and to attain to a knowledge of one's self. But can knowledge in such a subjective field ever claim objective validity? Is it not at best a kind of personal knowledge, valid only for the self? If this is so, the psychology of consciousness would have to be excluded as a foundation for any scientific psychology, as indeed many investigators maintain, the most uncompromising in this respect being the Behaviourists. In opposition to this view, we have the opinion of the Solipsists, that only personal inner experience can claim real validity, that this personal knowledge is the only trustworthy kind of knowledge there is, and that any knowledge of an external world can never be more than an illusion. In both cases, however, conviction is based on a pre-conceived attitude, which is used as the starting-point for judgment. Thus from the outset a piece of metaphysical conviction is involved in the attempt to deal with experience. It is better not to start with an intuitive conception of what experience is as a whole, but with an exact description of what actually happens.

What would be the criterion of objectivity for a student of the psychology of consciousness, who set out on his research with objectivity as his aim? Let us take, as an example, the view of Husserl that every object in the external world is given to us against a background of horizons, so that we can never have it as an isolated experience. Why should such a view claim objective validity? Intuitive insight brings its own evidence, but this is not sufficient where thought is concerned, for here insight must be tested against other views and ideas bearing on the same subject, and, where possible, be confirmed by repeated recognition. The investigator will thus, by introspection, subject this view to constant questioning, as to whether it is regularly confirmed at different times and in relation to different objects. Other views, if he is

[1] This disposes of the question as to whether in consciousness there are two modes of activity, or only one, viz. conscious perception. Both are true. There are different ways in which the self is experienced which are capable of intuitive comprehension, but only one way of perceiving relationships.

unable to reconcile them, must likewise be investigated and tested afresh, to see if they will allow of modification to bring them into line with the totality of thought-forms. It is also part of the experience of the psychology of consciousness that communications from other persons enable us to confirm or question our own assumptions. The fact that the real existence of these persons is not assumed in the psychology of consciousness does not require the exclusion of this experience. Even in this branch of knowledge, comparison of one's own assumptions with the communications of others, concerning assumptions they have arrived at under similar circumstances, is of importance in reaching a conviction of objectivity.

The mode of testing is thus no different from that employed in the natural sciences. It is possible even to conduct experiments with one's self and with others. It is the kind of experience which is entirely different. Only those intuitions which relate to the ego are dealt with; all else is set on one side and left out of consideration. How far objectivity represents something different in the two kinds of scientific research remains to be considered more closely. In the psychology of consciousness, objectivity is, from the outset, admitted to have a subjective character; it has to be extracted from subjective experience, discovered within this. This has, however, nothing to do with the relative or absolute character of objective conviction. It is thus possible to maintain that a well-founded science may be derived from subjective experience, in which certain constant facts and laws are established which lay claim to objective validity. Thus we see that the psychology of consciousness is a science with a very special field of experience as its object of study.

Let us now compare this conception with that other one, which regards psychology as one of the natural sciences. For the adherents of this latter conception, the experience on which psychology is founded is of exactly the same character as that investigated in all the other sciences dealing with the external world, except that a different sphere of facts is selected for investigation. A psychology of this kind sets out to study phenomena of the external world in the same way as do the sciences of physics and anatomy, and any psychological understanding and explanation is primarily an understanding and explanation of other people. Only subsequently may they be applied to one's self. According to this conception, only experience of the object can be described as objective experience. In this respect, only the behaviour and expressions of other persons would be amenable to exact comprehension. Hence the Behaviourists, the most consistent defenders of this conception, see in an exact description of man's behaviour the only possible scientific basis for all psychology. It then becomes a part of biology, for, according to this conception, there is no essential distinction between human and animal psychology.

Let us look a little more closely at this point of view. If we ask ourselves in what way psychological convictions arise in ourselves, and how they have arisen in humanity as a whole, it certainly seems quite plausible that perception of other individuals may have provided the first stimulus for psychological explanation. And, indeed, we are stimulated to psychological considerations every day because of the behaviour of other people. If we try to fit these facts into our scheme of the functions, we might put it somewhat as follows: Intuitive judgments, in selecting certain relationships from instinctual experience, will often have as their content the relationships existing between other individuals, and between other individuals and ourselves. If this kind of intuitive discernment is elaborated into ideas, thus giving the possibility of thought concerning our fellow-men, this will furnish the building-stones for a psychological understanding and explanation, in which certain images (visual at first, but later primarily verbal) will become associated with certain modes of behaviour. In this way there arises a recognition of psychological forms, which for a long time remains naïve, uncritical, and (as in every science) closely bound up with intuitions, and which is only gradually subjected to testing and arrangement, as a result of mutual communication. There seems to be no doubt that the earliest psychological knowledge is pre-occupied more with the behaviour of our fellow-men than with introspection. Also, one might concede that the way in which these intuitive judgments are developed into a science cannot be shown to be in any way different from the manner in which biology, or indeed any of the natural sciences, has developed. In every case, certain relationships are selected by means of intuitions, from the unity of the world as it presents itself to us, and are given a separate existence. They are then tested against other illustrations of the same relationship, so that gradually a world of objects and of determined and determinable relationships arises. The totality of the body of settled knowledge becomes enormous, while the mode of testing and perceiving it undergoes refinement. The interrogation of nature by means of experiments grows ever more exact. All this may be applied to the study of mankind, even though, in comparison with the investigation of inanimate nature, it has only comparatively recently been done in any systematic way. Today, however, we have without any doubt a science which may claim the designation of a natural science of psychology, and which is elaborating and will continue to elaborate, with ever increasing exactitude, its own peculiar methods of research.

We have now landed ourselves in a difficult situation. We have two quite different kinds of psychology, working on quite different methods, and to some extent opposed to one another, and we have justified both of them, and have recognized them both as scientific. We shall not only have made both kinds of psychologists into our opponents, but my readers will, moreover, perhaps feel this point of view to be confusing and scientifically dishonest. I might try to save myself by an attempt to explain both points of view psychologically, and by maintaining that the psychology of consciousness corresponds to an introverted, and the natural science of psychology to an extraverted, attitude. No doubt we shall find convinced supporters of the first conception among introverts, and of the second among extraverts, although this will not always be the case, for other factors are also at work. But this is not only not a solution of the problem of the two psychologies, on the contrary it rather declares it to be insoluble, for it suggests that there is a different kind of truth for different types. This, however, does not appear to me to be correct, for, after all, the classification into introverts and extraverts only signifies a reference to certain emphases in individuals. We will not, therefore, make use of this excuse, but will try to find a way of reconciling the two kinds of psychology.

One difficulty certainly arises from the fact that in our minds the idea of natural science has quite involuntarily become a somewhat rigid and dogmatic conception, providing us with a certain support, and, in consequence, a standard of comparison for much that is less certain. The objectivity of natural science appears as something absolutely unassailable, so that we no longer even enquire how this conviction has come into being. It would, however, be useful here to examine psychologically how this conviction has developed.

Neither ontogenetically nor phylogenetically do we find in men an objective conception of nature in the sense that natural science of the present day has it. On the contrary, the conception of nature that we find in children and in primitive man appears rather, in comparison with our conception, as a projection of subjective experience. Objects are endowed with a soul, with sex, and are considered as exerting influence on one another, as men do. Animals also are seen much more humanized than would accord with our mode of judgment. Primitive understanding and explanation of natural phenomena doubtless occur by means of empathy or identification. Hence the world appears to primitive man and to the child as unquestionably alive. What is this empathy, regarded psychologically? It is a kind of intuition, for it means the comprehension of a whole in its relationships. But all intuitions are not expressions of empathy. There is something extra, namely, the experience of the self. In empathy, a relationship is understood as if the self had a part in it. This kind of concrete intuition by means of a projection of the self into the object is probably the original form of intuition, and even now it still plays a large part, especially in intuitive people. Abstract intuition seems to me to be a later acquisition. Thus it is possible to defend the view that both context and object were first comprehended by means of empathy, long before any thinking or causal explanation were possible.

Even in the most abstract conceptions of natural science we can still trace vestiges of empathy. When certain bodies are regarded as attracting or repelling each other, or as producing energy, a projection of ego-experience has a part in the idea. How, then, has this emphatic understanding of nature gradually become dehumanized, until it has become an abstract explanation of causes? This question is, in my view, identical with that of the origin of thought. From the world of experienced associations, won through the projection of the self, has arisen the world of objective relationships evolved by means of abstraction and examination. As I have already demonstrated (p. 53), thought begins with doubt, arising from contradictions in the practical consequences of certain views which were arrived at intuitively. These views, by friction with one another, then come to be modified, whereby the process of abstraction arises in its most primitive form. Much of the content of an intuition may be confirmed, but only a part of the whole, and that only subject to conditions, is demonstrably correct. This process still has great significance, and every development in science is founded on it. By means of this process, that which is subjectively determined by empathy is in most cases proved to be untenable. We have all had experience of this, when, for example, we think we have, by some projection of ourselves, understood an animal, and have subsequently had to recognize that its behaviour is to be understood as the result of quite a different set of circumstances. Concrete intuition was a bridge which now breaks down. By this bridge, however, we have reached the experience of a connection, and usually, moreover, even the recognition of a false intuitive judgment will have brought with it a positive gain. What remains, in the form of an abstract from the subjective experience, will always be recoverable in the same way. The concrete experience of the intuition is reduced, through friction against fixed and tested knowledge, to an abstract judgment. The essence of thought consists in an adjustment of certain contents to the total fixed deposit of earlier experience, whereby reductions and abstractions come into being. The original empathetic experience is then in the extreme case of theoretical physics reduced to a few fundamental properties such as matter, energy and direction. Instead of an association that is experienced, one that is arrived at by calculation, based statistically on accumulated experience, comes more and more into the foreground, as the main factor. The association that is experienced remains, however, in spite of this, the fundamental fact from which all concepts of associations and matter are derived, by means of ever-increasing abstraction from concrete intuitive experiences.

Workers in the field of natural science, with their concepts and methods ready-made for them, have, as a rule, no recognition of this fact. For them, their fundamental concepts and classifications are just as objective as are the facts which they are investigating. Only in recent times has it been more and more clearly discerned—particularly in certain schools of philosophy, but also in some sciences—that the fundamental concepts and forms in the arrangement and classification of material are subjectively determined. Nernst's postulate that probably all natural laws are statistical in character has already attained almost classical importance in the history of science.[1]

It appears thus that even the objectivity of the natural sciences is not absolute and determined from without, but is rather a task to be understood only as conditioned by subjectivity, and perhaps never to be more than approximately accomplished. Control of objectivity in our hypotheses has thus to be ensued not only by means of an ever more exact examination of the external world, but also by examination of the methods of classification and of fundamental concepts, that is to say, of the subjective aspect.

Many investigators will admit—if they recognize this aspect of scientific control at all—that, in theory, this problem of the development of objectivity from subjectivity exists, but having done so, they will frequently cease to pay much attention to it, regarding it as of little practical importance. It is also conceivable that it is not of equal importance for all sciences. In psychology, however,

[1] W. Nernst, "Zum Gültigkeitsbereich der Naturgesetze", *Die Naturwissenschaften*, Heft 21. (No English translation.)

it most certainly cannot be neglected, without causing a great deal of confusion. Only by recognizing the subjective aspect of all scientific methods is it possible to envisage the organic unity that exists in the two kinds of psychology: the psychology of consciousness, and the natural science of psychology. For we realize then that this paradox is not characteristic of psychology alone, although it is of particular importance here, and that it has often been emphasized to an impermissible degree, so that it has appeared insoluble. If we are to establish this more thoroughly, it is necessary for us to look at the problem from a somewhat different angle.

When, in any science, an hypothesis is postulated, this hypothesis may be tested and controlled in three different ways:

First, its validity in relation to the facts on which it is founded may be examined. How far, for example, must the relationship which has been grasped intuitively be limited to certain circumstances? How far has the selection of ultimate causes from experience been correct? and so on.

Secondly, one may investigate the mental condition of the person who makes the hypothesis, in order to test its validity. Was he intoxicated, or excited, or inhibited by prejudices, or too stupid to grasp the situation? In such cases, it would indeed be an extraordinary accident if the hypothesis nevertheless turned out to be correct.

Thirdly, one may test the internal structure of the hypothesis. The facts may be correctly understood, but something may be deduced from them for which there is no true justification. The form of the argument proves to have a flaw. Here a general knowledge of scientific form is the basis of criticism.

These different modes of testing hold good for every science. In practice, however, they are not of equal importance in every science. It is expected of a worker in natural science that he should have learned to think correctly, and to exclude his subjective impulses in his observation, so that in describing his perceptions and his experiments he lays stress almost exclusively on the first mode of testing. All the same, experience will soon show that even here the second mode—and, indeed, very occasionally the third mode—has not become entirely superfluous. Originally, subjective influences were much more openly discussed, even in natural science. Today, such discussions are more often held in private. In psychology, this restriction has not yet become so general.

In psychology, however, the second kind of criticism is of special importance. Certainly it does not stand alone in this. It shares this situation with all the sciences which have reference to humanity, such as history, the state, religion, art, etc. Some people doubt if it is possible to achieve any objectivity, of the kind aimed at in the natural sciences, in these domains. If one studies the development, from the historical point of view, of the objectivity which obtains today in the natural sciences, the conviction very soon arises, that we are dealing with a difference, not of kind, but of degree, and there follows the hope that humanity will find the way even here, if not to an absolute, at least to a very much greater objectivity. We will now proceed to examine how far such a process is likely to complicate our notion of objectivity.

It is, however, possible to maintain forthwith that a psychology of consciousness is indispensable not only for the examination of hypotheses [1] in regard to their logic and their form, but also for the exclusion of subjective influences on these hypotheses. That this is often overlooked by workers in the field of natural science, is the consequence of a certain mechanization in their methods, and of a superficial scientific attitude. They have become accustomed to handing over the checking of their hypotheses in many cases to instruments. But the human element can, even so, never be wholly eliminated. What happens in the mind of the student of natural science as he examines the findings of his instruments? Does he not also examine himself? Does he not have to eliminate his own wishes, to check his own pre-conceived opinions? Sometimes his instruments will help him in this, but sometimes they will not. He must have some knowledge of himself, and only the psychology of consciousness can give him this, for, as a science of one's own personality, it alone enables us to see and control ourselves objectively. The more consciously and the more scientifically he does this, the better able is he to exclude sources of error. Moreover, he must constantly make use of his philosophical knowledge and critical capacity, for these give him the power of judgment in matters of form and intellect. This is true in equal measure for the student of natural science and for the psychologist, whether the latter is working as a student of natural science or as a psychologist pre-occupied with his own consciousness. (It is for this reason that logic is a pre-requisite in all the sciences.)

The criticism of subjective influences, with their clouding of judgment, is almost as important for the maintenance of object-

[1] This examination then belongs no longer to psychology, but to the realm of philosophy. The psychology of consciousness, however, provides the material from which the philosopher gains his insight and builds up his concepts.

ivity in psychology as is the control of facts. And the psychologist will get even less help here from instruments alone than does the physicist or the chemist. Hence training in objective perception must be even more careful in the case of the psychologist than it is normally expected to be in the natural sciences. And in this training, the psychology of consciousness must always be an important factor, although this is not recognized by many investigators. The question may, however, be asked as to whether the rôle of the psychology of consciousness is confined in psychology, as it is in the case of the natural sciences, to this work of control or criticism. We must therefore consider more closely this problem of objectivity in psychology.

So far, the result of our investigation has been that we have seen that every objective observation represents an abstraction from a subjective experience, in natural science just as in the psychology of consciousness; and that various modes of control and criticism make a true objectivity possible. Immediate instinctual experience of the world, of men and of ourselves, and the immediate intuitive grasp of relationships in these spheres, is something quite different from the world, mankind and one's self as seen objectively in thought, and particularly in their scientific settings. Thought has, from immediate instinctual and intuitive experience, created something which is quite different. The relationship between immediate experience and objectified experience has been very variously regarded by different investigators. For some, the objectified experience of thought is the true reality, while for others, these thought-images are merely instruments, a net thrown over reality, to enable us to ensnare it; only a world of "as if . . ." The psychologist need not concern himself with the metaphysical problems that arise here. One thing, however, is clear to him, namely, that, from the psychological point of view, objectified experience is a more recent achievement. Whether it grasps the true meaning of the world, or is of pragmatic significance only, at any rate it has been gradually evolved by man from other modes of experience. And the psychologist asks himself how this process of objectification takes place psychologically, and what it is that determines whether an objectification is to be considered true or false.

We saw that originally all conscious comprehension probably occurred by means of concrete intuitions, through a projection of the self into the objects concerned. This does not apply to all conscious *experience*, for instinctual experience of the world involves no intellectual comprehension. But we also found that the natural sciences systematically excluded anything subjective. This means that this original mode of comprehending the world is later systematically reduced in all those aspects which are not subjective. The object, after having been comprehended first of all as a subject, now assumes in this way a dehumanized objectivity. Even one's fellow-man, by means of a further dehumanization, comes to be regarded, under the term "person", as practically a thing. Abstraction in natural science turns everything in the world into objects or things. This tendency is not found at all in the beginning of science. Compare, for instance, a description by the alchemists of some chemical process, with the description in a textbook of chemistry. Does this materialization come about only through abstraction from intuitive insight, or is there another factor involved? I believe that there is an additional factor, which may explain both this extreme materialization and atomization, and also the belief in the absolute validity of this conception of the world. This factor is connected with instinctual experience.

Instinctual experience is the original basis of all experience. It is more immediate than intuitive experience, because it is always there and it offers the most dependable contact with the environment. Although intuition may often, through insight into relationships and possibilities, give support where instinctual action offers nothing, nevertheless nearly everyone in his ordinary behaviour is initially guided by instinctual experience. Intuitions, deliberations and feelings contribute important amplifications, and these may with many people play a very important part. But it is from the instinctive sphere that we derive our experience of continuity both in the world of sensations and in our own being in its relation with time (Bergson's "*temps vécu*"). Thought is occupied first of all with the fixing and arranging of relationships and facts, selected by intuition from the instinctive sphere, in accordance with their proved value. But there follow, however, other intuitions, by means of which we perceive in a comprehensive vision[1] the individual structures of these thought-products in their context, and thus arrive at a comprehension of totalities in the structure of a science or of a conception of the world. After an increasing number of isolated experiences have been established as scientific facts, the possibility of thought concerning them, perceived intuitively, awakens an ambition to include the whole of instinctive experience in controlled systems of facts and relationships. Experience is no longer isolated and classified for practical purposes only, but

[1] The Author uses the term "*Überkuppelnde Intuitionen*" here; literally "over-spanning intuitions".—TRANSLATOR'S NOTE.

we want to be able to give an account of every possibility in the way of experience—"art for art's sake". In this way, there arises the modern scientific conception of the world, which adheres as closely as possible to all that can be confirmed or foreseen in the world of instinctual experience. The more possible it becomes to survey experience by means of stable thought-images, thus rendering adaptation a matter of calculation, the more superfluous does intuition become; for every possible intuition is anticipated in this conception of the world. Hence it appears much safer to stick to this controlled experience than to try to discover relationships afresh for oneself. Thought-structures, adhering closely to instinctual experience, furnish a system which includes every possible association. These structures are not identical with instinctual experience. For instance, they exclude as far as possible all that is qualitative. But they prove to be superior to, and more trustworthy than, immediate experience, and hence they are for many people (particularly those of thinking-type) more essential than this.

In order to comprehend every possible relationship, it is necessary to analyse experiences in as great detail as possible. Hence we get an atomized conception of the world, with fixed mechanical relationships. The more comprehensive vision provided by intuition [1] has rendered possible the recognition of certain structures appertaining to the sphere of thought, and in accordance with these everything is arranged and classified. These structures then tend to assume a mechanical character, from which every human element is excluded. Finally, we get a very reliable, very comprehensive, somewhat rigid picture of the world, which is imposed upon us because of its practical validity, and because of the fact that we all make use of it.[2]

In this way, what was originally a practical method of grouping

[1] See Translator's Note on p. 264.

[2] All the products of intuitive insight, of feeling and of thought may, in fact, be transferred into the instinctive sphere, to become habits there making for further mechanical adaptation, without any real insight, feeling or thought. Many investigators do not distinguish this mechanical habit-thinking from living thought. This kind of thinking, expressing itself, for instance, in routine knowledge, is, from the point of view of conscious orientation, more akin to instinctual behaviour than to thought, although it arose in the beginning from a true act of thought. There are plenty of people who are capable of making use of thought-forms in the service of a kind of instinct-training, but who are less capable of themselves making deductions concerning relationships. Since our education provides us with thought-systems, this kind of instinct-training is, in fact, part of the development of all thought-forms. Learning by heart belongs to this instinctual, technical aspect of thinking.

and classification, and should have served to stimulate fresh insight and freer activity, has become something absolute, extraordinarily intimidating and inhibiting to intuition, and tending to an ever-increasing mechanization of human behaviour. It certainly puts into man's possession the sum-total of knowledge in regard to species, but it reduces his capacity to work on this himself, because he is no longer expected to make his own observations, but has to accept a ready-made body of objective knowledge. With such a state of affairs there is no longer any demand for control, by means of examination of subjective influences, of opinions alleged to be objective. In this way, the objectivity of natural science is simplified by means of a convenient, but not always permissible, mechanization.

Let us now return to psychology. Here we also find the influence of this fixed kind of scientific objectification, embracing the whole of experience. To some psychologists, it appears as the highest aim to relate their knowledge in some way to this fixed, objectified world. In this case, objectivity means for the psychologist merely that he associates his perceptions with "things". He attempts this by means of general hypotheses (such as that of psycho-physical parallelism), which then take on the authority of a creed; or by a general relation of mental structures to physical make-up (such as Kretschmer has attempted); or by an exact observation and, where possible, measurement of the physical manifestations or performances which accompany mental activity (as is done in experimental psychology). All these points of view have, of course, their value, theoretical and practical, but what they seek to prove goes far beyond this value, and is connected with metaphysical pre-suppositions which are not, or are at most only partially, discerned. That it is possible to isolate mental material and see it objectively, appears fundamentally incredible to these investigators, and, consciously or unconsciously, they seek support in that conception of the world which the natural sciences give.

This is, however, not very psychological, since from the psychological aspect this scientific conception of the world can only be regarded as a creation, evolved gradually in the human mind from a wealth of subjective experience. Although it is perfectly true that we accept this conception more or less ready-made, and that it has enormous practical and intellectual significance in the whole of our conscious life, yet it is definitely not primary, and it can only be regarded as absolute from a metaphysical, not from the psychological, point of view. The psychologist must therefore allow for a certain relativity in his estimation of this conception of the world, which will come all the more easily to him, in that, since Einstein's work, even the physicists take a similar point of view. But it follows from this, that the main emphasis will now no longer rest on the problem of objectivity, but on that of objectification. Thus it has become fairly obvious that two modes of objectification in natural science can be distinguished: (*a*) a more complicated kind, which examines not only the system of facts, but also that aspect of it which is concerned with forms and with the psychology of consciousness; and (*b*) a simple form, which attempts merely the placing of what is discovered within the conception of the world which has already been objectified. And it will be clear that this latter simple form is not very suitable for psychology, for the very reason that the latter is a young science in which intuitions are of considerable importance. Much more important is another circumstance, however, and this we must now consider.

I do not think Bergson is right, when he maintains that intuition can understand only living, and intellect only inanimate, nature. The inventor of a machine, when he suddenly perceives certain connections in the reactions of matter, having previously surmised something of the kind quite intuitively, has employed his intuitive function on inanimate nature. All perception of relationships is connected with intuition. And all abstraction and classification in a system of knowledge points to thought, whether living or dead matter is involved. When thought has evolved fixed ideas in some field, that which first appeared as intuition may be accepted in the form of thought by people who have never themselves intuitively perceived the associations involved. They appropriate these products theoretically and practically. In doing so, they may come to a living perception of the subject, supposing they learn to grasp the connections intuitively, but it may remain for them a matter of rote-learning. This latter mechanical mode of appropriating the results of research is, however, much more possible in the case of inanimate than of living things. So far, Bergson is right. Mechanized thought has far-reaching uses in the control of a machine. But when a mother attempts to make use of educational views, which she has accepted as a result of her belief in an authority, without any intuitive comprehension, she is not likely to get much practical advantage from them. When it is a question of living nature, and particularly when it concerns our fellow-men and their affairs, we are usually dealing with very complicated contexts, which must be perceived afresh in all their variations if they are to be rightly understood. Intuition must always prepare the way here for the classification which thought enables. This may, however, also occur in natural science, and is not specific for psychology. In psychology, there is something else, namely, that these intuitions are not simply abstract observations, but concrete experiences of empathy. What does this mean?

We come here to a point which has been particularly emphasized by Jaspers.[1] He has drawn a sharp distinction between the understanding that results from empathy, and plays a great part in psychology, and the reasoned causal explanation, which is characteristic of the natural sciences. So sharp is the distinction, indeed, that there appears to be no bridge between the two. According to him, causal explanation only exists in the natural sciences, and understanding by means of empathy only in psychology. It will be clear from my reasoning that I cannot follow him here. I regard an understanding by means of empathy as the starting-point of all natural science, and I esteem causal explanation as admissible in psychology. In my terminology, understanding through empathy is comprehension by means of concrete intuitions, and reasoned explanation is comprehension by means of thought-structures. And it seems to me to be true for all science that all thought-structures originally developed from intuitions (some at first from concrete intuitions, others directly from abstract ones). Nevertheless, Jaspers is to some extent correct in his differentiation. For while, in the natural sciences, intuitions can be readily separated from ego-experience, in psychology many of them remain in concrete form, and understanding through empathy is seen here as a constant necessity, while in other fields it has in most situations been resolved into other forms of intellectual comprehension. Objectification, which has become in relation to nature something more or less mechanical, and usually presents itself only as an historical problem, remains, therefore, in the psychological field (as also in the mental sciences) a real problem. We may ask ourselves daily: How far is my insight into this or that person objective? Here, if anywhere, we learn that there are limits to any objectifying comprehension, that it stands for an ideal which is never quite attained.

The difference between objectification in psychology and in the natural sciences, such as chemistry and physics, lies also in the fact that the process of abstraction from the concrete intuitions by which the world is comprehended has, in psychology, not only

[1] Jaspers, *Allgemeine Psychopathologie*, 2nd Ed., 1920. (No English translation.)

been carried much less far than in the natural sciences, but that, from its very nature, it cannot be carried so far. But this also means, at the same time, that even when the attempt is made to carry objectification as far as possible, it assumes a particular form which it shares with the mental sciences. For objectification relates here not only to the object concerned, but to one's personal attitude to the object.

Let us take, for purposes of comparison, a scientific explanation and an act of empathy. When I reflect how the pictures in a film give the illusion of a continuous movement, and in explanation picture to myself the extent in time of a visual impression on the retina, my thoughts move in objective images which entirely exclude my own subjective experience. Perception of movement is in physiology regarded as the experience of any individual, not as my personal experience. If, however, I follow the content of the film, and make psychological observations concerning it, I am likewise objectifying, but my subjective experience is the means to this objectification and cannot be entirely excluded. Concrete intuitive perception, being simultaneously ego-experience and object-comprehension, is thus objectified from two sides. We already know these two kinds of objectification as phenomenological and scientific objectification, but up till now we have regarded them as two modes of exclusion. Here, however, they are not mutually exclusive, but complementary. *All psychology, as also all mental science, objectifies not one side of experience only, but requires the objectification of both sides in reference to one another.* While the natural sciences employ the psychology of consciousness only as an aid in excluding inappropriate material, in psychology and the mental sciences this process of exclusion has an important, positive significance of its own, namely, ego-experience as that aspect of empathy which gives it meaning in the process of objectifying. My description of the content of a film pre-supposes the possibility of a certain form of experience. Hence I can only talk about it with people who also have the same experience, or who are able to objectify it, so that differences in our subjective experience can be compared.

This task of the objectification of subjective experience, as part of psychological objectification, has only recently been defined, and its significance is still not properly appreciated by some investigators. While this kind of objectification has been recognized as a problem and dealt with by the mental sciences, chiefly from the phenomenological aspect, it is in its psycho-analytical aspect that it is most prominent in psychology. This has come about more by chance than by deliberate intent, and consequently the psycho-analysts themselves are for the most part not clearly conscious of the problem. It will be worth while, therefore, to consider this problem somewhat more fully, since the co-operation of psycho-analysis and phenomenology in its solution is likely to be very fruitful.

Phenomenology in the field of psychology attempts to objectify the subjective aspect of personal activity, by elaborating inner observations derived from intuitive insight concerning this activity, and then classifying them. By this means, fundamental differences may be understood, which subsequently prove to be of great importance in the understanding of other people. In this way, their attitude is objectified by means of distinctions discovered in ourselves. Psycho-analysis works in another way. It secures its objectifications of subjective attitudes, in the first place, from other people, not from personal introspection. Psycho-analysis is a method, derived from psychotherapy, by which all the isolated occurrences in the way of behaviour and speech revealed by patients are understood (they themselves being unaware of their significance), and subsequently, by means of an objectifying of these intuitions concerning others, built up into a body of knowledge concerning their problems. Thus it is here not our own subjective attitudes, but the ego-activity of other people, from which, when it has been intuitively understood, observations are abstracted and arranged in a systematic body of knowledge. In this manner, Freud has been able to develop an entirely new psychology of subjective attitudes. He has investigated the history of peculiarities in these attitudes, and has been able to explain them as determined by experiences and by groups of instinctual drives. As a result of this work, the objectification of subjective attitudes has become possible in a way quite different from introspection, and psycho-analytical psychology has thus evolved another kind of psychological objectification from two aspects, the aspect of surmised contents and that of ego-activity.

Our next question must concern the relationship between phenomenological and psycho-analytical objectification of ego-activity. Some psycho-analysts hold the view that this kind of objectification, drawn direct from the object, is the only reliable and objective kind, and that psycho-analysis represents a natural science of psychology and is able to dispense with introspection. This does not strike me as quite correct, because it would mean that an important part of the process in objectification is overlooked. It is true that psycho-analytical views represent deductions relating to other people, while phenomenological views have the activity of the self as their subject-matter. In this way, there is a resemblance to natural science. But, as I have already explained, it is not possible for natural science to dispense entirely with introspection, since abstraction from intuitive insight pre-supposes some control of subjective activity. This is, of course, no less true of the concrete intuitions which the psycho-analyst arrives at through his empathy. These have to be controlled, not only by comparison with other experiences with the same patient, and with the totality of our knowledge of mental contexts, but also by the prevention of any subjective projections on to the patient. Freud has indeed not overlooked this fact, from the practical point of view, for he requires that every analyst must himself be thoroughly analysed before he takes up this profession. In this way, the analyst attains a knowledge of his own subjective attitudes, and is thus able to exclude them in his observation of his patients. When this analysis of the analyst has once taken place, it seems, according to the theory of psycho-analysis, that the objectivity of the analyst's intuitive understanding of the patient may now be assumed. If this were so, the status of the worker in natural science would be attained, of whom it is also assumed that he observes objectively. But two objections may be raised to this. In the first place, we are never quite sure, even in the case of the worker in natural science, of his absolute objectivity, and there is therefore still need for constant introspective control; and in the second place, such control is doubly necessary in the case of empathy, because here a subjective attitude can never be entirely excluded.

The psycho-analyst is thus not in a position to dispense with introspection, because he needs it for inner control in correct objectification. Moreover, for abstract representation of objectified experience, phenomenological control is a necessary factor. And in the third place, this control seems to me important for the objectification of one's personal point of view. The latter does not, it is true, play a very important part in practice, but in systematic expositions it is necessary to be able to compare one's own position with that of others, since otherwise a personal point of view will develop into philosophical dogmatism. This relative attitude to one's own point of view is only possible with the aid of phenomenological introspection.

If phenomenology is indispensable to psycho-analysis, it is also true that phenomenological observation can only be entirely fruitful if it is supported by psycho-analytical observation. For, in the first place, the objectification of the attitudes of other people covers an infinitely larger field than the phenomenological objectification of one's own attitude could ever offer. Moreover, it furnishes an intuitive understanding of subjective attitudes which would otherwise remain obscure. But most important of all is the fact that it provides the only possible control from without of introspective observations, for these are expressed to the analyst and by him understood and objectified along with previous utterances and actions of the patient, while at the same time they are to some extent arranged in a phenomenologically verifiable context. Thus, although some of the results of this work have no reference to phenomenology, yet, on the other hand, they do provide a wealth of material which may be understood introspectively. This proves, moreover, that one's own ego-attitude may be objectified not only from within, but also from without. In this important function of psychology, both methods are mutually complementary.

Psychology has thus in the realm of science a peculiar, and indeed central, position, since abstraction from concrete experience can, from its very nature, never be completely accomplished, and hence certain aspects of experience, neglected in other sciences, can never be entirely disregarded. There are boundary regions where psychology overlaps to some extent the natural sciences, phenomenology, and the mental sciences. But as soon as it identifies itself with any one of these branches of learning, it ceases to be psychology.

Natural science excludes the subjective aspect of experience, and this is permissible, because the subjective attitude of the student in this field is simple and unambiguous, so that, in relation to the complexity of objective description, it may be safely neglected. But when experimental psychology describes merely the experiences or the reactions of the subject in relation to some specific stimulus, without taking into account his mental attitude, then it becomes the physiology of sensation, and ceases to be psychology. However simple the subjective attitude may be, it must be referred to in psychology.

Phenomenology excludes the objective side of experience. This may be done without loss, where the objective aspect is so simple or unambiguous that in objectification, compared with the ego-aspect, it plays no part. But when only inner relationships and processes are observed, without any reference to the concrete person existing in the world, it is impossible to count this kind of study as psychology. Psychology, as a natural science, and phenomenological psychology are thus both boundary regions of psychology, which can never themselves be described either as exclusively a natural science, or entirely a matter of phenomenology.

The mental sciences also deal with both objective and subjective aspects of experience, but they are not on that account identical with psychology. For they seek only what is collectively true, and exclude purely personal experience. Abstraction is also carried much farther than in psychology. When jurisprudence deals with the question of a personal sense of justice, it becomes psychology. And *vice versa,* when the psychologist treats of justice, art or religion as structures having a separate existence, apart from the concrete experience of the individual, he has ceased to work as a psychologist. But there is a borderland of psychology where it encroaches upon mental science, just as it does on natural science and on phenomenology.

The essence of psychology thus consists in the study of concrete experience, with its inter-relations between objective and subjective influences, from which ultimately all established objectified forms are constructed. These forms are assumed by the other sciences to be objective, but for the psychologist they are subjectively conditioned, and the abstraction that has made them possible is a problem for study. Hence the psychologist can learn from everyone, but it follows, too, that his findings are of importance for all the other sciences.

There remains still a further important problem to discuss, which is of extreme significance, especially in this present critical phase in the history of psychology. If in psychology (and in the mental sciences) objectification concerns not only the objective aspect of experience, but also its subjective aspect, we may ask how far objectification is thereby restricted in its aims. With this kind of objectification the possibility of shared experience is presupposed. In law, too, an article can only be understood from the point of view of certain ego-attitudes, and in art the work of an artist only speaks to us when we are in a certain frame of mind. In so far as we understand this, we are in a position to attempt the objectification of this subjective aspect of experience. But we learn that this understanding frequently lets us down. Then we are inclined to regard the other fellow as abnormal or crazy, we reject the law as senseless, and the artist's work appears to us as distorted and without significance. Not only does an aspect of the objectification of subjective experience become impossible in certain cases, but we may be inclined, on the other hand, to ascribe a position of importance in objectification, and consequently, in theory, to personal subjective attitudes which control our own lives. The result of this is seen in the fact that there are a variety of psychologies and a variety of tendencies in the mental sciences. The objectification of subjective experience is here from the beginning based on differing points of view.

We are now in a position to give more precision to our problem. We saw that both phenomenology and psycho-analysis attempt, though in different ways, to objectify the subjective aspect of experience. Are their methods ahead of other psychological methods in this, or does there exist a whole series of possible modes of scientific observation? And how far is it indeed in any way possible to deduce objective facts and rules from what is entirely subjective? We shall have to consider the problem of objectification a little more closely.

What is implied in the objectification of the subjective attitude which is part of some experience? In the case of a purely scientific observation it implies something fairly unambiguous, and this subjective attitude may, therefore, in the further objectification demanded by the natural sciences, be taken for granted and neglected. In the case of a political conviction or of a religious belief, such a subjective attitude implies something much more pivotal, affecting the existence of the whole personality. One may be able to grasp intuitively this attitude, by means of an act of identification, but in order to make a true objectification of the experience, it will be necessary to give central importance to the fundamental orientation of the personality, and this demand gives to all psychological observation a particular kind of stamp. This holds, not only for attitudes universally considered as basic, such as concern morals or religion, but for those individual attitudes arising from affectively overwhelming experiences, such as are seen in pathological conditions, such as delusions of reference, litigiousness and paranoia.

In psychology, we find in such influences, arising from basic attitudes and affecting the whole of theoretical objectification, the source of many scientific tendencies which work at cross-purposes with one another. These tendencies have for their adherents a much more convincing appeal than have any other kinds of psychology. In this way, certain comprehensive intuitions[1] concerning the essence of existence are taken as the starting-point for a system of thought, and as a result, "observations" concerning individual intuitive experiences take on immediately a certain colouring. How far is all objectification of ego-activity subject to such influence, whereby certain aspects of this activity are from the outset con-

[1] See Translator's Note on p. 264.

sidered more essential, of greater value and significance than others? Is it an illusion to think that we have found a point of view which will enable us to overcome this subjectivity (as, for example, the phenomenologists and psycho-analysts think)? Would the only honest, practicable possibility be to permit the determination of psychology by an attitude born of an all-comprehending intuition, i.e. by a metaphysical conviction? [1]

It seems to me that we need here a further distinction. If it is a question of understanding the life, the mode of existence, of an individual, this seems to me to be only possible if one sets out from such a basic attitude. It is for this reason that a painter of genius can with a few strokes conjure up the essence of an individual, better than a hundred photographs. Such an intuitive comprehension probes more deeply into the mystery of an individual life than any psychological description. In the same way, a fairly universal basic attitude, shared by several people, can usually be better elucidated as such, than by means of intellectual abstractions. Yet thought comes into play here also, attempting objectification from the standpoint of this basic attitude (as, for example, in theology or in some aspects of jurisprudence). Some people, with their concrete, practical lives, are more at home with reasoning of this kind than with abstract contemplation, which seeks to avoid any subjective starting-point; just as a literary and psychological biography gives a more lifelike picture of an individual than a series of experimental psychological investigations concerning him. The more the description of an individual's psychology gains in general validity, the more does the essence of the said individual elude one. The only possible way to avoid this seems to be to base one's objectification on a certain basic attitude.

Is it, however, the function of psychology to comprehend in this manner the essence of the individual? Is not abstraction the essence of all science? The natural sciences, after all, only provide the means for a survey of a given concrete material in its connections; they have to accept this material itself, and can do no more than describe it; they cannot explain it, they can only expound and examine its connections with other given material. Originally, matters concerning metaphysics, taste and religion were intermingled with scientific observation, and this may indeed have made science appear much more living to its enthusiasts than it appears today, for it must have seemed in those days to give a more direct

[1] Dr Robert Wälder in his lecture on "Die latenten metaphysischen Grundlagen der psychologischen Schulen" approaches this point of view (*Abhandlungen aus der Neur. Psychiatrie, Psychologie und ihren Grenzgebieten*, Heft 61).

access to the mysteries of nature. Natural science is today more modest and timid in this respect, but this does not mean that the relationship between man and nature has ceased. In many respects, this relationship is more intensively sought than before. But the search takes place, for the most part, outside the sphere of natural science, in travelling, sport, etc. Natural science can indeed give access to nature, but its usual means of approach is by way of thought.

A similar, but more modest rôle is played by psychology in psycho-analysis and in phenomenology. It has given up the attempt to understand the essence of an individual or of his basic mental attitudes. Like the natural sciences, it seeks to describe only structures and relationships. Both tendencies (psycho-analysis and phenomenology) are doubtless used by adherents for the propagation of metaphysical conceptions, but that was not the intention of their creators. Have these forms of psychological observation, then, no general attitude specific to themselves, no definite, basic point of view? Do we not also find here a metaphysical and philosophical point of radiation in the background, comprehensible only by a comprehensive (*überkuppelnde*) intuition, but beyond that impossible to vindicate? Is not the attempt to objectify subjectivity even here under the influence of a basic point of view of our own? The answer to this question seems to me to be, that even here there is a certain basic point of view, which, if it is compared with other basic attitudes, must be understood intuitively before it can be objectified; that, however, the essence of this attitude is the exclusively scientific determination to leave this personal attitude out of the picture. Looked at from the point of view of a philosophy of life, this mode of observation has no advantage over others, but from the point of view of scientific method it is the only purely scientific one.

It is certainly true, as we have seen, that the mode of abstraction in objectification in the two sciences is different. Phenomenology draws its abstractions from the objectification of personal introspective experience such as one might enter in a diary, by availing itself of the control offered by knowledge concerning forms of ego-activity, and neglecting anything that cannot be so unequivocably determined. This criterion is then applied to the introspection of others. Psycho-analysis draws its abstractions from the objectification of the experience of others, in so far as it has been made accessible by means of empathy, by examining the intuitions thus obtained concerning attitudes of the ego in others, in the light of a mass of knowledge concerning such attitudes in one person, and the historical connections relating to such attitudes in others. In both cases, there is an effort to objectify subjectivity in a system which admits all objective knowledge, but aims at complete independence of any basic principle or attitude. This is only possible if all these basic attitudes are regarded as relative, to be objectified themselves in regard to their structure and references, but without, of course, any possibility of pronouncing on their value for the individual.

But how far can one investigate the inner forms, the structure, of a personal attitude from the phenomenological point of view? How far can one, by empathy, truly feel the relationship of such a personal attitude with other personal attitudes in another individual, without oneself sharing the same attitude? Can, for example, a non-Catholic ever truly understand the structures and associations of the specifically Catholic mentality? And what criterion have we, by which to judge whether these attitudes have been correctly objectified or not?

Here we come to the question as to what are the limits of a scientific psychology. In answering such a question, we must be very cautious, for these limits may be displaced, as experience expands during the development of a science. It is possible that the present-day formulations of psychology are rejected by Catholicism, because they seem to pay too little attention to essential matters, while these, in a more subtle form, will come to be recognized as of universal validity. The formulations of a creed, moreover, also develop, and, in doing so, are to some extent influenced by scientific formulations. In any case, the psychologist must here take into due consideration the fact that the correct objectification of the attitudes of other persons is a very difficult task, and one for which his capacity for intuitive empathy is occasionally insufficient. If he is so presumptuous as to deny his own limitations in this respect, it may easily happen that he will present a caricature in the belief that it represents a true portrait. The soundest criterion here will be, not only whether he has been able to adjust every possible known fact to a single view, free of contradictions, but also whether he has gained the agreement of others, and particularly of those whose attitudes and reactions he has described. In psycho-analysis, as also in phenomenological investigations, considerable weight is attached to this agreement. In the study of collective mental structures, this kind of control is much more difficult to secure. The psychologist finds himself, indeed, frequently compelled to forgo a description of structure or an explanation by means of associations, in spite of his intuitive conviction, simply because the material offering comparison and enabling a correct classification under psychological heads is still too incomplete. Here we find, therefore, a second limit to psychological understanding, but one which seems in this case to be only a temporary one.

Although I thus admit that a psychology which is based upon a certain basic attitude—for example, that of the Catholic faith—is in a position to get at a deeper understanding of certain manifestations associated with this basic attitude, yet it is true that scientific value can be ascribed only conditionally to such a psychology. Its findings must indeed be taken seriously by a psychology which is independent of this attitude, but they will then need to be rearranged with a view to a more generally valid formulation, and perhaps formulated in a different way. What they lose during this process in intimate conviction for those who share the same basic attitude, they will gain in helping towards mutual understanding. A purely scientific psychology, confined to the observation and classification of psychological facts, can, therefore, never itself be a philosophy of life nor determine basic attitudes towards life. Science can never be a substitute for life, but it can serve life, quite apart from the purposive use to which scientific findings are put.

CHAPTER II

THE UNITY AND TRANSCENDENCE OF CONSCIOUSNESS

I

I HAVE in this book described certain mental types as determined by various modes of conscious experience. This conception gives rise to problems, to which it will be worth while to give special consideration.

The first problem concerns the various forms of consciousness, compared with consciousness as a unity. The concept of unity in the psyche frequently gives rise to confusion, because no distinction is made between phenomenological unity and the structural unity of the psyche, when objectified. These concepts are indeed associated, but their foundation is different.

From the phenomenological point of view, unity is found in the various kinds of ego-activity: first of all, in the consciousness of the moment, where the ego itself provides the unity, since it experiences itself as a unit directed to the contents of its consciousness. In the second place, there is for this experience a continuity in time, since we are aware of a unity between what we remember in the past and what we are experiencing today, a unity that is also projected into the future. In the third place, this ego-experience also embraces a qualitative unity, since my experience of myself in relation to a given object is always of myself in a certain state of mind or attitude. These attitudes of mind vary, but my experience of myself in them is felt to be continuous.

The concepts of the self, characteristic of the "natural science" type of psychology, must be distinguished, on account of their different mode of objectification, from the experience of the self, referred to above, which would be described as phenomenological. They are not based on an immediate experience of unity. A connecting totality is grasped intuitively, and from it the concept is abstracted. At first, no essential distinction is drawn between such a concept of another individual as a self and other concrete intuitions. As I showed in the previous chapter, abstraction of the object is only partially successful in this case. One might speak here of "the other self", when actually two opposing concepts would be combined. This "other self" offers no basis for our self-experience. It is the projection of a unity.[1] From the ideational point of view, it has the structure of an objectified concrete intuition, in which certain relationships are indicated. For this reason, it is possible, taking different intuitions as starting-point, to present different types of "other selves" objectified in this way, for example, the biological self, the bodily self, the social self, the personality, the character, etc. These different contexts may also be applied to one's own objectified life, when one observes one's self as "another self". But this is quite a different experience from the immediate experience of the self.[2] It is an experience in the realm of thought, with certain objectified totalities as its object.

As it is our intention to investigate phenomenological objectification here, we will not consider the selves which are the result of objectification along the lines of natural science. The problem is now how to express in abstract form the relationship between unity and variety in conscious experience. The central problem is here that of the unity behind the qualitative variety in experiences of the self, since the types of conscious orientation which have been described are actually founded on the possibility of such qualitative variety in experience. For this reason, we are bound to give primary consideration to this problem.[3]

If we are aware of variety in our experience, and yet the unity of our ego—which can only be experienced in this way—is not disturbed thereby, we can only objectify this experience in ideational form as a multiplicity in unity or as a structural totality. It is now our business to make use of intuition and of our phenomenological experience, to understand how we come to see these various possibilities of consciousness as a structural unity. This unity is certainly not present in immediate subjective experience. But there is always within and around us a great deal that is not separately discerned, until intuition selects certain associations and makes it possible to raise questions. We are not dealing here with entirely

[1] The unity of the concrete intuition which arises as a result of empathy may be described as one borrowed from the unity of self-experience.

[2] In the opinion of some workers, there is something more real in these objectified "other selves" than in experience of the self as introspectively perceived. In my view, both kinds of intuition are of essential significance.

[3] The momentary unity of self-experience may also be questioned; for example, we may enquire how far this unity may be suspended because of a split in the mental attitude; or how far its continuity in time may be interrupted by, for example, a phase of depersonalization. I am not attempting to consider these difficult phenomenological problems, which have been intensively studied by Oesterreich in his book on the "*Phänomenologie des Ich.*" It is possible that further insight into the unity of qualitatively various ego-activities will help in the further solution of these questions.

new distinctions. Functions, such as thinking and feeling, have, for example, been for a long time considered separately. But, as far as I know, these functions have until now never been studied as a unity. Jung has indeed attempted such a study, but it lacks phenomenological clarity. There is much in my study which is related to his views, by which I have, of course, been influenced in many ways. But I propose here to attempt the elucidation of the problem in my own way.

We are dealing thus with the question as to whether there is a unity in the qualitatively various forms of self-experience, and a unity in the varieties of conscious orientation in regard to the world and to one's self. Let us begin with the latter paradox.

I experience myself always as existing in the world, and my consciousness is able to occupy itself as much with the world around me as with myself within it. It is a question of the emphasis in attention. The other aspect is always more or less there, but there are states of consciousness in which it is almost entirely the world which is the object of attention, and others in which it is practically exclusively one's own attitude. In both directions we experience, however, a limit to our consciousness. Experience of the world is limited by the world unknown to me, a limit which gradually passes over into that of the world which I can never know. Experience of the self has as its limit that part of myself which is unknown to me, which self I am as unable to comprehend in its entirety as I am the world. If we represent the field of consciousness as a circle in which the dark unknown world surrounds consciousness of the world, there will lie within this circle a similar dark region adjoining the consciousness of ego-activity—the unknown self. Since our field of consciousness extends backwards and forwards in time, it may at any moment be represented as a transverse section through a thick-walled tube (conscious experience).

We may now classify the type of individual by introducing the concept of a mean field of consciousness in which it is possible to show the main orientation of a certain individual within this series of consecutive fields of consciousness. To do this, we first divide this field of consciousness by means of a circle into two unequally thick rings, separating consciousness relating to the world from consciousness relating to the self. In this way, the difference between an extraverted and an introverted individual may be shown in this mean field of consciousness. Although in both types states of extraversion and of introversion will occur, and the field of consciousness be occupied alternately by more of the world or more of personal ego-activity, yet in the course of their lives it will, on the whole, be true that the mean field of consciousness will in the extravert be occupied more by the world, and in the introvert more by his own states of mind.

It is possible to show something more by means of such a diagram, namely, that boundaries of the unknown world and of the unknown self are not equally sharp in the two types. The extravert is conscious that there are many influences coming from the external world which he does not understand, but of which he could understand more than he does. The frontiers of his world are open. The other frontier, which borders on his self, appears to him, however, as much more closed and absolute. He takes it for

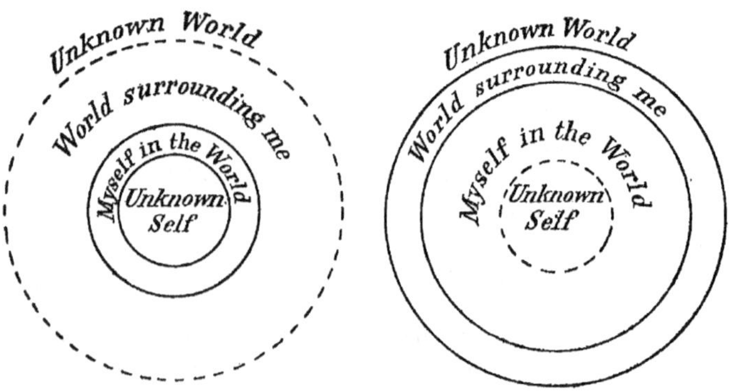

A. In the Extravert B. In the Introvert

Diagram of the Mean Field of Consciousness

granted that there is very little scope for comprehension in this direction. In the introvert, it is exactly opposite. His own attitudes and activity are almost always present in his mind, and there is always something more for him to know there. The frontier is not closed. But the world appears to the introvert from the beginning as pretty well unknowable. It is possible, of course, to learn something about it, but very soon the frontier becomes a rampart, impossible to penetrate.

We can also make use of this same diagram to show the qualitative differences in the forms of conscious orientation seen as a whole, by marking off various regions in the field of consciousness. If we super-impose the changing fields of consciousness of an individual one upon the other, it will yield his mean field of consciousness. If we bring together in this way every possible field of consciousness in different individuals, we shall get a general scheme of all the possibilities in the way of conscious orientation. We have distinguished four functions or forms of conscious orientation, and we should therefore divide the circle of the field of consciousness into four sectors.[1] It is not a matter of indifference how we do this, for we remember that we have recognized certain relationships between the forms of conscious orientation.

The whole of consciousness rests on instinctual experience, where impulse and the world-as-given react upon one another, and the meaning of the world is bounded by that of instinctive life. Above this basic layer floats, as it were, the intuitive sphere of consciousness, in which certain connections in experience are discerned, without being directly deduced therefrom. Experience of the self is felt here as inspiration, the world as a mass of possibilities and opportunities, and the essence of life as spirituality, which is the source of all inspiration. Between these two spheres of consciousness, which in themselves have no continuity with one another, lie the spheres of thinking and feeling (which in my opinion originally developed from the inter-action of instinct and intuition).[2] Thinking has a directly continuous relationship with the instinctive sphere as well as with intuition, because it exercises control over insight arrived at intuitively, and organizes its products in a system. We get, therefore, intuitive thinking, occupied with forms, intuitively conceived, and with possibilities of thought, and "materialistic" or technical thinking, directed more towards the perceptions that arise from sensations, and on practical matters. The subjective aspect of experience appears in consciousness as the will to control by systematization, while the world is felt as an ordered, systematized and objectified world, whose ultimate meaning appears as a directing mind revealing itself in Law. Feeling is also immediately connected with instinct and intuition, since through it affective, instinctual experience is ordered in such a way that it can be grasped intuitively. Moreover, we find evidence of this mediation between impulse and value through feeling in the existence of an intuitive kind of feeling controlled by spiritual and ethical values,

[1] We may postpone here the question as to whether the possibilities in the way of consciousness are, in fact, equally great for every individual, the difference lying only in the different mode of realization. In any case, the same diagram does not appear to me to be valid, for example, for a savage, since in his case thinking and feeling would occupy only narrow sectors, while the sphere of intuition, and above all that of instinct, would occupy the greater part of the area.

[2] Whether one puts thinking on the right and feeling on the left in the diagram, or *vice versa,* is of little importance. I have followed the plan of the body, in which the left side is associated with the heart, the right with the dominating hand.

and an instinctual kind, controlled by moral and sensuous factors. In the experience of the self, feeling appears in consciousness as the will to right behaviour; as experience of the world, it means the experience of obligation in certain circumstances. From the point of view of feeling, the meaning of life appears as spiritual order under the domination of Love.

It would seem in place here to draw attention to the fact that

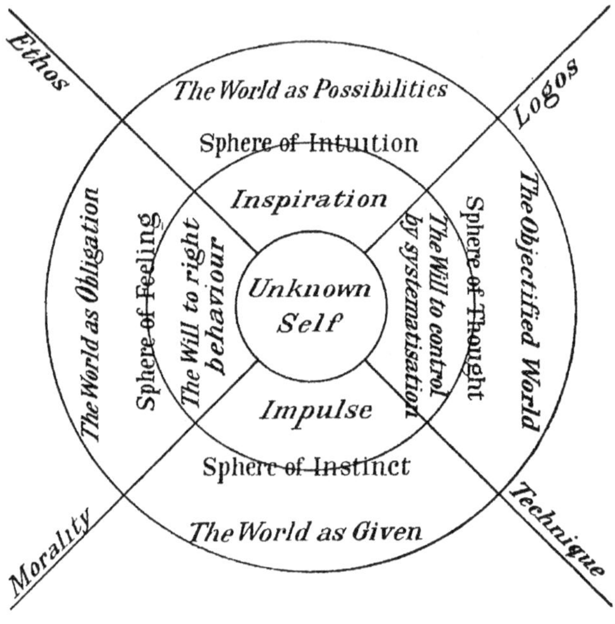

Diagram of the Possibilities in Conscious Orientation

in the possibilities of conscious experience there are two kinds of polarity, namely, a polarity in the mode of grasping the facts of the world and of our selves, and a polarity in the ordering of what has been grasped. The first kind of polarity, that between instinct and intuition, appears as the sense of contrast between life and spirit, projected on to the world. The second kind of polarity, that between thinking and feeling, appears as the opposition between Law and Love in the individual and in human relationships. The first opposition strikes us as cosmic, while the second seems more human, but both are felt to be of absolute value in the metaphysical background of life.

Within this scheme of the possibilities of conscious orientation, it is now possible to expand the diagram of the mean field of consciousness of a given individual, already given for introversion and extraversion. Although we assume, naturally, that every individual possesses all these possibilities of experience, and, indeed, experiences them all under certain conditions, nevertheless only a part of them is a more or less constant possession of the phenomenological self. A large part remains obscure as possible experience, and is in consequence put to less use in conscious life. Conscious orientation is directed, both in the world and in the experience of the self, particularly on to those forms which possess greater clarity

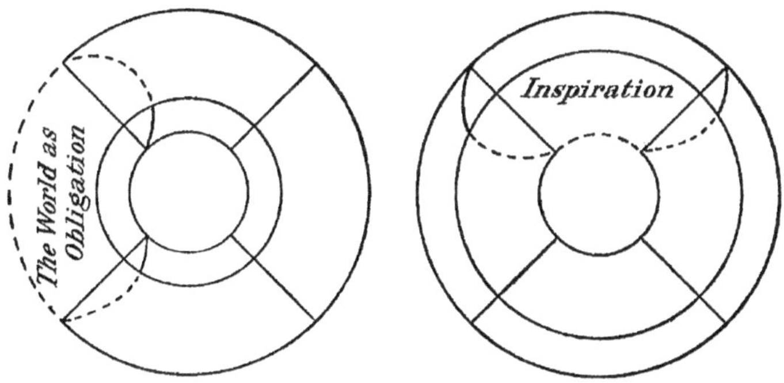

Extravert of Feeling-type Introvert of Intuitive type

Diagrams of the Mean Field of Consciousness as Limited by Type

and differentiation. As a result of this, we get considerable differences in the conscious experience of individuals. One feels more at home in some of one's experiences than in others. This familiar part of one's experience is that fairly well illuminated field which the self experiences as its content. (In so far as this awareness concerns self-experience, the objectified contents of this experience are described as the conscious self.)

The most important mode of orientation in a given individual is indicated by this delimitation of the mean field of consciousness. At the same time, the influence of the world and of the self varies according to whether extraversion or introversion is the more marked. For example, in an extravert of feeling-type there is more conscious experience of the world than of the self, and this world appears as a mass of relationships and obligations forming the very essence of life in a human community.

In an introvert of intuitive type, his own inner activity has the strongest influence in consciousness, and is experienced as inspiration. These inspirations often appear to arise from the unknown self, but occasionally they are attributed to a spiritual power external to the self (as with the daimon of Socrates).

In a similar way, it is possible to demonstrate on this diagram other typical limitations. Further elaboration along these lines may be left to the reader. I should, however, like to throw some light on the complication which results from the effect of polarity, by demonstrating it in the diagram. At the same time, I shall also manage to show on the diagram the effect of secondary functions.

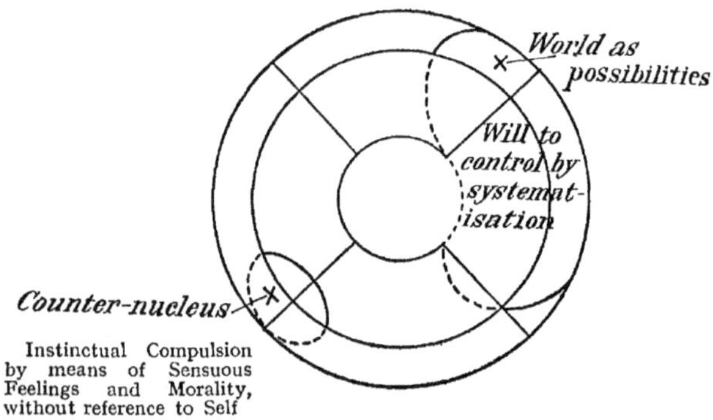

Thinking Introvert with Intuition as Subsidiary Function and with Polarity

Let us take, as a first example, an introvert of thinking-type, with intuition as a fairly well developed secondary function and with strong polarity. Conscious orientation is in such a case directed chiefly on the subject's own systematic thought-activity, and this more in regard to the aspect of form than that of matter. Logical forms are experienced as something vital, originating in the self, and intuition makes it possible to arrive at a new vision of spiritual relationships. (This may happen on very different levels, as I have demonstrated in my description of this type.) In regard to the world, such an individual is hampered in his vision by seeing it for the most part through the spectacles of his own opinions and conceptions. It is true that when he is in a more extraverted mood his intuition will act more freely, and for this reason the world will occasionally appear, even to this individual, what it constantly looks like to an intuitive extravert, namely, as a mass of possibilities and tasks.

To this normal mode of orientation for the type there is now added an entirely different kind of conscious experience, the result of strong and frequently repeated experiences of the effects of polarity. The content of these experiences is feeling, and feeling which is closely bound up with the sensuous instinctual life, and bearing on objects in the world. Their significance for the personal self is much less clear than is their outgoing intention. Every introvert of thinking-type probably has occasional experiences of this kind. Usually they are quickly forgotten, although for the moment they may exert a powerful and bewildering influence. But if they occur often in the field of consciousness, they may not only for a time break up the habitual form of conscious orientation, but even to some extent alter and destroy it. These experiences form a kind of "counter-nucleus" in the mode of orientation. Sensual feelings and conventional moral evaluations may then give rise to tensions, in spite of the fact that they are felt to be something foreign to the self. In the case of characters with much polarity, there then arises the need to deal with manifestations of the counter-nucleus in accordance with the standards of the dominant function. Abstract thinking concerning conflicts and problems in feeling is in consequence stimulated. In cases where the conflicts in feeling are under the control of repressed complexes, an obsessional neurotic character may be developed, but where there is greater freedom in thought, we get a morality founded on principles and reason, capable of giving rise to fresh insight into the life of feeling. The ordinary orientation of the introvert of thinking-type may, as a consequence of this kind of complication, undergo considerable alteration.

From the various possibilities to which polarity gives rise, I will select one other example, an extravert of intuitive type with feeling as his secondary function. The mean field of consciousness of such an individual would be mainly occupied by the world, which reveals itself as a mass of possibilities and relationships, offering a constant succession of tasks to be performed. These tasks are, in such a case, mainly related to matters concerning feeling-relationships. Where extraversion is marked, there will be dependence on chance ideas and encounters, giving rise to a changeable, somewhat superficial enthusiasm for all kinds of opportunities in the way of self-expression and personal relationships. These people often possess a remarkable ability in the presentation of ideals and plans in a vivid manner, making use of their personal relationships to realize them. Owing to the charm which often characterizes these people in whom feeling and intuition are combined, and to the persuasive force of their intuitions, they are often capable of exerting powerful influence. When in a state of introversion, their subsidiary function manifests itself in a more independent form, so that one finds in their inner orientation a striving after a right attitude, such as one might find in an introvert of feeling-type, but here it is less predominant. As a rule, too, the inner attitude is determined by aims that are the product of the subject's circumstances and are grasped intuitively.

This average or mean mental attitude may be further complicated by the effect of a counter-nucleus in the field of consciousness, if the instinctive side of the personality is constantly intruding on

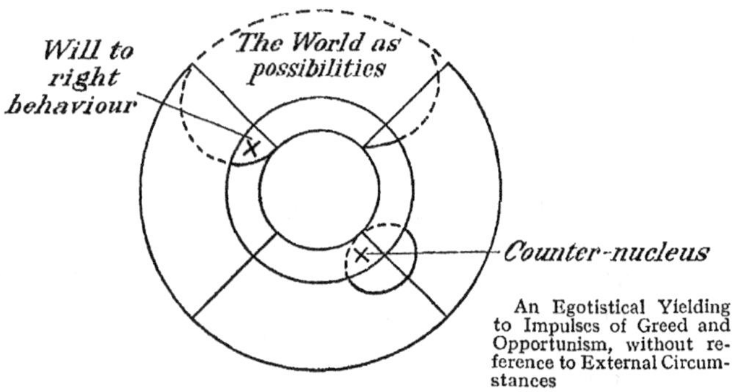

Intuitive Extravert with Feeling as Subsidiary Function and with Polarity

the habitual conscious experience. Other intuitive extraverts also may occasionally experience such a strange mixture of simple, egotistical greed and cold, calculating opportunism, characteristics in marked contrast to their usual disinterested enthusiasm. They very readily forget such experiences, however, together with the actions to which they give rise. But if this mode of orientation constantly obtrudes on the field of consciousness, their habitual confidence is disturbed, and the need arises to come to terms with this "other side" of the personality. This is no easy task, for this counter-nucleus is an indication of something that does not fit in with the habitual view of the world, something that is as a general rule depreciated and in sharp contrast to the prevailing ideals of the person concerned. At the same time, there is often a vague consciousness of the connection of these manifestations with the unknown self, and for this reason a sense of inferiority in regard to this self arises. If these manifestations are linked up with complexes, there is usually a defence set up against them by means of neurotic anxiety and compulsive precautionary measures. It may happen, however, that the effect of polarity is to extend the sphere of activity, by giving more value to the instinctual, practical aspect of life, with the result that artistic work, and even technical and social work, is undertaken.

I must here emphasize once more that only the general characteristics of conscious experience can be shown by means of this diagram of the mean field of consciousness. It does not explain the contents of this experience. Description of type presents the stage for mental happening, but does not determine the parts played by the actors. To understand the contents (for example, of certain neurotic manifestations), or the mode in which certain problems are solved, a different, more dynamic approach must be made, such as will enable us to look at these mental structures from the historical point of view. This approach has been specifically elaborated by the psycho-analysts. It should be noted, however, that these contents are also modified by the field of consciousness in which they appear. And, finally, I would urge once more that the less well illuminated parts of the field of consciousness must not be confused with the unconscious of psycho-analysis. When critics of psycho-analysis raise the objection to the concept of the unconscious, that it is not a question of unconsciousness, but unawareness, their observation has much more bearing on what I mean by this dark region of consciousness, than on the unconscious of psycho-analysis. We are, as a matter of fact, never quite unaware of this dim region in the field of consciousness, but we find it difficult to find our way about in it. This is true, not only for contents concerning the activity of the self, but also for external phenomena, of which we may also remain only dimly aware. The psycho-analytical concept of the unconscious means something quite different, namely, that phenomena, of which the subject is aware—whether clearly or vaguely—are not regarded as part of the activity of the self, and so not reckoned as part of the objectified self, although closer investigation shows that they can only be properly understood and explained in connection with this activity of the self. The main problem is here the separation or association of certain objectified contents in relation to the objectified image of the self. That which does not seem to the person concerned to be part of his own objectified self, while to the observer it is connected therewith, forms, in the category of objectified mental facts, the region of the unconscious. Hence this region is part of the psyche as objectified according to the methods of natural science, not of the psyche as objectified phenomenologically.[1]

I will summarize the findings of this first part of our investigation as follows: Experience of the unity behind the qualitatively various forms of ego-activity has given us insight into a certain context of possibilities in the way of conscious orientation. The different ways in which I realize the contents of my field of consciousness are grouped into functions which stand in a certain relationship with one another, and by means of these I am able to classify my experience both of the world and of my self in certain categories.

There is still something to add concerning the concept of the self. Experience of the self is unified. Whether in pathological conditions it may be experienced as split, or may disappear, is a difficult phenomenological question, with which I shall not concern myself here. Normally it is unified. From the phenomenological point of view, the self may be described as the totality of ego-activity in so far as it has become conscious. In this totality we have to distinguish: (*a*) the fully conscious self, in which we have a fairly comprehensive view of our activity (in the diagram of the mean field of consciousness this is the clear part of the inner ring); (*b*) the dimly conscious self, in which our own activity strikes us as more or less incidental (the dark part of the inner ring); and (*c*) the unknown self, of whose boundaries we become aware when we realize that we are able to understand only a part of our activity.

[1] Freud regards this kind of activity of the self, which is by the person concerned unrelated to the objectified self, as an expression of the "Id", and distinguishes these objectified phenomena from those which belong to the objectified self, which latter he has named the "Ego". These distinctions have, however, nothing to do with those made in phenomenology. Freud's "Ego" has no direct connection with the experience of the self as studied phenomenologically. It is a kind of intuition, clarified and reduced to ideational form, by means of which a certain kind of context within the self is objectified. Distinctions such as these, where one group of scientifically objectified facts is ascribed to one cause, and another group to a different cause, are in the realm of science not only permissible, but necessary. Freud's primarily physical conception of this "Ego" is from this point of view also comprehensible, since it is a fact that the psyche, from the point of view of natural science, is objectified as being closely bound up in the unity of the body and its manifestations. Difficulty will only arise if this scientifically objectified "Ego" is confused with experience of the self, or with the concept of the self, as objectified phenomenologically.

II

There is a second problem, which, associated to some extent with that of the structure of the field of consciousness, is concerned with the various degrees and modes in which consciousness is transcended. In so far as consciousness always has reference to something beyond itself, it may always be described as transcendent. Even when, in introspection, consciousness is apparently occupied only with the self, it has reference to more than the contents of this consciousness, to wit, the activity of the self, the intentions and the laws of the subject's own being. All this is indeed, to some extent, expressed in these contents, but not in its entirety.

In addition to the problem of the formal definition of this transcendence, there arises that of its constitution. Introspection teaches us that there are different degrees of transcendence. There is not always an equally strong reference to that which lies outside conscious experience. When undertaking a logical investigation, our activity is directed to the logical structure of our own thought. In an action determined by feeling, it is directed to the other person. In a fantasy, however, it is uncertain how far the reference really is to the person who is the object of the fantasy, or how far one is really referring to one's own purpose in the fantasy. There are thus degrees of transcendence, but it is not easy to determine these degrees more exactly. The question occurs as to whether perhaps the degree of transcendence coincides with that of extraversion or introversion. It certainly seems obvious that an outstandingly extraverted state would furnish a marked degree of transcendence in regard to the world, just as an outstandingly introverted state of mind would transcend in the direction of its own activity. This seems to suggest a rivalry between the world and the self. The more we are pre-occupied with the world, the less is the factor of our own activity represented in consciousness, and the more extraverted may the condition be called. When, on the other hand, a philosopher is pre-occupied with phenomenological observations, or when a poet expresses his feelings in images, consciousness is concentrated on the activity of the self, and we are dealing with an intensely introverted state of consciousness. In such a state, the world may almost disappear. To this extent, degrees of extraversion and introversion coincide with degrees of transcendence. Is this always the case?

In studying this question, we find, first of all, that the situation is usually not so simple as we have described it. If we observe the course of consciousness for a time, we shall see that there are variations, both in the intensity of transcendence and in attention. The scientist, making an observation, may be occupied with thoughts which do not refer to the object, but to his own activity (for example, the reflection: Shall I be able to continue my observation undisturbed?). The poet may be deflected from his feelings by the crying of his child, or by hearing the preparations for his meal. If such disturbances in conscious activity become very obtrusive, extraversion may be completely transformed into introversion, and *vice versa*. What change in the degree of transcendence does this involve? It is naturally not to be expected that the poet, even though, from a practical point of view, his attitude is determined by the arrival of a meal, will now have his attention as intently riveted on this as it was on his own feelings. Hence there arises a state of distraction. This word means the turning of the attention on to several objects at the same time, with a diminished degree of transcendence. The scientist, while controlling his inner state, may during some observation in the external world be deflected to some emotional problem, and here also distraction may arise.

The problem of distraction brings us to the question of the significance of fantasy in these cases. Distraction may mean that an intensive pre-occupation with some internal or external object may disturb the attention given to another external or internal object. The distracting factor may, however, be a more or less distinct fantasy. Fantasy is peculiar in that the fantasied images possess a very slight degree of transcendence. Attention is, it is true, directed inwards, but the reference is not to one's own being. Even the fantasied images [1] are themselves not the real subject of reference, although they may play a part in this. As far as transcendence is concerned, fantasy remains in consciousness as a fluctuating quantity. This is true both for introversion and for action based on fantasy (such as play), where the tendency is certainly towards external reality, but the latter is not really meant. We find such actions in hysteria, and more especially in schizophrenia, where what is really meant is only vaguely intimated by means of a symbol. Freud has demonstrated, however, in his *Psychopathology of Everyday Life*, that there are all degrees of transition between this kind of behaviour and normal mental life. Both in introverted and in extraverted states there are very different

[1] Jung calls these images archetypes, and in his treatment he teaches his patients to refer to them specifically. By taking them seriously, he reveals the importance of the inner world as revealed by them, and thus they stop being " mere fantasies ".

degrees of transcendence. There is a continuous transition between what is really meant in the internal and in the external world, and what is only apparently meant. A high degree of transcendence might here be compared with apperception, were this concept not confined to intellectual activity. Also, there is more in the concept of apperception than is meant in the degrees of transcendence described here. This brings us to a further problem.

In some states of consciousness, attention is directed simply on to objects in the external or in the internal world. But there are more complicated states, in which both external and internal worlds are simultaneously involved. We learned in the first part of this chapter that both the world and ourselves are constantly present in our consciousness, although in different states of mind the influence of one or the other aspect varies very considerably. The transcendental aspect of consciousness is, however, usually directed either inwards or outwards, but there are situations when reference is actually both to self-activity and to external objects at the same time.

If I consciously and with intention concentrate on some physical performance or upon the observation of some scientific experiment, my reference is to my own attitude as well as to the object. There are situations in which the performance passes straight from the subject to the object, and others in which we are not only conscious of the object, but feel a deep penetrating influence from it, and are conscious, moreover, that this is happening to us. When this happens, we feel it as something out of the ordinary.

The concept of apperception (as opposed to perception) conveys something of the tension of this situation, and the division into passive and active apperception corresponds to what we have described as being directed inwards or outwards. Thus, in addition to varieties of intensity in transcendence, it is also possible to assume differences in power of penetration, by which I mean apperception of the inter-action of the two aspects (directed inwards or directed outwards) of consciousness. I should like to apply the description "penetrating" to this form of transcendence.

We have discovered that consciousness expresses itself in acts which bear different qualities, and this leads us to a further peculiarity of transcendence, namely, its definite form. The various functions of conscious orientation refer to their contents in different ways. If a man experiences another person by means of his sense-organs, his attitude to him is different from that of someone who understands something about him intuitively, or from that of someone whose attitude to him is determined by thought or feeling.

In the same way, self-conscious activity varies in character, according to whether one is occupied with one's suffering, or one's actions, or is concentrated on some inner vision, or is plunged in one's own feelings or thoughts. The act by which consciousness is transcended, the form in which a reality is grasped, is different in each of these cases. We may now ask ourselves if these different ways of transcending consciousness are connected with other peculiarities which we have differentiated. It has already become evident that in all the functions it is possible to distinguish tendencies to introversion and to extraversion, so that the direction (outwards or inwards) in transcendence does not depend upon its form. But what about the penetration of transcendence in the various forms? Is it associated with certain functions? Do we find it, for instance, more readily in thought, where the concept of apperception is also most applicable? We must go into these problems rather more thoroughly.

Thought is probably the function which has been most fully investigated, hence it would be as well to begin with it. Extraverted thinking brings a systematizing and objectifying attitude to bear on experiences of the external world. The systematic forms employed for this purpose are present in consciousness in a more or less latent fashion, and assert themselves in the course of the thought-process. It cannot be said that these thought-forms originate in the self. It is, therefore, quite possible to direct one's thought upon the external world, without the development of any penetrating power in the transcending consciousness involved. On the other hand, introverted thinking can give rein to ego-activity in the way of classification and objectification, without there being any real pre-occupation with the external world at all. The world is taken "as if" it were there. If transcendence takes on a penetrating quality in these cases, it is felt to be a special experience, which is a rarity with most people, and quite unknown to many. When it happens, the extravert will feel that his classification is not only in his consciousness, but proceeds from his very self. It comes as a kind of revelation, uniting what is within and what is without, and at the same time he experiences in a special way his own thought-activity. The introverted thinker will experience this activity as something quite ordinary, but he is more astonished to find that his own thoughts are accepted as of general validity. It is this success in reaching the external world which gives him the feeling of a special experience. The compelling power that lies in the fact of the universal validity of his thoughts may suddenly lay hold of the introverted thinker. In my opinion, it would be a mistake to describe such experiences as not belonging to the sphere of thought (as being feelings, for example). These different degrees of penetration belong to the essence of thought.

We shall find similar conditions in the sphere of feeling. Extraverted feeling has reference to the external world, and is directed in its personal attitudes and values by a hierarchy of symbols in consciousness. The influence of the self in this process is usually not taken into account. It is possible, for instance, for such an extravert to fall in love, without his feelings penetrating into his own being. But other feelings may arise, which possess the quality of penetration, and when this is so, they are felt to be something completely his own, giving his life some different and deeper significance such as he has previously never known. Here also there is a new relationship between what is internal and what is external. In the case of the introvert of feeling-type, the experience of penetration is again reversed. The personal and private quality of feelings are here assumed as a matter of course. Feeling-attitudes, arising from the self, reach consciousness, but are for the most part not expressed, and establish no contacts. What to the extravert appears entirely natural, is here, if it happens, a rare experience. It seems that feeling, like thought, may often taken place entirely within the sphere of consciousness, without any recognition of its meaning as a relationship between the world and the self. Both functions, however, only reach their full fruition and meaning when they have reference both to the internal and to the external world. The transcendence that has penetrating power is, in fact, the original form, while one-sided transcendence must be regarded as a later product of mental experience, whose nature it is to prepare the way for union between what is within and what is without.

This original meaning of consciousness is more evident in the two older functions, intuition and instinctual experience. In the case of intuition, the external world may be seen in the light of some comprehensive (*überkuppelnde*) vision to have a meaning, which nevertheless does not and cannot be held to arise from the self. Such ideas are often the residue of something read, or of some encounter with other people, and the impression of originality may be deceptive. But there are intuitions which seem to come from within, like a flash of lightning, to illuminate the world around. These "penetrating" intuitions sometimes give the impression of inspiration or clairvoyance. Such experiences seem to me to be commoner with intuitive persons than is the corresponding experience with thinking- or feeling-types. At the same time, intuitions of this penetrating kind are for most intuitive extraverts a somewhat rare experience. As a rule, the outstanding thing in consciousness is for them their relationship with the external world. In introverted intuition, we find again the opposite state of affairs. Introverted intuitions have reference to the internal world, and the influence of these, reaching consciousness, provides a nucleus of images and convictions. Sometimes these are projected to form a would-be external world, like the spirit world of primitive man, but they do not really establish contact with reality. It is, however, possible for intuitive insight to arrive at a profound comprehension of real external contexts. While introverted intuitions deal, as a rule, with the inner world—the resultant vision being then frequently projected into, or set up behind, the external world, in the form of "the other world"—this kind of insight may in rare cases throw such a light upon the essence of men and things, that both inner and outer world are seen in their true relationship. Although in practical psychology such experiences must be subjected to critical examination, since mistaken value is often ascribed to them by the individuals concerned, it must nevertheless be admitted that extremely important intuitions may arise in this way.

In the sphere of instinctive experience, the transition between one-sided and penetrating transcendence seems to me to be more continuous than in the other functions. In describing the peculiarities of instinctual experience, I have suggested that the external field of experience, with its emphases, and the activity of the self are felt in consciousness to be bound together in a unity. If any part is, in some observation, selected and seen in isolation, then in my estimation we are no longer dealing with instinctual experience as such. The fact that, in the sphere of instinct, transcendence always has a penetrating quality, brings us to the view that the transcendence of consciousness is originally two-sided, and that in the simpler states of consciousness, moreover, we nearly always experience, and are referring to, both aspects in conjunction. In instinctual experience, attention is not evenly distributed over the field of experience, even though the whole of the latter is always represented in consciousness. The emphasis may be on the internal or the external aspect, according to whether the personal condition is one of tension, or of rest, or of well-being, or whether a definite object is engaging the attention. Hence it is possible to distinguish here states of greater or less introversion or extraversion, but transcendence seems to me to be less one-sided than in the other functions, because the relationship between subject and object is always represented in consciousness.

Thus from our discussion of transcendence we have found that it may, in connection with the various functions, appear in forms both one-sided (directed inwards or outwards) and two-sided or penetrating, and that in instinctual experience, which we may call the original form of consciousness, the penetrating form of transcendence is predominant. From these facts we might deduce that those forms of conscious experience which have penetrating quality are the most primitive, and that the one-sided form is a later development.

We have still not given a sufficiently full picture of the various forms in which transcendence in consciousness may be experienced. For instance, it may be asked how far in introspective experience the various functions are perceived in sharp distinction from one another, and whether it is not possible for them in some way to be represented in combination. I suggested in my description of the functions that they continually pass over into one another, that, for example, feeling may intrude into one's thinking activity, and may indeed supersede the latter, and so on. There are thus transitional forms and states, which may only be described as mainly under the control of one of the functions. Here also we may find a kind of distraction in conscious orientation, similar to that which we found in the mingling of introverted and extraverted states. Moreover, we have seen that in practice it is quite possible, in certain connections, for two functions to work together. Thought, for instance, is quite prepared to admit the reality of instinctual experience, and in the same way it can enter into living combination with the intuitive perception of relationships. But it cannot simultaneously admit experience of feeling, because it is of its very nature to disregard any subjective attitude, while it is just subjective attitudes which count in the experience of feeling. The polarity that exists between thinking and feeling, and between intuition and instinctual experience, has been suggested in the diagram of the possibilities of consciousness (p. 284). It may be asked whether the simultaneous activity of polar functions can only involve distraction of transcendence, in contrast to adjacent functions, where, in certain circumstances, their combined activity may result in an intensification.

These problems have directed our attention to certain states of consciousness which are marked by a special form of transcendence. There exist modes of orientation which cannot be classified without further discussion under any of those which have been described, but which have in certain circumstances considerable importance. There is, for instance, aesthetic experience, which is more or less accessible to most people in the form of artistic appreciation, but is probably most intensely realized in artistic creation. It does not seem possible to me to class this kind of conscious attitude, without more ado, under any of the functions we have defined; and no more possible to explain it as a special attitude determined by fixations. If one goes into the phenomenology of this kind of artistic perception, we can trace connections with both instinctual and intuitive experience. It is obvious that art pre-supposes instinctual experience in those to whom it appeals, and avails itself of the emphasis on this kind of experience to hold the attention. Colour effects, beauty of form, sound, emotional expression are all things which appeal to instinctual experience. At the same time, it is obviously true that the artist exercises choice, and occasionally only makes use of a form in order to suggest certain associations. The symbol is of great significance in art, from symbolic art, where this significance is predominant, right through the various domains of art down to the handicrafts, where the criteria of instinct have the greatest influence. A painting usually expresses something, even when its only intention has been a simple joy in flowers, animals or landscape. The way in which the flower or the landscape is seen may at the same time reveal some mental attitude. For this reason, even a mere building, whose purpose is purely practical, may have a style suggesting the spirit of a period, so that even in the most practical forms of art-expression we find something of an idea, and some representation of a vital meaning. On the other hand, it may be said that an art which represents life exclusively through abstract symbols, thereby losing contact with instinctual experience, ceases to be art. It is not only modern art, with its abstractions, which approaches this limit; the intellectualized, conventional, anaemic art of the end of the last century also shows the same danger. We may therefore suppose that instinctual experience and intuitive comprehension stand in art in a vital relationship. Before we go further into this question, we must define its scope rather more precisely, through a study of the significance of thought and feeling in aesthetic experience.

It seems to me that thought is only indirectly related to aesthetic experience and the development of art. On the technical side, it always plays a certain part in any artistic expression, and reason may introduce abstract ideas, by filling the work of art with representations which illustrate its connection with reality. But as soon as reason dominates, the effect is not to induce artistic intuition, but to paralyse and deaden both experience and creative activity. Only when thought is absolutely subordinate to artistic perception, is it able to intensify aesthetic experience and amplify its expression.

Aesthetic experience is usually assumed to be connected rather with the sphere of feeling than that of thought. But it seems to me that even here a predominating attitude of feeling would be a disturbing factor in artistic experience. As I have already shown in great detail, feeling erects emotional structures in accordance with standards which are more or less fixed. Might it not be possible to regard aesthetic feeling as one of the plastic expressions of feeling in general, in which case artistic experience would be part of the life of feeling? This does not seem possible to me, owing to the presence of different standards in the two cases. Feeling is directed towards human relationships, and its standards are closely connected with these. Even where feeling is directed towards animals or inanimate objects, it is primarily derived from human relationships. The criterion of artistic experience is the possibility of grasping and expressing a significant context in concrete form. The meaning here is much less abstract, much more closely connected with concrete representation and a concrete attitude, than it is in the more abstract intuitions which we specially associate with the concept of intuition. The meaning of an intuition requires, however, no clear-cut abstraction before it can be expressed, and things can often be represented in art which are not capable of any precise formulation. In art, it is not possible to speak of criteria, in the sense that one does in the case of feeling or thought, since there is a lack of definite standards. In artistic expression, the essential question is whether the material offers sufficient meaning. In some forms of art, this meaning can be clearly seen; in others, it is only vaguely indicated.

Feeling is, like thought, ill-adapted for supplying the meaning of an artistic representation, because it is too much tied to definite forms peculiar to itself. In thought and feeling, meaning has become fixed, expression conventional, and a given material, the material for artistic expression, can only have a meaning in so far as it corresponds with these collective criteria. Only where the expression of feeling is so spontaneous that the universal aspect of feeling is entirely absorbed into the personal experience concerned, where its true expression, its presentation, appears as the most important factor—only in such a case is feeling related to art. For the artist, feeling is the occasion, but his essential concern is even here the relationship between form and content. If he gets no farther than feeling, he overlooks his real function.

Hence it may be said that when art expresses thoughts or feelings, it transforms them into an intuitive experience, and into an extremely concrete, not to say primitive, intuitive experience, where meaning is intimately bound up with form and material.

In this close connection between the form, consisting of an instinctual experience, and the content, consisting of an intuitive meaning, we have, in my view, the essential characteristic of artistic experience. If we apply this to the problem of transcendence in consciousness, we shall find ourselves able to expand our view of the possibilities in regard to this experience of transcendence. In addition to direction, degree and penetration, we may now contemplate the possibility of polarity in this experience. We have suggested that penetration is a more primitive form of transcendence than one-sided direction, particularly in instinctual, and to some extent also in intuitive, experience. We may now add that, in its original form, the transcendence associated with intuition is not only penetrating, but has a polar character.

Here we come up against further problems. We found that polarity existed, not only between instinct and intuition, but also between thought and feeling. Is it possible in these latter functions, also, to speak of polarity in transcendence in certain states of consciousness? Thought and feeling are later developments than intuition, and, moreover, they have not developed from one another, in the way that we may say intuition is founded upon instinctual experience. It is, therefore, not permissible to assume that relationships existing between instinct and intuition also exist between thought and feeling. The latter functions are more differentiated, and introversion and extraversion are in them more easily seen in isolation. Moreover, in individuals of these types who are characterized by polarity, the opposition between the two functions is even more clearly evident. Is it possible to find a conscious attitude in which thought and feeling are intimately combined, such as we found in the case of instinct and intuition, in artistic experience? There certainly is a sphere where thought and feeling meet, namely, when we are dealing with the question of reasonableness. We recognize reasonableness as an important cultural product, as a result of which, conscious orientation is subjected to the control of collective human standards. The word reasonableness has, however, not so much to do with a definite experience, such as might be equated with an artistic experience, as with an average attitude in consciousness, as a result of which, opposites are held in equilibrium. Another form of conscious experience, in which thought and feeling play a large part, is the understanding, as a whole, of another person. Here one does get the impression occasionally that thought and feeling are one. Yet it seems to me that in this case the essential factor in this form of all-inclusive understanding is derived from a comprehensive (*überkuppelnde*) intuition. It seems to me that although polarity between thought and feeling plays a large part in consciousness, it is not possible to assume a transcendent experience of this polarity in any particular state of consciousness.[1]

A further question arises here, as to whether other forms of polar transcendence, apart from aesthetic appreciation, may be distinguished. In my view, the answer to this question is that polarity is of importance in all creative mental activity, and I find the possibility of such conscious creative experience in three further forms, viz. (*a*) philosophical insight, (*b*) the perception of new ethical values, and (*c*) religious experience. The first two forms seem to me to have a similar structure to that of artistic perception, except that in the first case, intuition is bound up with the origins of thought, and is directed towards the comprehension of reality, while in the second case, it provides a fresh vision of ideal modes and standards of behaviour in the sphere of relationships. The creative factor in both cases lies in the fact that both the reality of instinctual experience and a personal intuitive insight come to expression simultaneously. The awareness of meaning is here more precise than in the case of artistic appreciation, and is confined to a certain sphere. Not only are the world within and the world without seen in their relationship, but the two modes of experience, inner and outer, the experience of fact and the experience of meaning, are seen in their inter-relationship. The findings of thought are not applied in philosophy in the same way as they are in science. They incite the philosopher to study the inter-connections of these various products of his thought, in order by this means to get at the essence of the world and of life. From whatever facts he originally sets out, he strives to reach in the end an experience of unity between fact and vision. Such an experience must necessarily include much more than the tested products of his thinking. It extends beyond the bounds of thought, which is what gives rise to abuse of philosophy from critical and one-sided thinkers. In my opinion, thought returns in philosophy to its original function as mediator between instinctual experience and intuition; it makes use of all the unrelated knowledge gathered in the course of centuries to envisage and experience a unity in all these varieties of experience. The feeling of transcendence in consciousness is in this experience directed towards both matter and meaning, both the external and the internal world, which together, as Husserl has truly seen, represented for

[1] This does not necessarily mean that these kinds of experience could not be included in a more comprehensive form of transcendent experience. I shall return to this later in discussing ethical, philosophical and religious experience.

the early philosophers a single domain. Although I doubt whether there is in consciousness an experience of polarity between thought and feeling here, it seems to me that philosophical experience, in which the direction of transcendence is determined by polarity, as it is in aesthetic appreciation, must be distinguished from other forms of thought, on account of this polarity of transcendence.

There seems to me to be a similar polarity of transcendence in the experience of ethical values. Feeling was originally the mediator between two spheres of experience: between the existing relationships between people, and the image, personally and intuitively perceived, of what those relationships ought to be. Insight into this mediating significance of feeling has not so entirely disappeared as it has in the case of thought, although even here the fixed criteria of feeling are usually treated as if they were something of independent origin. Moreover, it makes a great difference in conscious experience, whether we are moving in the sphere of feeling, or whether we are, in our vision, perceiving these opposites in a living unity. Vital ethical experience includes simultaneously the facts of the actual attitudes and relationships of men, and the spiritual laws and ideals which determine the structure of these facts. For the psychological comprehension of this experience, there is a difficulty in the fact that an "ethical attitude" may mean two things: on the one hand, the intuitive realization of norms, and on the other hand, the experience and actual realization of these in one's own life of feeling. In the former case, transcendence is certainly penetrating in character, but has no polarity in direction; in the latter case, the world of what is is impregnated with the sense of what ought to be. What is sensed in this way appears as literal truth, an obligatory task, an absolute claim. One might put it this way: that in living thought there is always something of the philosophical attitude, in which relationship appears as a matter of ordered objective forms; and, similarly, in living feeling there is awareness, however vague, of the compounding of two opposing aspects of experience. From this it follows that there is no clear-cut boundary-line between the experience of polarity and the ordinary forms of consciousness, with their more exclusive selection of one aspect of experience. In the more complicated conscious experience of polarity, there is a greater tension between the opposites concerned, and it is less defined, and more creative, than the ordinary forms, which are more precise. The transcendence of polarity appears to be the earlier form.

We have found polarity in three forms of transcendence: in artistic, philosophical and ethical experience. What is its significance in religious experience? The psychological conceptions of religious experience may be divided into two groups, those which represent it as a special form of experience, and those which regard it as a conclusion drawn from other experiences, i.e. as more indirectly founded. Freud, who maintains religion to be an illusion,[1] may be taken as an example of the second group. For him, religions are a form of defence—and, moreover, a mistaken form—against one's own instinctual drives and against life's troubles. Religious experience has no place in his psychology. In opposition to him, one may take as an example of the second group, William James, who in his book, now become a standard of reference, *The Varieties of Religious Experience*, takes as his starting-point a special kind of experience, which he designates as religious. It is not possible to go thoroughly into this problem here, but, for our question concerning the modes of consciousness, only the latter conception need be considered, since we are not dealing now with the possibility of drawing true or mistaken conclusions from the various forms of experience, but only with the investigation of the fundamental forms of consciousness. My view is that of William James, and it seems to me that he and many other scholars have shown in a convincing manner, that in the domain of religion the starting-point of psychological study is to be sought in a special kind of experience. I will try to describe briefly the characteristics of this experience, so that we may then consider it in connection with the problem of the various forms of transcendence.

To James, the essence of all religious experience is a feeling of discontent, that something is wrong with our way of living; and this state of dissatisfaction then finds a solution in a relationship with a higher being, which includes the world and is thus able to provide an experience of safety and of union with the world and with men. This unity may be experienced in mystic ecstasy or in pious acceptance of daily tasks. In the phenomenon of conversion, we can see most clearly the transition to a different attitude, which is not, it is true, identical with religious experience, but which represents a certain preparedness for this experience, and an attempt to maintain its after-effects. The essential thing here is the special experience, which is felt to be something independent of the will, more in the nature of a gift (the "grace of God"). This central experience is difficult to describe, and is very variously indicated by means of symbols.

The development of the psychology of religion has, since the time of James, brought to light much that is of prime importance

[1] Freud, *The Future of an Illusion*.

in regard to the meaning of these symbols and their place in religions. Among these symbols, that of father and mother play a large part, so that Freud and his followers are inclined to see the origin of all religion in the family situation. The facts to which they have drawn attention are, in my opinion, true and significant, but they throw light only on the development of certain religious forms, not on religious experience itself. That the father and the mother have become symbols may certainly be explained as a result of disappointment with the actual father and the actual mother, leading to their replacement with mightier, and more loving, parents. We may question, however, whether the relationship which is sought in religion can be equated, without further discussion, with the original relationship with the parents. One might indeed ask, whether whatever it is, which causes the child to idealize his parents and to see in them something higher than himself, is not really itself an attribute of the religious life, and an indication of a special kind of orientation. Psycho-analysis, concerned, as it is, chiefly with mental contents and the investigation of their inter-relationships, has occasionally paid too little attention to the differentiations of phenomenology, which do give us a clearer grasp of the forms of conscious experience. In addition to the problem of the origin of religious symbols, and of their connection with the rest of the life of men and of humanity, there is the further problem of the experience which is indicated by means of these symbols. Hence it is important that any investigation of religious forms should be supplemented by another kind of investigation, that of religious experience itself. Since James brought this question into the forefront of the newer psychology, students in various countries have made important contributions to it.

A full exposition of the development of this aspect of the psychology of religion would require a whole book. For my purposes, I must be content with a few suggestions. I will begin by reminding you of Rudolf Otto, who in his book, *Das Heilige*, speaks of "motives derived from an intense and absolutely single-minded excitement".[1] He designates this experience as "numinal" and as the "*Mysterium tremendum*". In assuming that the positive element in this is exclusively an emotional experience, I do not think he is quite right, even though the fear involved may point to an emotional attitude. In my opinion, however, this represents only part of the experience, and does not represent its real meaning. Otto seeks a fuller understanding of religious experience in the

[1] He even adds: "Anyone who has never known, or is incapable of, this experience is requested to read no further."

elements of fear, of almightiness, of energy and mysticism. He illustrates these elements in many examples, and suggests that what he calls the "numinal" factor must be regarded as a primary spiritual faculty, impossible of explanation from other mental factors. This element is demonstrable in the earliest manifestations of religion, as Otto indicates in various examples.

Martin Buber has approached this problem from a somewhat different angle. He attempts to formulate a distinction, from the phenomenological point of view, and in relation to immediacy of experience, between religious and other kinds of experience.[1] He points to a contrast between two different forms of relationship in conscious experience, which he defines as "I—you" experience, and "I—it" (or I—he or I—she) experience. It is not possible to relate this kind of antithesis to that between the different functions, or to that between extraversion and introversion, but there is, nevertheless, something essential in it, connected with the problem of the differences in the experience of transcendence. Introspection will convince us that the antithesis between "encountering" an object, and its mere experience, is found everywhere. One can put it still better by saying that it is not possible to identify "I—you" experience with any particular state of consciousness. Any other experience seems to be a more limited, one might almost say a rigid, fixed after-effect and abstraction of an "I—you" experience. Buber finds this fuller, immediate "I—you" experience in three spheres: in life with nature, in life with men, and in creative mental work. Encounters with nature are familiar to most of us from childhood. These encounters are rather different from instinctual experience, which is the child's guide, at first uncertain, later ever more certain, from birth. They are also different from the "Aha!" experiences of intuition, by which purpose and association are first revealed to the child. The state of tension, characterized by astonishment and emotional feeling, consequent on "I—you" encounters is not transformed into any judgment, nor is it made use of in any practical activity. For Buber, the outstanding characteristic of this experience lies rather in its comprehensive completeness, which is felt both in what is encountered and in the outgoing of the self towards it. "The relationship with the 'you' is immediate. Between the 'I' and the 'you' there is no abstraction, no foreknowledge, and no fantasy."

This kind of immediate experience, which, according to Buber, passes over, without break, into other forms of experience, seems

[1] Martin Buber, *Ich und Du*, 1923, and *Zwiesprache*, 1932. (No English translations.)

to be the more primitive form. "A relationship is the beginning of all things." "The very first impressions and stimuli, awakening the mind of primitive man, are those which reveal an association, or come from the experience of an opposite. They are the product of the state of mind when associations and opposites are realized." His speech expresses this. In the course of history, both of the individual and of humanity, an ever-expanding "it-world" is developed from "I—you" encounters. "The development of the capacity for experiencing and applying to some use is generally accompanied by a diminution of man's capacity for experiencing relationships."

We may accordingly assume with Buber that in the history of the individual, and in the development of human modes of consciousness, there is a phase, preceding the development of the differentiated functions, characterized by a more indefinite, but at the same time more comprehensive, form of transcendence. A comparison of the differentiated functions with Buber's "I—you" relationship reveals further how, in the main, creative activities in consciousness are derived from the latter. It is not possible to go further into Buber's interesting discussion, but we must study a little more closely the question of the connection between "I—you" experience and religion.

Buber describes religious experience as "that immediate relationship to a 'You', whose nature it is that it can never become an 'It'". This relationship is, moreover, something which happens to us, and nothing is excluded from it, although it is not possible to find in it any single thing in isolation: "To look away from the world will not bring you to God; to gaze at it will not help you to Him; see the world as in Him, and you stand in His presence." "God is indeed entirely that 'other', but He is also entirely the 'self': He is the whole of present experience, internal and external. He is indeed the *mysterium tremendum*, who in His appearance casts us down at His feet; but He is also the secret of the obvious, closer to me than myself."

"Man's sense of a 'You', disappointed as he is in finding that all his individual 'you'-experiences become 'it'-experiences, directs the strivings of his most essential 'I' beyond all these, but not beyond his own eternal 'You'. Not that he is seeking something: there can in truth be no search for God, for there is no place where He cannot be found." "It is as though, when going on one's way, one wished that this might be *the* way; in the strength of this wish, one's striving comes to expression. Every experience which reveals a relationship to Him is, as it were, a viewpoint, from which one gets a vision of ultimate fulfilment. In all this, one has no share, and yet one is part of it, because one is expectant. Expectant, but not seeking, one goes one's way; and so nothing can disturb one."

Buber shows again and again that religious experience is not external to ordinary experience, but that it includes it in a higher totality of experience. For this reason, it is impossible to designate any particular element as essential to it. "Some people are inclined to regard, as the most essential element in the relationship to God, a feeling of dependence, more recently and more exactly described as the feeling of being God's creature (*Kreaturgefühl*). Although it may be right to select and define this element, yet to emphasize it without describing other elements to counter-balance it, is to mistake the quality of the complete relationship." Every "I—you" relationship is experienced in the form of this comprehensive awareness, even though it is also characteristic of it, that it is constantly broken up into isolated experiences. "Every actual relationship in the world is exclusive; something else breaks in upon it and destroys it. Only in the relationship with God are unconditional exclusiveness and unconditional inclusiveness one and the same thing, comprising the All."

Buber has drawn the attention of the psychologist to two important facts: first, that there are important differences in the way in which relationships are perceived, i.e. in the way consciousness is transcended; and secondly, that this special form of "I—you" relationship offers an approach to the understanding of religious experience. It is obvious, of course, that Buber's "I—you" relationship is different from the simple forms of transcendence, and that even the penetrating forms of the latter are too defined to be equated with this comprehensive experience. What is the relationship, however, of the polar kind of transcendence, found in aesthetic, ethical and philosophical experience, to this "I—you" relationship? These forms of conscious experience are indeed comprehensive, but even they seem to be more defined and more differentiated than the experience described by Buber. Also, there is nothing to correspond with Buber's three spheres "in which the world of relationships is constructed": life with nature, life with men, and life with spiritual realities. It is easier to see in states of consciousness, characterized by polar transcendence, a first differentiation of the "I—you" form. This differentiation has some connection with the above three spheres, in that certain kinds of experience with polar transcendence are more likely to arise in certain spheres, for example, ethical experience in the life with men. Buber's spheres seem to me, however, to have more to do with the content of experience than with its form. As far as form is concerned, aesthetic, ethical and philosophical experience differ from an "I—you" encounter in their mode of orientation. But that there is a connection with the immediacy of the "I—you" relationship is seen in the fact that both these states readily pass over from one to the other.

The relationship between an "I—you" encounter and religious experience is different. Here also "I—you" experience seems to me to be the more primitive, but the mode of awareness is in each case the same. Transcendence is in both cases more comprehensive than in the other forms of conscious orientation. In the religious form, it is indeed all-comprehensive. When a man speaks of God, he means more than an object, or a man, or a spiritual fact, even though in this last case the "You" of the relationship appears in the moment of experience to include the whole of being. It is as if, in religious experience, consciousness of the limitations of "I—you" experience were lost, as if there were a striving after an encounter with a "You" which would be a living, immediate relationship, not broken up into partial experiences of "its". It is probable that, in the history of mankind, religions first begin to exert powerful influence when the immediacy of the relationship they provide is threatened by the growing domination of separate forms of conscious orientation. Such a point of view enables us to understand why the religious man constantly seeks a comprehensive vision, under the inspiration of religious experience, of all his possessions in the way of isolated experiences and beliefs. It also helps us to understand the close relationship between religion and ethics, philosophy and art. It is true that these last modes of orientation are not immediately related to religious experience, but rather to the "I—you" encounter; but the way in which this is understood and represented has often an intimate connection with those religious forms in which a relationship with the absolute "You" is sought within some community. It is true that an "I—you" encounter may be experienced apart from a religious setting, and inspire a poem or a painting, a vision of life's meaning or a deed of ethical value, but nowhere is the "I—you" situation more strenuously sought, or the effects of its inspiration more constantly maintained and elaborated, than in religion. In religious experience, man seeks again that sense of the unity of consciousness in which the life of the world and the life of the self, each speaking with a single voice, come into intimate relation with one another. The psychologist, attempting to describe these important conscious processes, must be prepared to realize that these "I—you" experiences may be suggested, but can never be actually described. He will always be tempted to regard their after-effects, instead of themselves, as the reality. The dislike that many people, and especially religious people, feel in regard to psychology is probably connected with this fact. Naturally, any science only gives an abstraction from concrete experience, which must always appear feebler than the experience itself. This limitation is not upsetting so long as only certain details are being dealt with. But for people in whose lives these "I—you" encounters are of great significance, a description which is purely analytical appears very inadequate, when it is dealing with matters of the greatest importance.

The importance of the "I—you" relationship seems to me to lie in the fact that the foundation of all relationship is to be found within it, and I regard religion as an essential form of spiritual orientation, since in it man confronts universal being with all that he is himself. I cannot possibly go further into this question now, and I must even forbear to suggest in any greater detail the connection which the types of conscious orientation may have with religious experience, in so far as different expressions of the latter are derived from corresponding modes of the former. For our purpose, we must limit ourselves to the fact that there is a specific comprehensive kind of transcendence, indicating a special kind of relationship between subject and object; and that this form of transcendence probably preceded a further differentiation in modes of conscious orientation, and may still be of great importance in people aware of this differentiation, in certain states of comprehensive contemplation, when it may be the origin of important, conscious, creative impulses. Religions seek to develop this special kind of experience, which is held to be religious experience, and to foster its effects.

We have now come to an end of our investigation of the various forms of transcendence. It can only give us a general view of the problems involved. A fuller discussion would require a great deal more space than is at my disposal. It seems to me, however, to be extremely important in the study of the various forms of conscious orientation, to realize that it is not possible to classify in one group every form, but that there are forms which are more comprehensive, and that we shall gain a better understanding of the essential quality of the various specific forms by tracing their origin from those which are more comprehensive, than by trying to explain them the other way about. If we attempt to indicate the development of the more differentiated forms from the more comprehensive, by means of our earlier diagram, it will be necessary to make it clear that the more comprehensive forms should not be regarded as primitive. The contrast between primitiveness and differentiation in consciousness is not the same thing as that between "I—you" experience and differentiated orientation. It means the difference between the primitive and the differentiated working out of "I—you" encounters. It is in the life of men with creative minds that we find the influence on their conscious life of these "I—you" experiences. It would be truer to say that the loss of contact with these comprehensive forms of experience in men of highly differentiated orientation produces a certain poverty and rigidity. It would be possible even to account for the contrast between culture and civilization in the maintenance, in the former, of contact with "I—you" experience, and its loss in the latter. It seems to me to be of the greatest possible importance for the individual, and for humanity, that the separate modes of conscious orientation are repeatedly experienced in association with that creative form of experience from which they originally sprang—the encounter between the "I" and the "you" in which both are entire and one.

Let us now summarize the results of our examination of the various forms of transcendence. In doing this, we may start from the point of view that the differentiated forms have developed from others more comprehensive. In considering instinctual experience, we mentioned simple animal consciousness as one of the earliest forms of consciousness, noting how far removed it appeared to be from the more complicated forms of human consciousness. With the development of intuition comes an important change, not only on account of the more precise, more limited nature of the "Aha!" experience, but also because a more indefinite, more comprehensive form of conscious association now arises: the "I—you" encounter. From the contrast between instinctual and intuitive experience, and from the tension of these "I—you" experiences, there now develops in man a sphere of conscious orientation, which we may with Cassirer call the realm of symbolic forms.[1] The most essential factor in the conscious forms belonging to this sphere seems to me to be the reciprocal influence of instinctual and intuitive experiences. The contrast between these two types of experience is mirrored in the two categories of the natural and the super-natural (or magical and mystical), which are of such importance in primitive psychology. Modern men, even if they are not consciously entirely out of touch with "I—you" encounters and any magical or mystical point of view, find it extraordinarily difficult, as a rule, to reproduce from

[1] Ernst Cassirer, *Philosophie der symbolischen Formen*, 1925. (No English translation.)

the images of the primitive world the conscious experiences which they indicate. It is not permissible, however, to assume that this picture-language is nonsense. At any rate, something must have originally been meant by it, and this meaning will be most readily understood as concrete intuitions, a deposit from "I—you" encounters. From this phase of development subsequently arise, on the one side, the artistic, ethical and philosophical points of view, and on the other, the religious. There are, in addition, not only the simple instinctual, but also the intuitive points of view, having reference to certain special problems. In this phase of development, the image as sign and symbol plays the main part in the fixing of experience and insight. These images are in their origin closely connected with "I—you" encounters and with "Aha!" experiences.

This phase in the development of conscious modes of orientation gradually passes over into another phase, in which new modes of orientation come to exercise considerable influence. These new forms are those of thinking and feeling, which, originating in the tendency towards philosophical and ethical adjustment, come to have independent standing. The established, more or less universally valid forms of these conscious modes of orientation serve to give them ever-increasing significance. We may suppose that originally acts of thought and feeling were closely associated with concrete intuitions, and have derived from this fact their potentially penetrating kind of transcendence. A further differentiation in the modes of consciousness is now possible. Even in the case of intuitions fixed in images, there is a possibility of not seeing beyond the images to the relationships they are meant to indicate. In this way, a world of images of mental forms comes into existence, whose meaning is more or less uncertain. The reason why the expressions of primitive peoples may sometimes appear nonsensical to us may be because the association between image and experience is inaccessible to us; but part of the explanation must be that these images never had any clear meaning for the primitives themselves. Imagination, that is, domination by images, is, as a rule, the product of a practical situation, but such images possess, even with primitive people, a certain independence, so that they are capable of dominating consciousness in their own capacity (for example, in the form of visions or dreams). This "inner life" of consciousness acquires a much greater importance through the development of certain images from the spheres of thought and feeling. Thought has been represented as a kind of trial acting, but it is not usually explained how such activity in mental forms comes to be possible. If an act in consciousness is more than a simple repetition of an earlier act, or than a realization of a perceived possibility, but rather represents a testing out of the various situations in reality, then there must be some image, more or less objective, of this reality in consciousness. This objective reproduction of reality is, however, a late product in human development. That independence in conscious experience which permits us to calculate the effect of our actions in an objective world of thought has developed in the course of centuries from the realm of magical symbolic images, and is the product of their collective elaboration. The forms of consciousness which have developed under the influence of thought and feeling come to have a much more impersonal significance, and, at the same time, are much less immediate, than the connection between the self and the world. The penetrating forms of conscious experience become less marked in those forms in which the world or the self speak primarily to that which has become the great mediator: our *consciousness*. In this way, forms of conscious experience arise which were previously not possible. These forms I have indicated as being, in the first place, simply representations in thought or fantasy, having little relation to the world or to the self (in spite of being originally derived from both), and but slight transcendence; and in the second place, conscious processes characterized by a one-sided transcendence, and involving a relationship between the world and consciousness, or between consciousness and the self, without involving the other pole of consciousness. For example, an event stimulates only ideas and fantasies which remain entirely impersonal and apparently have no effect upon personal reactions. Or, on the other hand, thoughts or impulses may arise within ourselves which seem to have nothing to do with the world. Thinking and feeling may play for quite a considerable time within a field that is "only mental". There is a certain possibility of transcendence here, which has reference to stimulus and to a far distant goal, but it controls mental events only within certain distant limits (for example, in a reference to reality or to personal ideals). Under the influence of thought and feeling, the conscious mind detaches itself more and more from the experience of a relationship, and develops personal laws for the life of the spirit, which come to exert an increasingly strong influence on both experience of the world and of the self, by taking the place of simple immediate experience. With the appearance of the "I—you" relationship, the unity of instinctual experience was already lost to consciousness.[1] "I—you" realization does indeed bring with it the experience of another, but the relationship remains, and

[1] This transition is probably represented pictorially in many early myths, for example in the story of the expulsion from Paradise.

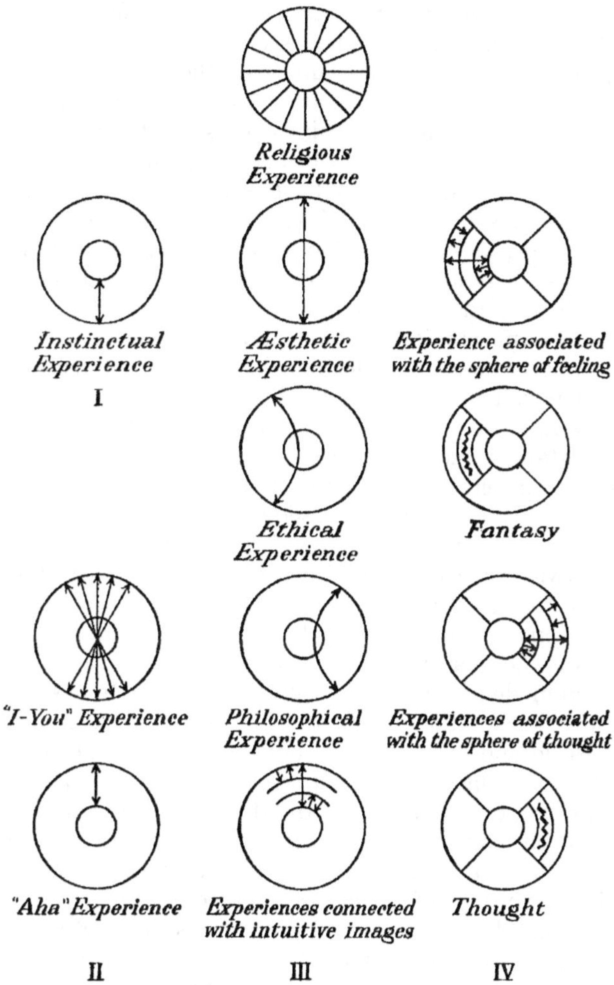

Forms of Transcendence

I. Animal Form of Meaning
II. New Forms from the Development of Intuition
III. Development of Symbolic Forms
IV. New Forms of Meaning through Thought and Feeling

may assume the form of a colloquy (as Buber calls it). The development of a personal world of thought and feeling offers, it is true, a fresh mode of orientation and a new security, but at the same time the unity of the world and the unity of the self are lost in the apprehension of manifold significances. "I" is threatened by "one" (compare "I think" with "one thinks"), as Heidegger has vividly expressed it; the world is experienced as something relative, which, in spite of the fact that it can be presented in a scientific and objective way, may be regarded from an infinite variety of points of view. So long as collective ideas and collective attitudes and moral forms possess absolute validity, the individual finds surer support in them than any personal experience can offer. In these days when all forms are liable to question, these collective forms are considered relative and are questioned as being "human—all too human". The value of more personal forms of consciousness, more immediately founded on experience and relationship, may, under these circumstances, receive greater recognition.

Speaking in general, it would not be right to say that any form of conscious experience had in itself the greatest value. Even though we may see in the "I—you" encounter the origin of all other forms (with the exception of instinctual experience), the more differentiated forms have, nevertheless, their particular significance for the situations to which they apply. The danger arises, however, that the man who is accustomed to employ with success a certain differentiated mode of conscious orientation is liable to over-valuate its importance in the whole conduct of his life and in his understanding of the world and of himself. From the description of functions in the first part of this book, it will be clear how the various modes of adaptation are determined, and the differences in transcendence, which have been discussed here, show that the experience of direct relationship, as well as its more special elaboration in certain circumscribed forms, is of importance. In order to give a survey of the situation, I have represented the various forms of transcendence in a series of diagrams, which is related to the earlier diagrams of the field of consciousness. These diagrams also indicate the relationship between the various differentiated forms of consciousness and the original unity of conscious experience. It seems to me to be of very great importance for the personal unity of the individual, as also for culture, regarded as the unified life-style of the community, that this original relationship should not be lost. Up to the present time, religion, more than anything else, has kept it alive and, quite apart from its possible metaphysical value, religion seems to me, from this point of view alone, to be of great significance for humanity. I am conscious that I am here touching on questions which go beyond the scope of this book, but it has been my wish, in so far as there is a close connection between religion and the structure of consciousness, at least to offer some suggestions as to how these questions may be regarded from the point of view of the types of conscious orientation.

CHAPTER III

THE PERSONAL EQUATION

Our discussion of the objective basis of psychology has revealed the peculiarity, that objectification is in psychology a considerably more complicated matter than it is in the natural sciences. In the latter, control of subjectivity is in the main negative, involving simply the exclusion of disturbing subjective elements. In psychology, on the other hand, the attitude of the worker has also to be objectified. As a result of insufficient appreciation of this fact—and its appreciation involves great difficulties—we have become accustomed to finding in psychology (as in the mental sciences) a whole series of different "tendencies". From the scientific point of view, this is not very satisfactory, and it is the task of psychology, by objectifying these various points of view, to bring about a greater consistency.

As I pointed out earlier, both psycho-analysis and phenomenology seem to me very important for the purpose of this objectification. Psycho-analysis has indeed in practice encouraged this striving for greater objectivity, by insisting on the would-be analyst undergoing a training-analysis himself, before taking up the work professionally. How far does he, by this means, attain a greater objectivity? The investigation of this problem is both practically and theoretically of the utmost importance for psychology. Hitherto no different qualifications have been required for the psychologist than for the student of natural science. Training for work in the natural sciences teaches the student to consider facts with a certain freedom from pre-conceived opinions, and to submit his experiences to some control. Sensory perceptions are decisive, and these may in the main be taken as the same for all men. Where sensory experiences are inexact, there is an attempt in all fields of science to replace them by instruments, which are, however, themselves only transmittors of sensory experience, and there remain in the end slight differences in the observations made. For example, the exact moment of the passing of a planet, seen through the telescope, is not exactly the same as registered by different observers. These small personal differences, which in the finer observations may have some effect, have in science been described by the term "personal equation".

The factor of the personal equation is, in the natural sciences, of very limited significance, but in psychology it is very much more important. Here it has so much influence, that the question may arise as to whether it is actually possible to attain in this field a real scientific objectivity. It certainly is an important step in the right direction, when the attempt is made to objectify one's own attitude, as is done, for example, in psycho-analysis. The good analyst will not only try to see the attitude of his patient clearly and to investigate its effects on his mental contents; he is also required to watch his own attitude with a certain suspicion, and to be aware of its effect on his relationship with his patient. In a personal relationship, this attitude can never be entirely excluded, but when it is known, it is possible to take it into account when arriving at any conclusion. Most men are, for the most part, unaware of this attitude; but a training-analysis should have enabled the analyst to deal with it consciously. Most important of all for this purpose is the resolving of that rigidity of attitude which is the product of unconscious fixations. This will make it possible for the analyst to realize his own personal equation in his observation and estimation of another individual.

Theoretically, there is scarcely any objection that could be made against this striving for objectivity, and in practice also it is certain that such an objectification of one's own personal attitude must improve psychological observation. But the problem remains, as to how far in practice this objectification of one's own attitude can be accomplished. And a further question is linked on to this, as to how far every possible aspect of the personal equation is dealt with in the psycho-analytical approach. The whole problem has received much less attention from the psycho-analysts than it deserves. This is probably because, in the psycho-analyst's view, subjectivity in attitude is entirely the result of complexes, and thus cannot be elucidated except by analytical treatment. Although it is not rare for analysts among themselves to attribute certain complexes to other people, or to each other, such an explanation is not, as a rule, regarded as more than an assertion. It is true that there are some excellent psycho-analytical biographical studies, which illustrate the possibility of such explanations on general lines, when adequate knowledge is available. But it seems to me, in the first place, that by no means all life-histories are so dominated by definite complexes that these latter provide an explanation of the whole pattern of the life concerned. And in the second place, it is very difficult to estimate, from the behaviour of an individual, how far this is influenced by complexes. Complexes have a limited effect: it is easier to explain from them a certain emotional attitude, than to deduce an individual's whole way of living. How wide of the mark an explanation of this latter kind can fall is illustrated by Maylan's "Analysis" of Freud's complexes.

Although I admit that there are people who can only be correctly explained from their complexes, this kind of personal equation seems to me to be important for most people only in certain "sensitive" situations. Even where such sensitive reactions bear an unmistakable neurotic stamp, one must be careful not to try to deduce from them the general characteristics of the subject's behaviour. They do not explain the main features of the personality-structure. The question, however, remains, as to whether it is not possible to evolve other kinds of personal equation, enabling us to correct our own subjectivity; and it seems to me that Jung, with his postulation of "psychological types", has indicated a further way here. I will give a short account of how the typical attitudes in conscious orientation require from the psychologist the consideration of a special kind of "personal equation".

When a physician conducts a physical examination of his patient, his type of conscious orientation exerts a certain influence on the proceeding. The instinctive individual lets his sensations speak first of all. His attention is riveted on the peculiarities he observes, and these guide him to the discovery of further data. On the other hand, the intuitive individual will start from an impression of the whole patient, and may occasionally arrive immediately at a suspicion of what is the matter. The man of thinking-type will proceed systematically and collect his data in accordance with a definite scheme, estimating these immediately in the light of his further discoveries. For the feeling-type, there is no peculiar method of examination. Feeling must rather be excluded; but in this case, the relationship between doctor and patient will be more vividly felt than in the case of the other types.

Each of these forms of experience needs to be amplified by the others, in order to satisfy scientific requirements. Isolated data are first rendered comprehensible by being fitted into a whole, which appears to be in part intuitively perceived, and in part built up by analysis and synthesis. Although, at the beginning, intuitive vision may be the important thing, this must be tested by the scientific elaboration of isolated data. And the scientific hypothesis will only come to life when it is amplified by special observations and applied intuitively on some special occasion. The education of the physician aims at this kind of co-operation of the various functions, but, of course, there frequently remain in the individual physician certain typical emphases, which may reveal themselves in his behaviour. In this case, it may be of considerable value to him to be aware of his personal equation in this respect, in order as far as possible to avoid one-sidedness.

Correction of this kind is far more important for the psychologist than it is for the natural scientist, because the effects of a one-sided conscious attitude are here much more far-reaching. Experience of one's own mental life is here the instrument for one's understanding of that of another. One may occasionally recognize slight indications in others of forms that are distinct in one's own mind. What is confused in one's own mind usually cannot be correctly understood in that of another, even though it may exist there in a very definite form. The answer of the earth spirit to Faust is often true here:

> "Du gleichst dem Geist, den Du begreifst."[1]

Thus one's immediate experience of one's fellow-man proves itself at once to be much more influenced by one's own personality than is one's experience of a natural object, and the way in which this experience is dealt with is likewise still more under this influence, since the different modes of psychological objectification are sometimes determined by typical attitudes. In the various schools of psychology, this influence can frequently be clearly demonstrated. One might even go so far as to say that the scientific conception of things mental has, as a whole, taken on a special stamp as a result of these influences. I will first try to elucidate this factor.

Men of different types are not all equally interested in scientific problems. Those of thinking-type are most attracted by such problems, and to these may be added those in whom thought as a subsidiary function has particular significance. Outstandingly instinctive or intuitive types are more inclined to practical activity, and feeling-types rarely go deeply into theoretical problems, unless perchance some feeling (e.g. for a loved person) influences them, or they belong to the rare polar type of orientation (see Part I, Chapter VI). This selection of the students prepared to work in the cause of science results, for the natural sciences, in the automatic exclusion of those less well adapted for this work. For psychology, this effect is not entirely favourable. Here even one's immediate experience of another person is partly determined by one's own predominating attitude, and this typical attitude is, in

[1] ("That spirit thou resemblest, whom thou dost comprehend.")

the case of the student, necessarily one-sided. As a result, certain spheres of mental life may easily be overlooked by the psychologists. The moment one's attention is drawn to this fact, one realizes in how many respects psychologists and psychologies are one-sided, and need amplification. The psychology of feeling is particularly seen to be very inadequate, but even intuition and instinctual experience appear usually in intellectualized forms. It is, in fact, often taken for granted that all mental activity consists of thinking. Certainly academic psychology has the best understanding of the laws of thought, and if medical psychology had not been developed out of human need, we should probably still not have begun to understand instinct and feeling. The psycho-analyst, having learned to be conscious of his experience in these spheres, has thereby opened up new perspectives for psychology. But even with him there is frequently that deprecating attitude of the intellectual towards feelings, which are accordingly only understood by him in their instinctual aspect.

If, after these more general observations, we turn our attention to the present-day condition of psychological science, we find there a mixture of tendencies and schools, which permit of no condensation into a single whole. For centuries, the prevailing psychological conceptions were borrowed from theological ideology, into which points of view derived from ancient times were woven. One particular conception of the world was expressed in every observation and speculation. Under such circumstances, it is scarcely possible to speak of science in the modern sense. In the last century, however, attempts were begun to base knowledge, in this field also, on a foundation of actual experience, and where this was done, the methods and schemata of the natural sciences were at first employed on this fresh material. Association Psychology regarded associated ideas as if they were isolated objects in nature. Experimental Psychology subjected facts to tests according to the pattern of natural science, and to a very large extent identified itself with physiology. Subsequently, all manner of different ways of understanding and confirming psychological facts were developed, and in accordance with these various standpoints, psychology has been split up into a whole series of different "tendencies".

Although I do not maintain that this recognition of a one-sidedness in conscious orientation according to type offers an explanation of all the varieties in outlook, this differentiation does, nevertheless, make it possible to get a better understanding of the one-sidedness in these points of view. An attempt to consider all the schools of psychology from this aspect would carry me far beyond the scope of this book. I shall only try to illustrate a few guiding principles.

We probably get the clearest picture of the possible variety in the approach of psychology to its material in the extremes of extraversion and introversion. The outstandingly introverted individual sets out primarily from his own standpoint, and will accordingly tend to consider the psychology of consciousness as the most essential foundation of experience. The convinced extravert sees in the experience of others the starting-point for his psychologizing, and hence he prefers, as a scientific basis for his psychology, the approach of the natural sciences. The different functions are likewise responsible for certain fundamental emphases in personal experience, which are, accordingly, likely to find expression in the various tendencies in psychology. The instinctive extravert will pay most attention to experiences associated with the organs of sensation. The behaviour of others, in so far as it can be noted and described, appears to him as the only reliable reality. Here we find the standpoint of the Behaviourists. Where instinctual experience is completely introverted, more consideration is given to personal internal structures and reactions. As a result, there is more interest in the structure of experience regarded from the subjective angle (e.g. as it is studied in "*Gestalt*" psychology) and in motivation and emotional impulses (as in McDougall's work). In work of this kind, facts are regarded in their human aspect, although they are not felt as personal. Extraverted intuition, when dominant, gives an entirely different picture of mental happening. The mind of another individual seems then to be comprehended immediately. (Scheler, for example, has defended this view.) Mental connections are regarded as self-evident, and a single happening carries conviction.[1] What is surmised as lying behind behaviour has more value than the simple description of facts. Any psychology whose aim is to *understand* has its foundations here.

Yet another picture is presented, when psychology appears to originate in introverted intuition. Its main truth is then presented in terms of a personal inner vision. In this case, super-personal value is often attributed to a single subjective experience. The essence of being is found in special occurrences. Introspection is subordinate to the experience of intuitive vision, its chief use being to help in the correct description of what is experienced. Even quite simple experiences are reduced to their essence, being regarded

[1] This seems to me to be the basis also of psycho-analytical psychology, in which, both theoretically and practically, the greatest importance is attached to intuitively perceived connections.

in a special light. This is the line taken, for example, by Spranger and Binswanger. They seek an immediate comprehension of the essence of spiritual existence, and in this resemble the philosophical approach of Heidegger.

With extraverted thinking, that which is "objective" and common to all men is what counts beyond everything in mental life; and where it is in control of psychological research, the more subjective and "irrational" aspects of experience are neglected. In my opinion, all observations, conceptions and deliberate recollection come under the category of universal thought-forms. In experimental psychology, we find these universally valid forms at the centre of every investigation, and this mode of observation is sometimes represented as being the only truly scientific one. But over against this we have psychological observation from the point of view of introverted thinking, where universally valid laws are sought first of all in personal experience. An inner need for logical order and for the construction thereof is felt to be the essence of mind. Phenomenology, as an attempt to regulate introspection in accordance with scientific principles, sets out from this point of view.

Psychological conceptions may also be determined by the attitude that takes feeling as its starting-point. In this case, where extraversion is predominant, the mind is seen as first of all offering possibilities of moral orientation. Although this form of orientation plays a smaller part in scientific psychology today than was the case in bygone days, it still forms an important factor in practical psychology. Educational psychology occupies itself to a large extent with the education of the feelings, and, in comparison with a former intellectualistic period, the moral education of the citizen is today once more regarded as a problem. As a result, the problem of the origin of feeling has become a current one. In considering this, the extravert takes the existing forms as his starting-point, and hence arrives at a somewhat conventional psychology of morals, such as is represented, for example, by the Catholic Church. On the other hand, the starting-point of the introvert is more ethical than moral, and, as regards conventional values, is more inclined to take up a revolutionary attitude. He sets out from those moral values, of which he has inner experience. Here good and evil are felt to be the profoundest revelations of man's being. This view of mental life has, as a rule, more influence on practice than on theory. As far as theory is concerned, the danger for feeling-types is that they tend to regard men in the light of their ideals rather than as what they really are.

The influence of the mode of conscious orientation on psychological theory may in some outstanding cases be very striking, but in many others the situation is more complicated. The psychologist's selection of his preferred theory is not entirely determined by his own type. Chance influences, such as that of a teacher or of a fashion, are occasionally very important. Even a complex may play a part, as, for example, when a man supports an opinion which was specially attractive (or unattractive) to his father. It is surprising how completely unaware most men are of these factors, which in no way detract from the student's feeling of objectivity.

Regarded from the point of view of the type of conscious orientation, two further factors, which may in certain cases determine the student's attitude, remain for consideration, namely, the effect of a subsidiary function, and the effect of polarity. Most students of psychology, and most practical psychologists, are not guided merely by a dominant function. Since the effect of a subsidiary function is generally more noticeable than that of the predominating one, the emphasis on this former aspect may, in fact, be very much in evidence. In a student, thought will, as a rule, be either the prevailing or the subsidiary function, and will further be combined with either instinct or intuition. Besides the two important groups of introverts and extraverts, we shall accordingly find two further main groups. In one of these, the chief emphasis will be on thought and instinctual experience, and in the other, on thought and intuitive experience. Students belonging to the first group will insist on exact and repeated testing of observations. They will be slow in coming to general conclusions, and will often give an impression of being somewhat heavy-going. Psychologists of the second group take up a less critical attitude to individual facts, but they have a greater comprehension of essential relationships. Alongside isolated facts, they attach primary importance to experience which they share with others by means of a sympathetic projection of themselves (empathy). This makes them more in sympathy with literary psychology. There are also psychologists who, being unable to unify within themselves the points of view presented by the two functions, defend a duality in their conceptions. In Jaspers' work, for instance, we find causal scientific explanation (after the pattern of extraverted thinking) and empathetic understanding (by means of intuition) side by side, but completely unrelated. Those psychologists who keep their knowledge and their faith in separate water-tight compartments belong to this category.

The influence of polarity upon the psychological point of view adopted by the student is more complicated and less transparent. In this case, his conscious attitude is interlarded with interests and reflections which do not correspond with his usual mode of orientation. In most people, this kind of thing happens from time to time, without influencing the subject's general attitude to any great extent. It is relatively rare that the results of polarity in attitude raise a problem. When this does happen, there is an attempt to bridge over the paradoxes involved, which in art, and even in psychology, may be both stimulating and fruitful. Men of genius often give evidence of this paradoxical polarity. It is not to be wondered at, that the psychology of such a man reflects the oppositions in his make-up; and if he is given to the formulation of theories, he will bring these problems into scientific psychology. This phenomenon of polarity complicates many problems which otherwise appear simple. Insight into these complications enables us, however, to arrive at a better understanding of the mental make-up of many interesting and creative people. I will try to make this point clearer, by referring to the effects of polarity in the case of Freud and of Jung, emphasizing at the outset that it will be no more than a sketch, indicating certain peculiarities in their life and work, in relation to this particular question. It would, of course, be impossible to do justice to their personalities in such a brief description.

Freud and his pupils will be perhaps surprised if I describe him as an intuitive. Freud himself has indeed constantly emphasized the significance of thought and science as the most important foundation for humanity. I hasten, therefore, to add that I regard thought as a strongly developed subsidiary function in Freud. Why do I consider intuition as his primary function? Freud has himself, on occasion, expressly rejected the significance of intuition, but in doing so, he is thinking of intuition as one of the recognized principles in philosophy. My conception of it is a much wider one. In my view, intuition plays a part in many mental manifestations in daily life, and is by no means exclusively occupied with metaphysical problems. One must also bear in mind that Freud is an extravert, and that, accordingly, he is familiar only with the extraverted form of intuition. Freud, like most other students, counts the effects of intuition amongst the products of thought, and there is no doubt that in him these two functions are very closely combined in their activity. But there are also intuitive people in whom intuition works independently.

Extraverted intuition makes it possible for the psychologist to understand by means of empathy, and even in his earliest clinical histories Freud reveals himself as a master in this art. At the beginning of his scientific career, he stood alone as the man who had the courage to found psychology on the data gained by sharing the experience of another by means of empathy. The method of psycho-analysis, which he has since elaborated with ever increasing precision, provides further scientific conditions, and thus the control of the intuitive apprehension of another person. Freud has, it is true, always employed the criticism of thought in this process, and he has created his own scientific forms for the establishment and arrangement of his material, as perceived. But the intellectual system has never been the main thing with him. He is, indeed, not greatly interested in systems. The forms he has created are related primarily to intuitive experience, and he is ready to modify them as this is added to. Experience gained through empathy is always the most important basis,[1] and, in consequence, many psycho-analytical concepts, as, for example, those of narcissism, and the transference, need systematic precision. This shows how inapposite is the contention that psycho-analytical psychology is the product of the committee table. At the same time, it is obvious that systematic classification is not of primary importance to the creator of psycho-analysis. It thus seems to me to be evident in Freud's work that in him thought, as subsidiary function, is in control of intuition.

Although we may thus accept that many of Freud's peculiarities may be attributed to his conscious orientation as an intuitive extravert, yet there are other facts which do not seem to agree. I have repeatedly expressed the opinion that intuitives are the farthest removed from the sphere of instinctual experience. But for Freud instinctual sexuality has become the most important factor in mental life. Furthermore, it might be said that Freud was the first to create a real psychology of feeling, although he himself would not so describe his psychology. How has it happened, then, that he has directed his intuitive insight towards a field which normally has little attraction for an intuitive extravert with thinking as his subsidiary function? Moreover, what we know in general about Freud's life has little in common with such interests. Instinctual needs, the frills of daily life, outdoor recreative interests —these are not of great significance for this quiet-living scholar. Nor do feeling-relationships, or the expression of feeling in art, appear to have had any marked influence on his life. He has lived

[1] This has recently been very vividly described by Reik (*Surprise and the Psycho-analyst*, London, 1936). Strangely enough, he resists the use of the word " intuition ", although it must be in the mind of every reader.

the family life of a worthy citizen, and yet he has given us an understanding of the love-life and of sexuality in all their ramifications and deviations. In these studies of his, it is noteworthy that the concepts of love and sexuality, hitherto frequently represented as opposites, are always regarded as one and the same thing. Freud has doubtless done a valuable service for psychology in investigating the relationships between sexuality and every other kind of feeling, but the lack of conceptual differentiation, and the sexual terminology, have occasionally a bewildering effect.

These oppositions in Freud's mental make-up must, in my opinion, be explained as the result of polarity. When the illuminated side of consciousness is constantly turned towards the spheres of thought and intuition, the effects of feeling and of instinctual orientation remain, for the most part, in the twilit regions of the mind, and, as a result, are not sharply differentiated. If, however, in a case like this, the "other side" penetrates into consciousness, it may become a problem. In an introvert, this problem will be seen as belonging to his own personal mental life; but the extravert will see it primarily as a problem in the mental life of others. Since the forms in this dimmer side of consciousness are less well developed, they reveal themselves as more independent of education and tradition. There is, accordingly, a tendency to leave these more primitive forms alone and to prefer the more developed forms of orientation. When the student turns his attention to spheres which are of polar significance for him, he is apt to regard the simple and nebulous forms in these spheres as their most essential characteristics. Freud has taken up an entirely fresh viewpoint of that realm of mental forms in which instinct and the expression of feeling are related, and, indeed, at first he saw nothing but what concerned sexuality, although he has since given consideration to the other aspects of instinctual life. His derivation of the more complicated forms of emotional life from the more simple strikes me, moreover, as being quite correct. But it is characteristic of his personal outlook, that the matter of ideals—in my opinion, the second most important factor in emotional life—has only much later received some consideration in psycho-analytical psychology. It is also remarkable, that in this psychology ethics are not given any importance, but are entirely subordinate to the influence of thought, if they are not pushed on one side as superseded. This lack is the more striking, when one sees in Freud, as I do, a strictly moral individual, maintaining certain high ideals in his personal life, although he may not expressly support them in theory. Beside a certain suspicion in regard to traditional morality, I see here

Freud's conscious orientation as a source of certain emphases in his psychology.

In Jung, whom I should like to take as my second example, we find an entirely different make-up as regards conscious orientation. He himself describes himself as a thinking-introvert, and his work confirms this in many respects. The experience of his own mental life is for him much more of a starting-point than it is for Freud, and this soon led him to consider introversion, not as pathological, but as a normal phenomenon. His early work showed, to a greater extent than was the case with Freud, the influence of certain intellectual systems. His experiments in association reveal the influence of the experimental methods of that time. A certain preference for the concrete is also evident, and is, moreover, constantly revealed in his forthright language; and it is this which leads me to the assumption that Jung's subsidiary function is instinct. This need for concrete instinctual experience is seen also in his private life. He lives out of doors, travels a great deal, and welcomes all the pleasures of existence. In his scientific work, this factor leads to the exposition of much concrete detail.

Characteristic of Jung's mental make-up is an inter-action between a zest for interesting facts and fairly independent thought-processes, which constantly seek to arrange these facts in an orderly system. It is this make-up which led him from the beginning to direct his interest towards fresh, hitherto unexplored regions, such as the psychoses, or the psychology of primitive peoples. He has done pioneer work in these fields, and has approached many new problems. Many people may be surprised at the suggestion that with all this Jung should be regarded as a thinking-type. If he is compared, for example, with Kant, as a typical introvert of thinking-type, it is clear that, in his case, both thinking and introversion are less exclusively involved in his mental make-up. This may be partly connected with the fact that, in Kant's case, intuition appears as the subsidiary function, which emphasizes the abstract aspect of thought. Moreover, Jung's efforts to bring out and develop the other functions in himself has prevented him from always considering orderliness of thought as the most important factor. But in spite of this, a striving after a psychological system of his own prevails pretty clearly over all his work.

In Jung, also, we find important traits which do not obviously fit in with the make-up of a thinking-introvert with instinct as subsidiary function. Men of this type usually show a very practical and solid intellectuality, with, if anything, a disinclination for speculation. Jung, on the contrary, has from the very beginning shown a tendency to concern himself with the consideration of ultimate issues. As a student, he took an interest, for example, in spiritualism. This element is also seen in certain aspects of Jung's psychology. Side by side with scientific hypotheses concerning the energy of mind, concepts are found, such as those of archetypes and the collective unconscious, which are somewhat remote from actual experience, but are closely bound up with metaphysical speculations. Quite apart from the question as to whether Jung is right in these hypotheses concerning the nature of mind, we may, from the way in which they are set forth, surmise that the polar aspect of Jung's mind is at work in them. For an individual of thinking-type, with instinct as subsidiary function, the dim field of consciousness lies in the spheres of feeling and intuition. When influences from these regions make themselves felt, they will not be experienced in clear-cut forms, but, on the contrary, in forms which are nebulous and primitive. If this polar aspect of the mind should come clearly to the fore, we should expect to find intuitions laden with feeling in a primitive, that is to say, concrete form. As a matter of fact, we do find that with Jung these concrete intuitions are of great significance, both in practice and in theory. In treatment by the Jungian method, the awakening of intuitions associated with emotion by means of drawings, fantasies, visions and dreams, plays an important part. In his theory, these intuitions are represented as the product of archetypes and of special mental impulses, having a fairly concrete existence in the mental life of the individual concerned. Although I regard it as of very great importance that Jung has indicated the significance of intuition and feeling, his descriptions of the forms of these two functions seem to me to be inadequate, and I consider that the effect of polarity is responsible both for Jung's interest in them and for this insufficiency. Like Freud, Jung is too apt to consider the simple forms in these, for him, newly discovered regions, as their most essential expression. In demonstrating this one-sidedness, I am expressing no criticism of the work of these two scholars. My only aim is to illustrate how complicated the personal equation may become in special cases.

I hope that in this brief sketch I have suggested the significance of the type of conscious orientation for the problem of the personal equation. It might, however, help in the estimation of this book, if in conclusion I were to indicate quite briefly my own type of conscious orientation, in order that my reviewers may find it easier to take my own personal equation into account. I regard myself as an introvert of thinking-type, with intuition as subsidiary function. Hence my interest in phenomenological distinctions,

The effect of polarity in me gives rise to an interest in feeling in its relation to the instincts. Hence my appreciation of psycho-analysis. But I lay more emphasis on the feeling-life as a sphere to itself, and on the significance of morality. How far a personal equation must be held responsible for my conceptions I must leave to the judgment of my critics. I myself am convinced that all efforts towards objectivity have their limits. Life, moreover, is more than psychology, but this fact should not prevent us from aiming at a science of psychology as an instrument for life.

INDEX

F

J

K

L

N

O

P

R

S

T

www.ingramcontent.com/pod-product-compliance
Lightning Source LLC
LaVergne TN
LVHW011109300926
849160LV00008B/325
* 9 7 8 1 1 3 8 8 7 4 9 3 0 *